Pharmaceutical Care

Pharmaceutical Care

Edited by
Calvin H. Knowlton, R.Ph., Ph.D.
& Richard P. Penna, Pharm.D.

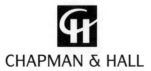

CHAPMAN & HALL

I(T)P® International Thomson Publishing
New York • Albany • Bonn • Boston • Cincinnati • Detroit • London • Madrid • Melbourne
Mexico City • Pacific Grove • Paris • San Francisco • Singapore • Tokyo • Toronto • Washington

Cover photo (*left to right*):
Janet Rossell, Patient, Mayor of Lumberton, Lumberton, NJ;
Orsula Voltis Thomas, Pharm. D., CDE, Pharmacist, Amherst Pharmacy & Health Education Center, Lumberton, NJ

Copyright © 1996 by Chapman & Hall

Printed in the United States of America

For more information contact:

Chapman & Hall
115 Fifth Avenue
New York, NY 10003

Chapman & Hall
2-6 Boundary Row
London SE1 8HN
England

Thomas Nelson Australia
102 Dodds Street
South Melbourne, 3205
Victoria, Australia

Chapman & Hall GmbH
Postfach 100 263
D-69442 Weinheim
Germany

International Thomson Editores
Campos Eliseos 385, Piso 7
Col. Polanco
11560 Mexico D.F.
Mexico

International Thomson Publishing - Japan
Hirakawacho-cho Kyowa Building, 3F
1-2-1 Hirakawacho-cho
Chiyoda-ku, 102 Tokyo
Japan

International Thomson Publishing Asia
221 Henderson Road #05-10
Henderson Building
Singapore 0315

3 4 5 6 7 8 9 XXX 01 00 99 98 97

Library of Congress Cataloging-in-Publication Data

Pharmaceutical care / [edited by] Calvin H. Knowlton and Richard P. Penna.
        p.   cm.
    Includes bibliographical references and index.
    ISBN 0-412-06981-4 (alk. paper)
    1. Pharmacy. I. Knowlton, Calvin H., 1949-- . II. Penna, Richard P.
    [DNLM: 1. Pharmaceutical Services--United States. 2. Delivery of Health Care--United States. 3. Pharmacy--United States. QV 737
    P534 1995]
    RS91.P43   1995
    362.1'782'0973--dc20
    DNLM/DLC   95-14254
    for Library of Congress   CIP

Visit Chapman & Hall on the Internet http://www.chaphall.com/chaphall.html

To order this or any other Chapman & Hall book, please contact **International Thomson Publishing, 7625 Empire Drive, Florence, KY 41042.** Phone (606) 525-6600 or 1-800-842-3636. Fax: (606) 525-7778. E-mail: order@chaphall.com.

For a complete listing of Chapman & Hall titles, send your request to **Chapman & Hall, Dept. BC, 115 Fifth Avenue, New York, NY 10003.**

Contents

The Nature of Pharmaceutical Care

Implementation of Pharmaceutical Care

Preface

Calvin H. Knowlton
Richard P. Penna

Why Was This Book Written?

Mrs. Smith: A Case Study

Mrs. Barbara Smith is a healthy 75-year-old woman who lives independently and maintains an active schedule which includes volunteer work, reading, and playing with her two young grandchildren. She drives her own car and depends very little on others for her day-to-day needs. The only medication she takes is digoxin, prescribed by her physician a number of years previously for a "heart irregularity". Constantly vigilant about her health, she visits her physician regularly and takes her digoxin religiously according to directions. Because of her extremely good health, she, her physician, and her family were astounded and surprised when Mrs. Smith developed a chest cold that rapidly progressed to pneumonia. Mrs. Smith required a week in the intensive care unit of her local hospital and two more weeks of hospitalization before she could return home. Even then, it was several months before she could return to her normal, vigorous schedule.

At first glance, one would attribute this episode to an unfortunate confluence of an unusually virulent bacteria with an elderly patient. But there's more to the story. Subsequent investigations determined that Mrs. Smith contracted pneumonia because she was malnourished. She became malnourished because she stopped eating. She stopped eating because she lost her appetite, and she lost her appetite because of a well-known side effect of digoxin. The dose of her digoxin was such that over time (perhaps years) small amounts began to accumulate in her blood until the drug began to exert its toxic effect (loss of appetite).

The point to this story is that no one—not Mrs. Smith's physician, not her nurse, not her pharmacist—thought to ask Mrs. Smith about her appetite even though the effect of digoxin on appetite is well known. These health professionals simply forgot! Simple greetings by physician, nurse, and pharmacist of "How are you?" were offered—and meant—strictly in their social contexts, not as health care questions.

This true story had a happy ending. Mrs. Smith recovered, and she is back to her usual, active life style, but now her physician and pharmacist closely monitor her medication. Of course, there was a cost. Medicare paid a handsome sum of money to the hospital and physicians who cared for her during her stay. Her family (not to mention Mrs. Smith herself) paid a substantial emotional toll as a result of her battle with a life-threatening illness.

All this financial and emotional cost and suffering could have been avoided . . . if someone, some health professional, had looked upon Mrs. Smith as a person who was taking a needed, but very potent, drug . . . if that someone had been concerned enough to worry about Mrs. Smith's therapeutic outcomes and ask a few simple questions periodically and especially whenever she obtained more of her digoxin.

The Response of One Profession

Pharmacy, like all health professions, is undergoing enormous change as the changing nature of the U.S. health care system makes its influence felt. As the profession most concerned with drugs (raw drugs, purified drug entities, formulated drug products), pharmacy began examining its societal role as the profession that must be responsible for assuring safe and effective drug use. For the past thirty years, pharmacy has explored the drug use process and has made some startling observations and conclusions. This book is about these observations and conclusions. It is about pharmaceutical care, a revolutionary philosophy of health care practice, a new way of dealing with the most popular therapeutic intervention used in health care. It's about the underlying trends in health care that make pharmaceutical care so critical to the successful treatment or diagnosis of illness. It's about what pharmaceutical care is and how it may be provided.

Our Health Care System Has A Drug Problem

The Extent of Drug-Related Illness

Several chapters in this book discuss in clear detail the startling statistics that demonstrate that drugs, for all their benefits, are associated with a major public health problem costing tens of billions of dollars annually. It's not the drugs themselves that are responsible for the morbidity and mortality associated with their use, it is how they are used—the drug use process (or lack of a process)—that is at the root of the problem. The evidence is very clear that when used within a systematic process that focuses on the patient and the outcomes of therapy in the patient, the drug use process becomes one of the most cost-effective health care interventions available. On the other hand, when used in the fragmented fashion so typical of today's drug use process, the results are a costly array of therapeutic failures, drug interactions with diet and other drugs, and adverse reactions to the drugs themselves.

Who's at Fault?

No one person or group of persons (professions) can be cited as causing our health care drug problem. Indeed, the evidence is quite clear that there is enough blame to go around for everyone: prescriber, nurse, pharmacist, and patient. Drug therapy goes wrong when:

1. The prescriber (physician, dentist, podiatrist, optometrist, physician assistant, nurse practitioner, or patient) decides not to use a drug when one is indicated, prescribes the wrong drug or dose, or prescribes a drug when no drug is indicated

2. The pharmacist does not get the drug to the patient when needed; the drug does not get to the patient's bedside in the hospital or nursing home; the pharmacist dispenses the wrong drug or the correct drug with wrong instructions

3. The patient refuses to obtain the medication or fails to follow prescribed instructions

4. No one monitors patients on medication for desired therapeutic end-points or adverse reactions or to determine whether the patient is taking the medication as instructed

What our health care system needs, therefore, is for someone—some group of health professionals—to step forward to take responsibility for assuring that these causes of drug-related illnesses are substantially eliminated and controlled. The best way to assure this result is for individual practitioners to assume responsibility for the outcomes of drug therapy in patients whom they serve.

Pharmaceutical Care, A New Health Care Discipline

Researchers and theorists within pharmacy have examined the nature and scope of the nation's health care drug problem along with its root causes. As a result of their findings, they propose that the public and the health care professions change their attitudes about the drug use process. They suggest that the same degree of attention be given to the drug use process as is given to the diagnostic process, rehabilitative process, or the nurturing process. They suggest that the best way that this can be achieved is for a profession to step forward and assume responsibility for the results (outcomes) of drug therapy in patients. This is the only way that all the functions that comprise the drug use process can be integrated into a safe, effective, and efficient systematic process that assures that the outcomes of therapy are the ones that are desired and expected by the patient and those caring for the patient.

They propose that a new philosophy of practice be adopted to assure that patients receive full benefit from pharmacotherapy. This philosophy of practice is called *pharmaceutical care*. It's a concept that in one sense is quite simple—a health professional must worry about the therapeutic outcomes in patients under his or her care. At the same time pharmaceutical care is quite complex. It involves issues related to interprofessional collaboration, quality of life, identifying and quantifying outcomes, performing various functions and tasks, ethics, competence, and the concepts of responsibility and accountability.

For Whom Was This Book Written?

Is Pharmaceutical Care Just for Pharmacists?

The adjective *pharmaceutical* when used to describe care, indicates that the care is associated with pharmaceutical agents, not the individual who provides it. Consequently, this new philosophy is not reserved for any one profession or group of professionals. While it is true that most of the underlying research and theory behind the concept were performed within the profession of pharmacy, it does not necessarily follow that pharmacists will step forward to provide pharmaceutical care. And "step forward" a profession must if it is to be granted the right to be held accountable by society for the outcomes of drug therapy in patients.

This book is written in the expectation that the pharmacy profession will accept the challenge and "step forward" to accept the public's mandate to provide pharmaceutical care. However, because pharmaceutical care is, by definition, collaborative, and because other professionals are involved in the drug use process, this book is intended for others as well. Moreover, it is entirely possible (and probable) that pharmaceutical care will be provided by a variety of health professionals.

Pharmaceutical Care is intended to provide information to practitioners (pharmacists, physicians, nurses) who are interested to learn more about improving the drug use process and how they can assume greater responsibilities in caring for patients with pharmacotherapy.

Potential Audiences

This book is intended to be a resource for all who have an interest in the use of drugs as diagnostic or therapeutic interventions in health care. While one would expect that a primary audience will be practitioners (pharmacists, physicians, and nurses), students are another major intended audience, especially pharmacy students. The editors recognize that, while pharmaceutical care is a part of every pharmacy school curriculum, there exists no organized resource on pharmaceutical care for students. Because the topic occurs in several places in a typical pharmacy curriculum, the editors intend that this book be used at several places in the pharmacy curriculum.

Introduction

Calvin H. Knowlton
Richard P. Penna

Why Pharmaceutical Care?

> Drug related morbidity and mortality was estimated to cost $76.6 billion in the ambulatory setting in the United States. The largest component of this total cost was drug related hospitalizations . . . (Johnson and Bootman 1995).

> Prospecting for revenue, pharmacies look beyond dispensing drugs. With insurance and other payment plans curbing prescription fees, some pharmacies are doing customer assessment and phone follow-ups to ensure that patients are sticking to a prescription's regimen. . . . The new services are part of a concept called pharmaceutical care, which calls for pharmacists to monitor, manage and enhance patient compliance with a drug therapy . . . (Wall Street Journal 1995)

> Twenty-five high risk patients were selected to attend a special asthma clinic that provided pharmacist-managed education regarding asthma and the proper use of medication. Regular telephone contact between the pharmacist and the patients continued after the initial education. The total number of Emergency Department (ED) visits for the 25 patients six months prior to the study was 92; the number of ED visits during the same months of the study in the prior year was 47. During the study period, there were only 6 ED visits (Pauley, Magee, and Cury 1995)

There are two messages (at least) portrayed by these quotations. First, there is a problem associated with the medication use process in the United States. Second, pharmacists are stepping forward to help resolve this problem. Blending the message in each of these quotations focuses upon the thrust and reason for this book: for many reasons the forces of change have provoked the profession to alter its societal mission and function. These forces include economics and adverse drug events, but they go beyond these two discrete challenge areas. The forces of change are both external of pharmacy (e.g., changes in demography, epidemiology, technology, economics, and ethics) and internal (e.g., pharmacists longing for expanded roles in health care and yearning to "get back to the patient").

Forces of Change: External

Patients are growing older and becoming more culturally diverse (cultural backgrounds influence attitudes about illness and drug use). Patients are seeking health care from a variety of practitioners who prescribe drugs as part of their therapeutic treatments. The average number of chronic illnesses per patient is increasing. Technology is affecting the nature and scope of information about medication that is available to the public. This same communication technology is facilitating patient data storage, transfer, access and analysis. Pharmaceutical technology is expanding the array of medications and the specificity, effectiveness, potency, and risk of medications.

Simultaneously, the ethical shift from provider paternalism to informed consent, patient autonomy, and empowerment has provided pharmacists with an opportunity to expand their role and to become a knowledge resource (e.g., health educator) for patients regarding pharmaceutical options and therapeutic insights. Finally, the increasing costs of particular medication regimens and the increased utilization rates for medication treatment have caused payors to attempt to control drug expenditures by limiting access to medications, requiring, for instance, that patients receive less costly "acceptable" alternatives.

This combination of externalities (demographic, epidemiologic, technologic, ethical, and economic forces) is creating health care situations in which ambulatory and institutionalized patients are being treated by multiple prescribers with highly potent and risky medications within an anachronistic drug use system. Such conditions are responsible for the increasing mortality and morbidity statistics associated with adverse consequences to drug therapy. This increase in negative health outcomes contributes to additional health care expenditures through hospitalizations, lengthened hospital stays, increased physician office encounters, more emergency room visits, greater use of diagnostic laboratory tests, and the prescribing of more medication (as was recounted in the true story in the Preface of this book).

Forces of Change: Internal

Self-satisfaction and economics are also important. The art of compounding is used sparsely in contemporary pharmacy practice. The task of repackaging and distributing seems insufficient as a professional calling. Optimizing the medication use process is a new and challenging role for pharmacists. Delivering pharmaceutical care is a new, authentic source of personal satisfaction. Furthermore, the economic reality within the profession is that dispensing fees, as the major economic resource for practice, are eroding quickly.

Thus, while this concept of pharmaceutical care is a revolutionary philosophy for the practice of pharmacy and for pharmaceutical education, its time has come. The vast majority of drug-related illness is avoidable, and pharmacists have been expanding their roles to include identifying, resolving, and preventing medication-related problems in the patients they serve by managing the drug use process. This is pharmaceutical care. It means managing the drug use process in collaboration with prescribers, other health care professionals, and patients, with the goal of optimizing therapy. Notwithstanding its newness, all major professional practitioner and educator organizations in pharmacy have adopted pharmaceutical care as the vision and mission of the profession.

Note, please, the focus upon the second word of the dyad—care. Pharmaceutical care truly is a revolution, in the literal sense. It calls for a rolling back—back to the patient and away from a fixation with the product. Instead of perching in the back of a pharmacy handling the drug products, pharmacists are moving out from behind barrier counters to areas in pharmacies designed to facilitate caring activities.

Sites, Systems, and Standards

The impact of these forces of change has permeated all aspects of pharmacy. Pharmacy layouts have been changed to accommodate the delivery of pharmaceutical care. New cognitive software programs have evolved to complement traditional pharmacy dispensing computer systems. Technician-driven dispensing (or robotic driven dispensing) models are replacing pharmacist-driven dispensing paradigms. Numerous new standards are in development to ensure and certify practitioner competency and to recognize pharmacy sites that have upgraded to support the consistent delivery of pharmaceutical care.

This book is intended to guide the reader through this wind tunnel of change for the profession of pharmacy. It is intended to confront and answer fundamental sociological and professional questions regarding this notion of reengineering an entire profession. These questions include: Where did we come from?, How did we get to where we are?, What is the nature of this change process?, Where are we going?, and What are the foundations and pillars to anchor and guide us in our travels?.

Coherence and Contingency

Whenever one discusses the future, and particularly when one paints the future in glowing detail, there is a risk that the focus on the new may appear to ignore or even to denigrate the past. We are very sensitive to this past/future potential polemic and have tried to be faithful and fair to those before us in the profession who were focused on the product.

Our attempt to ensure fairness should become apparent in the structure of the book. To provide coherence and a, systematic connection to pharmacy's roots we start with historical and philosophical perspectives that present the stable, constant elements of pharmacy: the abiding centrality of medication as a tool for preventing and treating maladies, and the role of pharmacists as society's medication mediators.

However, the term "coherence" suggests a fluid and flexible structure, rather than a fixed core of elements. And, following this model, the book next moves into the realm of contingencies (i.e., plausible futures). Contingencies are the various elements that impinge upon the profession's ability to move from product provision to pharmaceutical care. These elements are the various sociological, economic, and psychological situations pharmacy faces in its quest to assume more responsibility for patient care.

Outline of the book

The book is divided into three sections: Prelude to Pharmaceutical Care; The Nature of Pharmaceutical Care; and Implementation of Pharmaceutical Care.

Prelude to Pharmaceutical Care

The first chapter of the book introduces the concept of profession. It denotes that professions provide services that are unstandardized or adapted to the needs of individual clients. It further argues that pharmacy has lost three of its four traditional unstandardized roles: procurement, storage, and compounding of medications. The fourth role, dispensing medications, is in the process of relegation.

The second chapter presents the historical image of pharmacists from 17th century apothecaries to present. The author posits that pharmacy, through the adoption of pharmaceutical care, is returning to a high level of professional responsibility, after decades of existing in a commercial role.

The third chapter examines the "fit" of pharmaceutical care into the contemporary health care system. After a robust discussion of the context of the United States health care system, the author concludes that pharmaceutical care has arrived at a propitious time.

The fourth chapter describes the nature of the drug use process within the health care system. While the drug distribution process is effective and possibly efficient, the drug use process is in need of transformation. Extensive discussion ensues regarding some major trends (i.e., contingencies) that influence health care in general and the shift to pharmaceutical care in particular.

The fifth chapter addresses the issue of practice assimilation. The author asks, "How does pharmaceutical care 'catch on' in the profession of pharmacy." In exploring this question, the chapter traverses the field of "diffusing innovations" and investigates how the process (i.e., rate) of change is effected.

The sixth chapter, which ends this section, introduces the reader to the target for pharmaceutical care's influence: health-related quality of life. The link is made between capturing health-related quality of life measures and offering a strategy to monitor the effects of disease or condition management.

The Nature of Pharmaceutical Care

The seventh chapter changes focus and explores the philosophical nature of pharmaceutical care. To provide coherence, the authors trace the functional history of pharmacists from the age of medication compounder or preparer through the current age of quality drug distributor, and into the era of pharmaceutical care provider. The chapter examines the societal forces that are encouraging the functional shift and the scope of the pharmacy profession's response.

The eight chapter explores the nature of caring. Symbolic, and perhaps rhetorical, questions with which the authors wrestle include: What is meant by pharmaceutical care?, Is pharmaceutical care different than pharmaceutical services?, What is the difference between scientific decision making and professional decision making?, What does caring mean for pharmacists, and How does one go about establishing caring relationships?

The ninth chapter investigates the nature of pharmaceutical care vis-a-vis outcomes of medication therapy. The assertion is offered that pharmaceutical care focuses pharmacists on outcomes. However, the authors contend that outcomes, per se, are too vague in the pharmaceutical care lexicon of chronic illness. The contention is that the notion of therapeutic objectives is, perhaps, more meaningful. Provocative questions unearthed in this chapter include: What is the difference between the patient's illness perspective and the pharmacist's disease perspective?, and What is the relationship between pharmaceutical care and continuous quality improvement?

The tenth chapter reasons that if professional responsibility is an integral, proactive part of pharmaceutical care, then this expanded professional responsibility includes new duties of care. Pharmaceutical care positions pharmacists as more than merely passive observers of drug therapy. Pharmacists view pharmaceutical care as the means to go beyond roles of dispensers or advisors. Indeed, the authors assert, the pharmacists who deliver pharmaceutical care offer to be responsible for providing and optimizing medication therapy.

The eleventh chapter discusses head-on the need for pharmaceutical care. What is the evidence that a medication use problem exists in society? What is the evidence that society even recognizes medication misadventuring as a problem, or that society perceives a need to fix such a problem with what pharmacy is calling pharmaceutical care?

Implementation of Pharmaceutical Care

The twelfth chapter starts to move the nexus of the discussion toward the implementation of pharmaceutical care. Specifically, how are pharmacists reacting to the external forces of change? What are the most pressing forces? And how are pharmacists modifying their practices and routines in response to the movement toward pharmaceutical care?

The thirteenth chapter tells readers how pharmacists in various practice settings have reorganized their sites and functions to enable the provision of pharmaceutical care. The authors discuss what types of practice systems have been created to foster the new practice style and walk the reader through the systematic strategic planning process one might use to start a site reengineering.

The fourteenth chapter moves from site retooling to an exploration of the need for pharmacists, themselves, to gain some new competencies in order to deliver pharmaceutical care. The cardinal competencies revolve around honing patient assessment skills, patient monitoring skills (i.e., the caring skills), and interprofessional communication skills. The authors contend that pharmaceutical care demands more from a practitioner than a particular degree or a state Board of Pharmacy registration. It demands more than an accumulation of continuing education certificates. Pharmaceutical care refocuses capability from mere education or degree to the realm of competencies.

The fifteenth chapter broaches the issue of payment for pharmaceutical care. Payment reform ideas discussed include a shift from transaction-driven payment to capitation and an unbundling of reimbursement separating product cost reimbursement from compensation for caring activities. The elements of an ideal remuneration system are presented and explained.

The sixteenth chapter ends the section on pharmaceutical care implementation with an ethical read of the pharmaceutical care horizon. The author posits the question: How will the change to pharmaceutical care affect the moral nature of pharmacy practice? Discussion ensues on "What should I do?," and "What should I be?" In other words, what is required of the pharmacist who changes to a pharmaceutical care model?

Reengineering a profession is a major undertaking. Success requires grassroots adoption of a systematic change process. Fortunately, and with propitious timing, society has become aware of the flaws in the current drug use process; pharmacists have yearned for more patient care roles; and an economic imperative to reach beyond dispensing has occurred. This book examines the root causes and initial efforts of the pharmaceutical care reprofessionalization pilgrimage.

Contributors

Heidi M. Anderson-Harper, Ph.D.
School of Pharmacy
Auburn University
Alabama 36849-5501

David M. Angaran, M.S.
National ℞ Service Inc.
700 West Third Avenue
Columbus, Ohio 43210

David B. Brushwood, J.D.
College of Pharmacy
University of Florida
Box 100484
Health Science Center
Gainesville, Florida 32610-0484

Robert A. Buerki, Ph.D.
College of Pharmacy
The Ohio State University
500 West 12th Avenue
Columbus, Ohio 43210-1291

Kathleen M. Bungay, Pharm.D.
New England Medical Center
750 Washington Street
Boston, Massachusetts 02111

Donna E. Dolinsky, Ph.D.
Arnold & Marie Schwartz College of
    Pharmacy and Health Sciences
Long Island University
75 DeKalb Avenue
Brooklyn, New York 11201

Donald O. Fedder, D.Ph.
School of Pharmacy
University of Maryland
20 North Pine Street
Baltimore, Maryland 21201-1180

William A. Gouveia, M.S.
New England Medical Center
750 Washington Street
Boston, Massachusetts 02111

Amy M. Haddad, Ph.D.
School of Pharmacy and Allied Health
    Professions
Creighton University
2500 California Plaza
Omaha, Nebraska 68178

Hind T. Hatoum, Ph.D.
Director/Pharmacoeconomics
Searle
Box 5110
Chicago, Illinois 60680-5110

C. Douglas Hepler, Ph.D.
College of Pharmacy
University of Florida
Box 100484
Health Science Center
Gainesville, Florida 32610-0484

Gregory J. Higby, Ph.D.
American Institute of the History of
    Pharmacy
Pharmacy Building
University of Wisconsin-Madison
425 North Charter Street
Madison, Wisconsin 53706

Calvin H. Knowlton, Ph.D.
School of Pharmacy
Philadelphia College of Pharmacy and
    Science
600 South 43rd Street
Philadelphia, PA 19104-4495

Earle W. Lingle, Ph.D.
College of Pharmacy
University of South Carolina
Columbia, South Carolina 29208

Lucinda L. Maine, Ph.D.
American Pharmaceutical Association
2215 Constitution Avenue, N.W.
Washington, DC 20037

Susan M. Meyer, Ph.D.
American Association of Colleges of
    Pharmacy
1426 Prince Street
Alexandria, Virginia 22314-2841

Richard P. Penna, Pharm.D.
American Association of Colleges of
    Pharmacy
1426 Prince Street
Alexandria, Virginia 22314-2841

Michael T. Rupp, Ph.D.
School of Pharmacy and Pharmaceutical
    Sciences
1330 Heine Pharmacy Building
Purdue University
West Lafayette, Indiana 47907-1330

Carl E. Trinca, Ph.D.
College of Osteopathic Medicine of
    Pacific
College Plaza
Pamona, California 91766

Robert J. Valuck, Ph.D.
School of Pharmacy
University of Colorado Health Sciences
    Center C238
4200 East 9th Avenue
Denver, Colorado 80262-0238

Louis D. Vottero, M.S.
P.O. Box 270
Calais, Maine 04619-0270

C. Edwin Webb, Pharm. D. MPH
American Association of Colleges of
    Pharmacy
1426 Prince Street
Alexandria, Virginia 22314-2841

Bruce D. Weinstein, Ph.D.
Center for Health, Ethics and Law
1354 Health Sciences North
P. O. Box 9022
Morgantown, West Virginia 26506-9022

Prelude to Pharmaceutical Care

1

The Purposes of Professions in Society

Robert A. Buerki, Ph.D., R.Ph.
Louis D. Vottero, M.S., R.Ph.

Professions are found wherever humans live together in socialized groups. Professions emerged in the Middle Ages when specialized practitioners began to develop and provide an array of significant, unstandardized personal services that were central to human values. These services—such as health, education, religion, and welfare—were adapted to the needs of individual clients and required knowledge and skills that the typical client did not possess. Pharmacy is among the oldest of the healing professions and its practitioners provide unique, personalized services that meet the fundamental needs of individuals, communities, and society.

One approach to understanding the purpose of professions in our society is to examine these unique, individual service needs and how an organized body of professionals meets those needs. We will begin by examining the nature of professions in general. We will then explain how professions differ from other service occupations and from strictly commercial enterprises. Finally, we will examine the unique power professionals possess, as well as their special prerogatives, duties, and obligations, and explain why pharmacy is properly considered to be a profession.

What is a Profession?

The word "profession" means "to testify on behalf of" or "to stand for" something. Members of a profession define or *profess* their fundamental commitment to serving society. People who are professionals stand for something and avow not only to provide their clients with knowledge but also to use a particular body of learning to solve a specific range of human problems (May 1992, 28). In this context, pharmacists not only profess to be experts on drug therapy but also avow to help people make the best possible use of drugs.

Origins of Professions

In the medieval world, the term "professional" was not applied to lawyers, physicians, priests, or academics, who professed their commitment to apply their respective bodies of knowledge to the service of human need, but to monks, who professed their faith in God when they took up the contemplative life (May 1992, 28). In the West, we trace our professional lineage more directly to late medieval cities in Europe, especially Italy. As Europe became more urbanized, artisans broke away from the manor estates and took up middle-class occupations. Pharmacy was one of a number of occupations that developed guild-like associations during this period. (Sonnedecker 1961, 244). At about the same time, occupations that had been confined to the learned world of the medieval clergy became secularized.

Toward the close of the twelfth century, the physicians and pharmacists of Florence, together with some others, formed a single guild. Supervision was rigid. During annual inspections of pharmacies, guild commissions confiscated drugs not meeting the guild requirements and excluded the culprits from professional practice for varying periods (Sonnedecker 1976, 56–57). The separation of practitioners of pharmacy and organization into guilds was a prerequisite to professionalization; actual professionalization came more slowly. Historians date the legal recognition and regulation of pharmacy in the West, as an occupation separate from medicine, to the thirteenth century (Sonnedecker 1961, 244).

The Work of Professionals

In their practice, professionals use a variety of observable techniques and tangible goods. They also use intangibles, such as skill, knowledge, and previous experience, that often go unrecognized by members of the public. The end results of professional functions take the form of products, services, advice, opinion, and even a physical presence on behalf of another person or group (Mrtek and Catizone 1989, 24).

There is a uniquely *public nature* to the work of professionals. Professionals must use their knowledge not simply to display their virtuosity but also to serve human need. Moreover, professionals serve not only the needs of friends but also those of strangers. Professionals must act altruistically. The seventeenth century idea of "hanging out one's shingle" symbolized this readiness to "go public" and to serve the needs of the stranger (May 1992, 29).

Secondly, there is a *special nature* to the functions professionals perform. These functions are always more complex than the mechanical activities a client may observe. The seemingly simple chest tapping involved in auscultative percussion, for example, belies years of clinical experience. Moreover, it is not unusual for professionals to practice in relative isolation from the routines of daily life and provide their services to society itself in abstract ways (Mrtek and Catizone 1989, 24).

Finally, there is an *exclusive nature* to the functions professionals perform. Professionals, through a representative body of peers sanctioned by the state, are given the unusual authority to determine who may be permitted to practice and under what conditions. For example, state boards of medicine and pharmacy define the kinds of activities physicians and pharmacists are allowed to perform, outline the social privileges and professional prerogatives they may claim, and promulgate controls to guarantee that these privileges and prerogatives are not abused (Mrtek and Catizone 1989, 24).

The Societal Need for Professionals

Although many professions trace their origins to European medieval guilds, health professions in the United States emerged from other occupational groups. This emergence took place toward the end of the 19th century as a result of the development of complex urban society. These professions have since become integral parts of society. They have flourished simply because most people find modern life too complex to live without the benefit of expert consultation and specialized services (Mrtek and Catizone 1989, 25).

The services provided by professionals depend upon the application of formal knowledge, sometimes in highly modified form, to complex tasks and problems of immediate importance to clients. However, expertise in a profession extends beyond mere knowledge to include the skills, judgments, and experiences necessary to practice the profession at a level of competency determined by academics, regulators, and the public (Mrtek and Catizone 1989, 26).

The complex, ever-changing needs of American society in the mid-1990s provide a challenge to all professionals and a special challenge to health professionals. In the murky world of managed competition, does a health professional still declare, promise, or vow anything that would make a requirement of integrity clear and compelling? Should a profession be understood as a value-free collection of knowledge and skills learned by training and accessible to consumers or as a value-laden form of human activity constituted as much by the ends it seeks as by the skills it requires? (Lammers and Verhey 1987, 70)

The Inherent Power of Professionals

Professionals exercise power over their clients and over other professionals through the services they provide and the environment in which they practice. Expertise is sometimes equated with the power to control and master the formal knowledge of the profession (Mrtek and Catizone 1989, 26). Moreover, professionals often attempt to enhance their *power of knowledge* by transforming the formal knowledge base that is at the heart of their profession into an indecipherable argot of technical terms (Freidson 1984, xi).

Society grants varying amounts of discretionary power to each profession based on the value of the goods and services provided by the profession. These *powers of position,* once given, are very difficult to revoke. For example, pharmacists wield a certain power by controlling access to potent, often dangerous drugs. Physicians may wield power by deciding which types of patients they will treat. Society often has difficulty controlling or limiting such discretionary power even when this power exceeds the best interests of society (Mrtek and Catizone 1989, 27).

Society also grants each profession certain *functional powers* that can have a profound impact on the professional-client relationship. In pharmacy, these powers go far beyond the traditional power to dispense. They include: developing and managing systems of drug distribution that provide access points to patients and assure drug safety and compliance with legal and professional standards and providing other cognitive services solidly based in professional knowledge and skills. Health professionals should employ these powers to affect a "good outcome" for their patients as determined by their individual life-plans, their understanding of their illness, and their concept of what constitutes appropriate treatment (Brody 1992). With this in mind, pharmaceutical care encourages pharmacists and physicians not only to agree upon a therapeutic plan but also to share their functional power with their patients by including the patients in both the formulation and implementation of the plan.

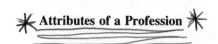

Attributes of a Profession

Dictionary definitions for the term "profession" more or less agree that a profession involves a specialized, intellectual learning which is used to render a particular service either by guiding or advising others or by practicing an art (Sonnedecker 1961, 245). A. M. Carr-Saunders and P. A. Wilson (1933, 284) point out that there is no single test or touchstone for professionalism, characterizing it as "a complex of characteristics." Roy Lewis and Angus Maude (1952, 64) have written that "a moral code is the basis of professionalism." Beyond this common thread of morality, however, the promulgation of a satisfactory definition of the term has progressed little beyond the six criteria proposed by Abraham Flexner in 1915 and elaborated upon by Isidor Thorner in 1942: 1) a relatively specific, socially necessary function upon the regular performance of which the practitioners depend for their livelihood and social status; 2) a special technique, competence in which is demanded, resting upon; 3) a body of knowledge embracing generalized principles the mastery of which requires theoretical study; 4) a traditional and generally accepted ethic subordinating its adherents' immediate private interest to the most effective performance of the function; and 5) a formal association fostering the ethic and improvement of performance (Flexner 1915, 904; Thorner 1942a, 308).

○ *Systematic Theory and Body of Knowledge*

A profession relies upon a body of knowledge organized into an internally consistent system of abstract propositions that describe its focus of interest. Theoretical knowledge and understanding underpin the technique of every profession (Sonnedecker 1961, 251). Moreover, as has been suggested above, patients use and benefit from this body of knowledge, even through they do not understand or use it directly (Mrtek and Catizone 1989, 25–26).

○ *Professional Authority and Special Privileges*

A profession serves society by doing for society what society cannot do for itself. In turn, society grants professionals special privileges when they demonstrate skill and knowledge. Professional discretion represents evidence of a social contract made by society to receive adequate professional services in return for the privilege of internal control. Some authors claim that professionals have abused and distorted the social privileges granted them through internal control and discipline (Mrtek and Catizone 1989, 27–28).

○ *Community Sanction and Social Utility*

A profession serves a socially necessary function. It provides a service that has a high social utility. This function is typically sanctioned through a system of professional licensure. This system of licensure is viewed by some social critics as a monopoly that screens and protects the profession from censure rather than protecting society. Others argue that the licensure serves as a positive influence for preserving professional commitment (Mrtek and Catizone 1989, 26–27).

○ *Ethical Codes and Internal Control*

A profession relies on formal and informal means of internal control and sanctions, traditionally codes of ethics and peer review mechanisms. A profession accepts responsibility to maintain a standard of conduct beyond compliance to law or demonstration of technical skill. Society expects a profession to generate its own statement of acceptable and unacceptable behavior, usually in the form of a formal code of ethics (Buerki and Vottero, 1989, 330–31).

○ *Professional Culture and Organizations*

Professions employ a wide array of values, attributes, norms, symbols, and argot which make up their culture. Professions also rely upon a network of organizations which foster the professional ethic and promote the improvement of individual professional performance. In addition to licensure, professional organizations often validate professional knowledge and competence through a collegially organized community of peers (Starr 1982, 15). Starr suggests that a professional's authority could be increased by membership in an organization that is generally recognized as being selective on the basis of consensually valid and professionally relevant competence criteria (Hepler 1985, 1301). For example, some professional associations have developed their own specialty certification programs.

The Process of Professionalization

Professionalism is a concept that develops around a given profession. Its basic characteristics include four aspects. The *psychological aspect* is comprised of an individual's personal sense of worth, ambition, self-esteem, and self-concept. The *social aspect* is how professionals evolve socially for a specific purpose. The *sociological aspect* centers on the profession's model, code of ethics, and theoretical knowledge base drawn from educational requirements. The *legal-ethical aspect* includes those laws and moral issues related to the public good (Sogol and Manasse 1989, 65–67). In contrast, *professionalization* is the dynamic process of becoming a professional.

Becoming a Professional

The process of becoming a professional begins with admission to a professional school. In professional schools, students are exposed to a variety of educational materials and problem-solving skills that will enable them to function within the current standards of the profession (Sogol and Manasse 1989, 68). Professional students gradually develop a professional self-image in the course of their training. This professional development consists of learning and assimilating the traits students will need in order to play the role of the professional after graduation (Buerki 1977, 29). Mary Jean Huntington (1957, 180) has shown that with each succeeding year in school, medical students were more likely to say that, on the occasion of their last contact with a patient, they thought of themselves as a doctor rather than a student. Similarly, Renée C. Fox (1957) has analyzed the development of medical students as they learn and assimilate the traits they will need to play the role of physician once they leave school.

Functioning as a Professional

True professionals behave in a manner that embodies both their professional technique and their commitment to provide individualized professional service. Professionals also subscribe to a traditional and generally accepted ethic which subordinates their immediate private interests to the most effective performance of their professional function (Thorner 1942a, 321). It is not unusual, for example, for a pharmacist to be called in the middle of the night to fill an emergency prescription. In a broader sense, professionals also use their knowledge and skill to benefit mankind. Many health professionals volunteer to serve on lay health advisory boards or participate in community health screening programs. Others, such as Dr. Albert Schweitzer, devote significant portions of their lives to providing health services in a missionary setting.

Professional Responsibility

Professionals develop a public and moral sense of responsibility to others by internalizing a clear sense of purpose, a strong commitment to serve the public, and a deep understanding of the ethic of the profession. This professional responsibility is reflected in the way professionals behave toward their clients and toward each other. The true professional will understand and practice the role virtues of their profession. Society expects its physicians to be competent, its lawyers to hold confidences, and its pharmacists to be trustworthy—role virtues all these professions share, to be sure. Professionals also strive to maintain their professional competence—generally through self-study or organized continuing professional education activities—in order to improve their professional service to the public.

The Special Nature of Professional Practice

As we have indicated, professions have developed around the provision of services that have three general characteristics: requirement of knowledge and skills that the typical client does not have; provision of personal services that are central to human values; and adaptation of these services to the needs of individual clients: that is, professionals provide unstandardized services (Larson 1977). Professionals must balance the provision of these services with the countervailing forces of professional prerogatives, authority, and autonomy.

Professional Prerogatives: Rights and Choices

Professional prerogatives may be defined as those rights that belong to specific groups or classes of individuals, as sanctioned by society. Professional prerogatives address issues within the professional's discretion which are not specifically addressed by the law. Within pharmacy, for example, many pharmacists draw attention to their "right" to decide whether or not to fill a prescription order and often speak of "exercising" or "not exercising" their professional prerogatives, demonstrating the voluntary nature of this activity (Buerki and Vottero 1991, 72). The concept of professional autonomy is a basis for exercising professional prerogatives. That is, professionals practice in a manner that cannot accommodate external interference. In daily practice, the knowledge and skills needed are esoteric, the tasks performed are complex, and the professional judgments made are sophisticated; thus, professionals could not practice effectively if they had to contend with such interference (Mrtek and Catizone 1989, 27).

Professional Discretion: Power and Societal Interest

Professionals not only exercise discretionary powers over their individual actions but also exercise self-supervision over the actions of their peers. For example, physicians' professional practices are regularly reviewed by peer-review committees composed of other physicians. Professionals also accept a social contract underlying their discretionary powers, balancing discretion and societal interest. Thus, pharmacists have the discretionary power to distribute certain dangerous or potentially habit-forming drugs within the community but typically exercise this power in a manner that is in the best interest of society. Some social critics have warned, however, that an unsanctioned expansion of these discretionary powers would be harmful to societal interests (Mrtek and Catizone 1989, 28).

Professional Autonomy: The Boundaries of Power

Society is reluctant to permit any profession to be completely autonomous. Full autonomy would provide professionals with a mechanism to define, control, and eventually monopolize the services of other interdependent professions to such an intolerable level that societal intervention would become inevitable. Thus, the virtual monopoly on prescribing medications enjoyed by generations of physicians is now shared by osteopaths, dentists, optometrists, and—in some states— by pharmacists. To avoid societal intervention, professionals typically seek to balance the relationship between their discretionary powers and the exercise of their professional autonomy (Mrtek and Catizone 1989, 28).

The Special Nature of Health Professionals

Health professions exist because there is illness. When they are ill, people are suffering an attack on their "wholeness," their humanity, and often their very identity. This vulnerability is unique in that a lack of health robs ill people of the ability to deal with their other vulnerabilities, such as the loss of personal freedom or privacy in a hospital setting. Moreover, because they do not have the knowledge or skills necessary to effect their own cure, ill people are forced to place themselves under the care of health professionals who have these skills. Unfortunately, these health professionals may also inadvertently bring harm to their patients (Pellegrino 1979). Health professionals should be alert to the sense of powerlessness that often accompanies illness and be prepared to respond to it (Brody 1992).

Pharmacy as a Health Profession

As health professionals, pharmacists make moral decisions that affect human purposes. Edward C. Elliott, director of the deeply probing Pharmaceutical Survey (1946–49), made this point clear when he concluded that "the profession of pharmacy is fundamentally moral in nature" (Elliott 1950, 4). More recently, Pellegrino and Thomasma elegantly encapsulated the moral dimension of the pharmacist-patient relationship when they declared that "any act which applies knowledge to persons involves values and consequently falls into the moral realm" (Pellegrino and Thomasma 1981, 178).

The Societal Need for the Profession of Pharmacy

For centuries, the profession of pharmacy has provided service of fundamental value to society. During the first half of the twentieth century, American pharmacy gradually lost three of the four professional functions that had characterized the work of pharmacists for nearly one thousand years—the procurement, storage, and compounding of drug products. At midcentury, pharmacists concentrated on the remaining professional function—dispensing drug products and managing the supply of medicines to society (Mrtek and Catizone 1989, 31). As drugs became more potent and federal and state legislation became more stringent, pharmacists took justifiable pride in being responsible and accountable for controlling drug distribution.

In the mid-1960s, pharmacists began to focus their professional attention upon assuring safe, effective, and cost-efficient therapeutic outcomes for their patients. By the late 1960s, the profession began to draw sharp criticism that it had become too commercialized (Francke 1969). By the mid-1970s, however, bolstered by challenging interprofessional practice settings and freer access to clinical data and other patient information, the profession opened a new clinical role for itself in the area of consultation. In recent decades, the societal need for both the distributive and the more highly specialized professional services provided by pharmacists has been well documented (Trinca 1991). Today, American pharmacists face the challenge of providing *pharmaceutical care,* which requires accepting responsibility for providing drug therapy for the purpose of achieving definite outcomes that improve a patient's quality of life (Hepler and Strand 1990a, 539).

The Evolving Societal Role of the Pharmacist

As we have suggested, at the turn of the century, American pharmacy began to move away from the path that had characterized its professional function since the earliest times, a function centered upon the knowledge and skills needed to compound drug products. The mechanized processes of industry and the emergence of new drugs placed the complexity of drug preparation far beyond the reach of the average pharmacist. Because drugs are inherently dangerous substances and the pharmacists' knowledge about their proper preparation, storage, and handling is greater than that of any other professional group, pharmacists began to develop a more technologically advanced role in quality assurance as it applied to drug distribution. This evolving professional function, as defined by society and the profession, ensured that the drugs provided to patients were safely and accurately dispensed (Mrtek and Catizone 1989, 29–30).

In recent years, pharmacy practice has experienced a gradual shift away from the technical paradigm, which emphasized drug products and their preparation, toward a more disease- and patient-oriented approach to pharmaceutical decision making. This shift in favor of more active, direct involvement with patient care came about more naturally in institutional settings than it did in community practice settings. Pharmaceutical decision-making has been strengthened by the institutional pharmacist's access to clinical data and the underlying interprofessional support of changing practice patterns and functions of pharmacists (Mrtek and Catizone 1989, 35).

Professional vs. Business Conflicts

The practice of pharmacy in the United States has always been associated with the merchandising of unrelated goods. The sale of general merchandise in drugstores was necessary in order to build an adequate cash volume to permit pharmacists to perform their professional functions. Moreover, having items besides drugs available in the pharmacy helped to establish the corner drugstore in the community. In one place people could obtain not only the prescriptions and other health goods needed in times of illness but also sundries and convenience items needed in times of health. The presence of departments beyond the prescription counter was not seen by pharmacists as deprofessionalizing when compounding was still an important part of their daily activities. Indeed, many pharmacists saw these departments as a natural extension of the prescription department. In 1899, pharmacist George J. Seabury noted, "Unlike the grocer, who is a . . . mere exchanger of articles that are daily requested of him, the pharmacist is expected, by his education and profession, to examine every article sold in his establishment and to be accountable for its quality" (Seabury 1899, 14). Over four decades later, sociologist Isador Thorner agreed: "Distribution may be in the process of becoming scientific and is being taught in schools of business administration but it cannot become a profession until the seller's interest is institutionally subordinated to that of the user of drugs. The grocer has no moral obligation to his customers parallel to that of the physician, lawyer or pharmacist toward his client" (Thorner 1942b, 617).

As the dispensing of prescriptions became a more centralized professional function of American pharmacists, however, many practitioners became torn over which of their functions—professional or mercantile—should assume primacy. Many sought to achieve an uneasy balance, a dilemma compounded by the commercial setting in which much of pharmacy is still practiced. The business and professional concerns of the pharmacist often conflict, and these conflicts can cause ambiguity in the way patients view pharmacists and their functions. Francke places the blame for this problem squarely on the appearance of the typical American retail drugstore: "The public can associate neither the drugstore nor the pharmacist in it as serving the health needs of society" (Francke 1969, 164).

The Professional Image of the Pharmacist

Pharmacists have also had to contend with the pressures of competing public and professional expectations. Some indication of how the public views pharmacy is given by public opinion polls conducted during the last two decades. These polls show that the public accords pharmacists a high professional standing in terms of honesty and ethical standards. It is significant that the prime source of influence on the views of individuals was their personal experience with pharmacists and the quality of each individual patient-practitioner interaction. It seems that pharmacists who demonstrate technical expertise and provide services consistent with their patients' views of professional services will be deemed professional. It is the collective judgment of the public that determines whether pharmacy is an occupation or a profession (Smith and Knapp 1987, 114–15; Hughes 1959, 447).

On the other hand, pharmacists have had to contend with negative public and professional perceptions of what was felt to be a diminished professional function. It is not clear whether this shift in perception arose spontaneously from within the profession itself or whether it was fostered by outside forces (Mrtek and Catizone 1989, 32–33). Pharmacists have also faced a variety of internal problems that affect their members and strain the fabric of their profession. These problems include interprofessional jurisdictional disputes over the control of drugs, the impact of technology, internal strains due to the evolution of practice, and the resultant differences in education, skills, and attitudes within the profession (Smith and Knapp 1987, 110–11).

The Covenantal Nature of Professional Relationships

The key ingredients of the notion of covenant are promise and fidelity to promise. A covenantal relationship is based upon the concepts of indebtedness and responsiveness (May 1983). The work of a health professional begins with a response to a patient's request for assistance or care. The patient thus provides the "gift" of a personal sanction to the health practitioner to initiate professional service. This "gift" creates a sense of indebtedness on the part of practitioners, providing them with an opportunity to perform their professional functions. Implicit in this covenant is the commitment to not only maintain a high quality of technical skill but also to safeguard patients from possible untoward effects related to their drug therapy.

Trust is also inherent in the relationship between health-care professionals and their patients. This condition is a reflection of the system of licensure that is imposed by society, a system that permits patients to place their most intimate thoughts as well as their bodies in the hands of professionals whose competency they cannot easily judge. In contrast to the practices of medicine and nursing, which are characterized by direct patient contact, the pharmacist often fills prescription orders in seclusion or partially shielded from the patient. Therefore, the patient must have even greater faith in the pharmacist's competence than he does in the physician's. As the practice of pharmacy expands to include more intense patient-pharmacist encounters, this trust will be increasingly challenged as patients have expanded opportunities to scrutinize and evaluate the professional services they receive.

Caring as a Professional Responsibility

Care and medicine have become closely identified, if not synonymous, in the minds of many. For example, medicine, nursing, and other health-related activities are often referred to as "caring professions." Care often appears to be a more important regulative notion for determining the basis and direction of health-related activities than might be morally justified. Care, however, is a significant notion that reminds us that medicine serves as one of the ways we can help others maintain basic physical and psychological integrity. Moreover, care directs our attention to the concrete patient in need without subjecting him or her to manipulation for the good of others. However, it is important that the care given the patient be based on the respect due each of us, well or ill, for otherwise our attempts to care can lead to sentimental or paternalistic perversions (Hauerwas 1978, 145–50).

Pharmaceutical Care: From Functioning to Caring

In a seminal 1989 paper titled "Opportunities and Responsibilities in Pharmaceutical Care," Hepler and Strand proposed a new philosophy of pharmacy practice that went far beyond the rather limited expectations of most pharmacy practitioners, even those dedicated to the patient-oriented practices embraced by the term "clinical pharmacy." They reviewed the alarming extent of drug-related morbidity and mortality in the American health-care system and concluded that this problem could only be addressed by a fundamental change in the pharmacist's professional function. They referred to this concept as *pharmaceutical care,* which they defined as "the responsible provision of drug therapy for the purpose of achieving definite outcomes that improve a patient's quality of life." They stressed that the practice of pharmacy "must restore what has been missing for years: a clear emphasis on the patient's welfare, a patient advocacy role with a clear ethical mandate to protect the patient from the harmful effects of . . . 'drug misadventuring.'" Rather than restrict the pharmacist's professional role to merely supplying and monitoring drug therapy, Hepler and Strand built upon concepts of clinical pharmacy to create "a process in which a pharmacist cooperates with a patient and other health professionals in designing, implementing, and monitoring a therapeutic plan that will produce specific therapeutic outcomes for the patient." Central to their shared vision is the establishment of a "mutually beneficial exchange in which the patient grants authority to the provider, and the provider gives competence and commitment to the patient" (Hepler and Strand 1990b, 8S, 12S, 15S). Leaders in pharmacy have embraced the concept of pharmaceutical care because they see within it an opportunity to respond to critical health-care needs of society and to recapture the sense of professional purpose which many feel has been missing from American pharmacy practice in recent years. These concepts are developed more fully in Chapter 16, The Ethics of Pharmaceutical Care.

Summary and Conclusions

Accepting the mandate of pharmaceutical care will greatly increase the pharmacist's responsibility to patients; discharging that responsibility will require philosophical, organizational, and functional change in the practice of pharmacy (Hepler and Strand 1990b, 12S). Today, the profession of pharmacy faces daunting challenges to its traditional functional autonomy. The profession has responded to these pressures by increasingly relying upon paraprofessional help, robotics, and computer-assisted patient information systems to manage its interpersonal patient-care functions. Just as pharmacy has learned it can no longer focus exclusively upon the safe distribution of drugs or even upon expanded clinical functions to justify its societal function, it may also learn it cannot solely rely upon the enhanced service mandate suggested by the concept of pharmaceutical care for its *raison d'être*.

Pharmaceutical care in its fullest sense involves professional care decisions beyond enhanced therapeutic outcomes. Practitioners who embrace the concept of pharmaceutical care will encounter increasingly complex moral and ethical situations which will require not only a deeper professional and personal commitment to patients as individuals but also a higher level of clinical knowledge as they deal with more complex patient-care decisions. As a result, the status of the practice of pharmacy will be further enhanced as a socially necessary health-care profession.

References

Brodie, D. C. 1981. Pharmacy's Societal Purpose. *American Journal of Hospital Pharmacy* 38 (12):1893–6.

Brody, H. 1992. *The Healer's Power*. New Haven: Yale University Press.

Buerki, R. A. 1977. Pharmacist Smyth and Druggist Smith—A Study in Professional Aspirations. *American Journal of Pharmaceutical Education* 41 (1):28–33.

Buerki, R. A., and L. D. Vottero. 1989. Ethics. In *Pharmacy Practice: Social and Behavioral Aspects*, 3rd ed., ed. A. I. Wertheimer and M. C. Smith, 329–49. Baltimore: Williams & Wilkins.

Buerki, R. A., and L. D. Vottero. 1991. The Changing Face of Pharmaceutical Education: Ethics and Professional Prerogatives. *American Journal of Pharmaceutical Education* 55 (1):71–4.

Carr-Saunders, A. M., and P. A. Wilson. 1933. *The Professions*. Oxford: Clarendon Press.

Elliott, E. C. 1950. *The General Report of the Pharmaceutical Survey, 1946–49*. Washington, D. C.: American Council on Education.

Flexner, A. 1915. Is Social Work a Profession? *School and Society* 1 (26):901–11.

Fox, R. C. 1957. Training for Uncertainty. In *The Student Physician: Introductory Studies in the Sociology of Medical Education*, ed. R. K. Merton, G. G. Reader, and P. L. Kendall, 207–41. Cambridge: Harvard University Press.

Francke, D. E. 1969. Let's Separate Pharmacies and Drugstores. *American Journal of Pharmacy* 141 (5):161–9.

Freidson, E. 1986. *Professional Powers: A Study of the Institutionalization of Formal Knowledge*. Chicago: University of Chicago Press.

Hauerwas, S. 1987. Care. In *On Moral Medicine: Theological Perspectives in Medical Ethics*, ed. S. E. Lammers and A. Verhey, 262–6. Grand Rapids: William B. Eerdmans Publishing Co.

Hepler, C. D. 1985. Pharmacy as a Clinical Profession. *American Journal of Hospital Pharmacy* 42 (6):1298–306.

Hepler, C. D., and L. M. Strand. 1990a. Opportunities and Responsibilities in Pharmaceutical Care. *American Journal of Hospital Pharmacy* 47 (3):533–43.

Hepler, C. D., and L. M. Strand. 1990b. Opportunities and Responsibilities in Pharmaceutical Care. *American Journal of Pharmaceutical Education* 53 (5):7S–15S.

Hughes, E. C. 1959. The Study of Occupations. In *Sociology Today: Problems and Prospects*, ed. R. K. Merton, L. Broom, and L. S. Cottrell, Jr., 442–58. New York: Basic Books.

Huntington, M. J. 1957. The Development of a Professional Self-image. In *The Student Physician: Introductory Studies in the Sociology of Medical Education*, ed. R. K. Merton, G. G. Reader, and P. L. Kendall, 179–87. Cambridge: Harvard University Press.

Lammers, S. E., and A. Verhey, eds. 1987. *On Moral Medicine: Theological Perspectives in Medical Ethics*. Grand Rapids: William B. Eerdmans Publishing Company.

Larson, M. S. 1977. *The Rise of Professionalism: A Sociological Analysis*. Berkeley and Los Angeles: University of California Press.

Lewis, R., and A. Maude. 1952. *Professional People*. London: Phoenix House, Ltd.

May, W. F. 1983. *The Physician's Covenant*. Philadelphia: Westminster Press.

May, W. F. 1992. The Beleaguered Rulers: The Public Obligation of the Professional. *Kennedy Institute of Ethics Journal* 2 (1):25–41.

Mrtek, R. G., and C. Catizone. 1989. Pharmacy and the Professions. In *Pharmacy Practice: Social and Behavioral Aspects*, 3rd ed., ed. A. I. Wertheimer and M. C. Smith, 23–57. Baltimore: Williams & Wilkins.

Pellegrino, E. D. 1979. Toward a Reconstruction of Medical Morality: The Primacy of the Act of Profession and the Fact of Illness. *Journal of Medicine and Philosophy* 4 (3):32–56.

Pellegrino, E. D., and D. C. Thomasma. 1981. *A Philosophical Basis of Medical Practice: Toward a Philosophy and Ethic of the Healing Professions*. New York and Oxford: Oxford University Press.

Seabury, G. J. 1899. *Shall Pharmacists Become Tradesmen?*, 3rd ed. New York: George J. Seabury.

Smith, M. C., and D. A. Knapp. 1987. *Pharmacy, Drugs and Medical Care*, 4th ed. Baltimore: Williams & Wilkins.

Sogol, E. M., and H. R. Manasse, Jr. 1989. The Pharmacist. In *Pharmacy Practice: Social and Behavioral Aspects*, 3rd ed., ed. A. I. Wertheimer and M. C. Smith, 59–88. Baltimore: Williams & Wilkins.

Sonnedecker, G. 1961. To Be or Not to Be—Professional. *American Journal of Pharmacy* 133 (7):243–54.

Sonnedecker, G. 1976. *Kremers and Urdang's History of Pharmacy*, 4th ed. Philadelphia: J. B. Lippincott Company.

Starr, Paul. 1982. *The Social Transformation of American Medicine*. New York: Basic Books.

Thorner, I. 1942a. Pharmacy: The Functional Significance of an Institutional Pattern. *American Journal of Pharmaceutical Education* 6 (3):305–19. Reprinted from *Social Forces* 20 (3):321–8.

Thorner, I. 1942b. Comments on "Pharmacy, the Functional Significance of an Institutional Pattern." *American Journal of Pharmaceutical Education* 6 (4):617–9.

Trinca, C. E. 1991. Does Pharmaceutical Care Respond to Society's Mandate for Professional Pharmacy Services? Paper read at the District IV NABP/AACP Annual Meeting, 16–18 November 1991, Columbus, Ohio.

2

From Compounding to Caring: An Abridged History of American Pharmacy[1]

Gregory J. Higby, Ph.D.

Arrival in the New World

During the 16th and 17th centuries, apothecaries on the European continent solidified their position as middle-class professionals. In England, however, the ideology of *laissez-faire* capitalism blocked the full development of professional control. Instead, a haphazard health care system emerged, composed of university-educated physicians, apprentice-trained apothecaries (who practiced a combination of medicine and pharmacy), and chemists and druggists, who came to control the drug trade. A large variety of barber-surgeons, apothecary-surgeons, and other healers also contributed to the nearly chaotic character of health care in early modern England. It was during this period of turmoil that English settlers came to dominate the North American continent. Thus, the foundations of the American health care system lie in the disarray of the English system rather than the stability of the continental European system.

The Pre-Professional Period (1620 to 1820)

There was little to attract physicians and apothecaries to the colonies of the British New World. The populace knew little about medicine and was often illiterate. For that reason, other people of authority—political leaders, clergymen, and midwives—commonly provided medical care. With the aid of home medical guides, New World men and women practiced both medicine and pharmacy. They diagnosed illnesses and made up and administered simple medicines. When physicians became common in the 1700s, pharmacists were still very rare. Physicians compounded their own prescriptions or had their apprentices do it for them.

---

[1]Based in part on an invited lecture delivered at the centennial celebration of the University of Minnesota College of Pharmacy on 12 October 1992.

Colonial Apothecary Shops

In colonial America, apothecary shops were only found in the largest cities. A major function of apothecary shops like Christopher Marshall's in Philadelphia (See Figure 2–1.) was to put together and service medicine chests for prosperous land owners and physicians. Early American apothecaries operated more as manufacturers and wholesalers of drugs and medicines than as retailers. Drugs and patent medicines could be bought from general stores, book sellers, and other merchants, who did not have the specialized skills necessary to operate a true apothecary shop. Because most physicians dispensed their own drugs, prescriptions rarely found their way to shops like Marshall's. Most of the compounding Marshall did was from old family recipes handed down over the generations.

The close connection between medicine and pharmacy is well illustrated by Jonathan Roberts, the first hospital pharmacist in colonial America. In 1751, the Pennsylvania Hospital was established in Philadelphia. At first, physicians in the hospital provided their own medicines, but after a large shipment of drugs arrived from London in 1752 it was decided to set up a pharmacy. Roberts was hired to handle the "shop." His duties, like those of hospital apothecaries well into the next century, required him to go on rounds, practice some minor medi-

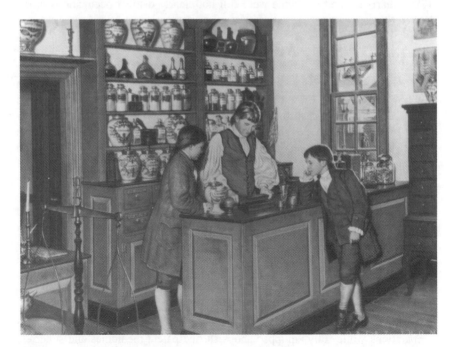

Figure. 2.1. Courtesy: Parke Davis

cine, take care of the hospital's accounts and library, and to perform odd chores along with managing the apothecary. When Roberts left the hospital in 1755, he was succeeded by John Morgan, one of the pivotal characters in the history of American medicine and pharmacy.

John Morgan held the Pennsylvania Hospital apothecary job for only 13 months before going off to Europe to study medicine. In 1765, having returned from Europe, Morgan proposed the separation of the practices of medicine and pharmacy. Morgan argued that physicians should write out their prescriptions, which pharmacists would then compound and dispense as had been the practice in Europe for centuries. This would discourage the over-drugging of patients, a common problem according to Morgan. Morgan did not merely suggest this division of labor, he brought his own pharmacist from Scotland and put his suggestion into practice. Although Morgan attempted to follow this model, he soon encountered problems. Patients were unhappy with the increased expense and inconvenience of receiving prescriptions from physicians that had to be filled by a pharmacist, and physicians relied heavily on the fees they received for the medicines they compounded and dispensed. By convention, American doctors diagnosed on credit but dispensed medicines for cash or for goods. Later in life, Morgan found his practice shrinking. He was forced him to open his own doctor's shop and practice medicine and pharmacy in one location. When he died in 1789, pharmacy and medicine were still not clearly distinct occupations in the United States.

Emergence of Pharmacy as an Independent Occupation

If Morgan failed to bring about the separation of medicine and pharmacy, when and how did it occur? From city directories and other documents, we know that apothecary shops and drugstores became more common in cities and towns after about 1810. Strangely enough, historians have not fully explained the emergence of the American drugstore. In their classic *History of Pharmacy,* Kremers and Urdang point to four roots from which the American pharmacy developed. First they cite the so-called "doctor's shops" of physicians like John Morgan. Second they describe the small number of shops operated by colonial apothecaries who specialized in selling drugs and related products, as much to physicians and landowners as to everyday customers. The third root was the general store, which sold opium to customers alongside flour without any legal restrictions. Finally they cite the drug wholesalers, who repackaged drugs and products imported from England for sale to physicians, apothecaries, general stores, and other outlets.

In the early 19th century, the offices of physicians contained a wide range of pharmaceutical furnishings. Some stocked just a shelf or two of standard preparations while fully equipped shops carried patent medicines and sundries. Some shop-doctors hired employee apothecaries, called "drug clerks." Graduates of medical schools had often missed out on the pharmaceutical training gained through a long apprenticeship and needed to hire someone with expertise to compound prescriptions. Even if they had sufficient expertise, successful shop doctors would often hire a drug clerk who would keep shop when the doctor's practice called him away. When they were successful enough to have a full, office-style practice, shop-doctors would often move and sell their pharmacy businesses to their clerks. This stimulated the growth of the retail drug trade. As a proprietor, a former drug clerk proudly took on the title of "apothecary."

Wholesalers and the Establishment of Corner Drugstores

Many of the most prominent early American pharmacies arose from the "front ends" of wholesale businesses. Under this system, wholesalers would fix up a public entrance to the warehouse where physicians and shopkeepers could place orders. Soon these front ends attracted walk-in customers interested in bargains or the freshest crude drugs. When new or exotic drugs came on the market, physicians would send patients to those wholesalers with the best trade contacts.

Nomenclature is another source of evidence that front-end wholesalers played an important role in the development of the American drugstore. Specialty retail establishments of the early to mid-19th century were called "shops." The term "store" was usually applied to businesses that carried a wide variety of goods, that is, a "storehouse." Apothecaries regarded "store" as a vulgar term, because it implied a lower class of retailing, such as the "general store." Wholesalers— called "druggists" in the trade—referred to their establishments as drugstores. When many of them moved into retail the name stuck.

Two additional factors not mentioned by Kremers and Urdang were critical to the pharmacy's development as an independent occupation and the development of its special environment, the American drugstore. The first is so obvious that we tend to ignore its significance. The services of apothecaries, regarded generally as a luxury in America during the Colonial period, came to be considered essential in the early 19th century. The best evidence of this change in attitude is found in the records of early American hospitals. The hospitals of the young republic usually employed medical apprentices as staff apothecaries. For example, the *Brief Account of the New-York Hospital,* published in 1804, states that

> A house Surgeon and Apothecary constantly reside in the Hospital.—these offices are filled by the students of the Physicians and Surgeons belonging to the Hospital, which affords an excellent school for the young men appointed to those places (Society of the New-York Hospital 1804)

By 1811, however, the position of apothecary at the New-York Hospital had changed. The job was held by a full-time pharmaceutical practitioner, tested before hiring on his prowess as a compounder of medicines. Instead of being obligated to go on rounds, he was required to stay in his "shop" at all times (Society of the New-York Hospital 1811)

The by-laws of the hospital passed in 1819 not only required testimonials on the applicant's behalf but also a $250 bond to ensure "faithful performance of the duties of his office, and that he will not cease to perform the duties of this office, without giving two months notice of his intention to leave his employment (Society of the New-York Hospital 1820)." In a little more than a decade, pharmacy services moved out of the hands of the medical apprentice and into the hands of a trained individual with professional responsibilities.

Dispensaries—clinics established to treat the deserving poor and supported by public or private largess—followed the same pattern as hospitals in the early 19th century. Full-time, responsible apothecaries replaced medical apprentices. By selecting mature apothecaries, the directors of hospitals and dispensaries obtained competent day-to-day management of their institutions. More importantly for the nascent occupation of pharmacy, full-time apothecaries provided reliable pharmaceutical services and probably encouraged prescription writing.

Beginning about 1815, study in medical schools began to replace apprenticeship as the standard system for the training of doctors. Physicians who gained their clinical experience in hospitals and dispensaries instead of as apprentices to physicians learned to write prescriptions rather than compound them. After graduation these young physicians wrote out more prescriptions—partially in emulation of their European-trained superiors and partially out of habit.

The years following the War of 1812 were transitional ones for the country's pharmacies. Physicians continued to dispense but began to take advantage of the slowly growing number of retail apothecaries. For example, the fee bill approved by the New-York County Medical Society in January 1816 contained a detailed section of "Pharmaceutical Charges," while in Boston, where there was more developed cadre of apothecaries, the local medical association omitted pharmaceutical charges from its fee bill. The physicians there were writing out prescriptions. Advertisements and city directories of the time indicate that the number of doctor's shops, was dropping off rapidly.

A small class of retail apothecaries presented no particular threat to urban physicians in the first decades of the 19th century, and provided several conveniences. New advances in chemistry and pharmacy added to the number of therapeutically active drugs available to physicians. It became difficult for physicians on rounds to carry all the drugs they needed to dispense. Well-educated physicians knew of the advances in pharmacy on the European continent and fostered pharmacy's progress in the United States.

About the same time, a change occurred in the American retail sector that would permanently affect the practice of American pharmacy. Specialized shops for all sorts of goods appeared as the major cities of the Atlantic coast prospered. Rather go to a general store for shoes, customers went to shops that sold only shoes. Apothecary shops fit into that trend. These early apothecary shops sold a great many more exotic items such as tropical fruits and spices, than shops in later eras. Apothecaries dealt with wholesalers and importers of exotic goods because these wholesalers and importers also handled drugs. In 1820, for example, one would usually go to an apothecary rather than a grocer to buy figs.

Summary of Pre-Professional Period 1620-1820

In the years following the War of 1812 a new, distinct occupation arose in American cities—the independent pharmacy practitioner. Before that time, *pharmacy,* that is, the making of medicines from drugs and other ingredients, was practiced primarily by physicians and their apprentices or by lay healers in the home. A complex set of economic, demographic, and other changes in the years following the war led to the emergence of American pharmacy practice and its unique location, the drugstore.

Period of Proto-Professionalism (1820 to 1850)

Two events occurred in 1820 and 1821 that make those years an excellent starting place for telling the story of American pharmacy's development as a profession. In January 1820, a group of about one dozen physicians met in Washington, DC and founded the *United States Pharmacopoeia*. Their objective was to "prevent trouble or uncertainty in the intercourse of physicians and apothecaries (Pharmacopoeia of the United States of America 1828, 3)." Apothecaries, however, did not participate in the preparation of the new standard. Physicians believed it was their prerogative to found the standards for medicines in the United States and did not invite official collaboration with pharmacists until 1850.

Founding of the Philadelphia College of Pharmacy

In 1821, some prominent physicians in Philadelphia, like the group in DC a year earlier, believed that it was their privilege to designate which apothecaries in their city were "masters" of the pharmaceutical arts. When their scheme became known to the pharmaceutical community in Philadelphia, outrage led to direct action. The apothecaries and druggists of the city organized the Philadelphia College of Apothecaries, which was soon renamed the Philadelphia College of Pharmacy. The initial objective of this local association was to head off the certification program being developed by the elitist physicians. The group was quite successful, and not only did the grand scheme of the physicians never get off the ground, the College of Pharmacy continues to be an active participant in the professional life of pharmacists in the United States today.

In contrast to medical schools, pharmacy schools of the early 1800s commonly held classes at night so that the apprentices could work in shops, warehouses, and manufactories during the day. To obtain a diploma, students were required to attend the same set of lectures twice, write a thesis, and pass an examination. Since the emphasis was on the knowledge and not the diploma, only about 1 in 10 students in the early decades of the Philadelphia College of Pharmacy actually graduated. Their real education came through work and reading the texts of the day—the pharmacopoeias and the dispensatories. The Philadelphia College of Science was nevertheless an important institution and it was no accident that the most important pharmaceutical book of the 19th century—the *United States Dispensatory*—was written by two of its professors, physicians George B. Wood and Franklin Bache.

Emergence of the "Pharmaceutist"

In the early 1830s, a growing number of pharmacists began calling themselves "pharmaceutists"—a shortened version of "pharmaceutical scientist." The rapid and profound advances of French pharmacy had made American physicians aware of new potent drugs such as morphine, strychnine, and quinine. In isolating these alkaloids, pharmacists had provided medical practitioners with potent plant drugs of reliable strength for the first time. Not only did this development attract the approbation of physicians, it increased the necessity for skilled pharmaceutical practitioners.

Discoveries such as the alkaloid, drew attention to continental pharmacists and American pharmacists began emulating them in other ways. In the larger East coast cities, pharmacists began participating in local scientific societies and discussion groups. Apothecary shops like that of Elias Durand in Philadelphia became gathering places for scientific investigators.

Relations with Physicians

The timing of the emergence of the American drugstore and the public recognition of the contributions of pharmacy was propitious. Physicians supported the appearance of pharmaceutists near their practices and welcomed them as subordinate colleagues. The pharmaceutists and apothecaries were few and did not compete directly with physicians for business. Moreover, they served as a check against unscrupulous drug wholesalers and other importers and helped to ensure drug quality.

The relationship between physicians and pharmacists varied over the next few decades. During the 1840s, medical schools increased their output of physicians, who flooded the markets in cities and towns. To survive, these physicians often reverted to setting up shop, selling drugs as well as advice. Pharmacists competed by doing the same. Then, during the 1850s, the borders between pharmaceutical and medical practice in cities became fuzzy again. Pharmacists began "counter prescribing," that is, recommending favorite preparations "over the counter" for customers. They also solidified their position as the prime sellers of patent medicines, which enraged physicians who saw nostrums as another competitor to their practices.

Nature of Antebellum Pharmacy Practice

Figure 3-2 is one of the oldest illustrations we have of an American pharmacy interior (circa 1836). Note that the work areas of the shop are right out front. This allowed the apothecary to get the needed light from the windows and allowed customers to watch him in action. This was important since many of his sales were simply crude drugs sold in bulk for home use. The customers liked to see the powder being weighed and wrapped. In addition, the front counter position permitted the apothecary to exhibit his skill in compounding. In contrast, the

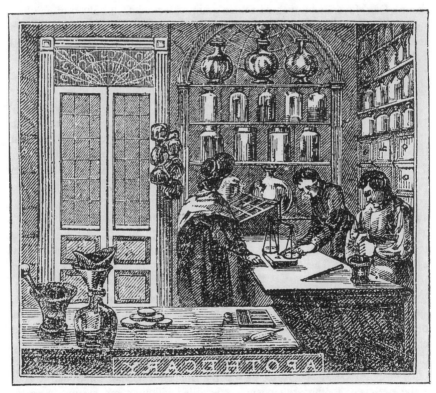

Figure 2.2. One of the earliest known depictions of the interior of an American pharmacy. From Edward Hazen, Popular Technology: or, Professions and Trades Vol. 1 (of 2), Harper and Bros., New York, 1841, p. 236, a book of vocational guidance that includes an essay on "The Druggist and Apothecary." Source of AIHP Photo: Kremers Reference Files, School of Pharmacy, University of Wisconsin.

pharmacist used a laboratory in the back, away from customer view, for the dirtier jobs of manufacturing.

In addition to medicines, apothecaries also sold the usual drugstore goods. In the 1830s, apothecaries started to phase out the sale of exotic food items such as figs, raisins, and citrus fruits. In cities they stocked fewer general articles such as glass, paint, and oils, and concentrated on patent medicines, fancy soaps, toiletries, dyes, and flavorings. Books were common drugstore merchandise in some parts of the country.

Pharmacy Practice at Midcentury

In some cases we have detailed records of the daily activities of midcentury pharmacists. For example, master pharmacist William Procter, Jr. filled six prescriptions on 27 February 1847, for a total charge of $1.20. The first was from a Dr. Mayer, who wanted fifteen grains of camphor dissolved in one-half ounce of ether, probably for his own use. The second prescription was for a tonic of ammonium hydrochloride and the syrups of ipecac, wild cherry, and balsam of Tolu, flavored with orange flower water. Procter asked fifty cents for this mixture, close to the maximum he charged for a single prescription. The third prescription Procter compounded called for a mixture of Dover's powder and potassium nitrate divided into six powder papers. Although this was an easy mixture to prepare, Procter charged 19 cents for it because of its expensive ingredients—opium and ipecac. The fourth prescription Procter prepared that day called for one ounce of uva ursi or bearberry and was probably ordered for a urinary tract disorder. Procter charged four cents for this package. The fifth prescription was quite typical for the time, calling for the combination of two crude botanicals, American columbo and valerian, with two chemicals, an iron salt and bicarbonate of soda, and division of the mixture into powder papers. This, was probably a stomach tonic. The last prescription called for zinc acetate to be added to a base of cerate of carrot. Procter charged 25 cents for this mildly astringent topical. The relatively high cost probably reflects the time required for preparation.

It is essential to remember that Procter, like most pharmacists of the day, spent more of his time manufacturing preparations than he did compounding or dispensing prescriptions. He made his own syrup of ipecac and syrup of wild cherry, as well as orange flower water and cerate of carrot. At that time, crude drugs such as columbo and valerian would be bought in bulk and powdered and otherwise processed according to the *Pharmacopoeia,* and pharmacists kept elaborate sets of apothecary jars and bottles filled with tinctures, syrups, extracts, and other preparations made on the premises. Pharmacists and their apprentices spent long hours powdering and sifting plant parts and, percolating, macerating, filtering, and bottling preparations. Many preparations were produced in bulk for physicians to use in the office or from their bags. Much of the occupational identity of pharmacists was wrapped up in this special activity that separated them from other retailers. However, like the hat makers, tailors, and other shop owners nearby, pharmacists gained much of their recognition from the overt skills they had learned over years of practice.

While prescription business continued to grow, patent medicines kept most pharmacies in business. Extremely popular since Colonial days, these secret remedies usually contained alcohol and either laxative ingredients or opiates and were not the largely ineffectual nostrums of later years. In contrast with other goods, patent medicines were traditionally marked up at 100 percent, which made them very popular with shop owners.

Opiates and laxatives were also popular in compounded prescriptions. Among the most common drugs in prescriptions were mercury or its salts, opium or morphine, hyoscyamus, ipecacuanha, china rhubarb, iodine, antimony, quinine, lead, and squill. The most common dosage forms were solutions, mixtures, and powder papers, followed by pills, plasters, and ointments.

Almost all of the common drugs, even South American drugs like cinchona bark, were imported from Europe. Pharmacists purchased them in bulk from wholesale druggists and examined them carefully for adulteration. Adulteration was usually benign and common examples included bullets added to bulk opium and sawdust mixed into a sack of powdered root or bark. In the 1840s, a new problem grew in importance and led eventually to a significant professional development—the founding of the American Pharmaceutical Association.

Drug Law of 1848

In the 1830s, drug exporters in Europe came upon a new way to make a little extra profit. Crude drugs like cinchona bark were soaked in a solvent to draw out some of the active alkaloid, then carefully dried and packaged as sound crude drug. The solvent would then be processed and the alkaloid extracted, resulting in a double profit for the exporter.

In the 1840s, European authorities started to crack down on this practice, so drug exporters began shipping the spent crudes to the United States. Some of these packages were marked "good enough for America." It is important to realize that the medicines of the 19th century truly worked on the body—they tended to be strong laxatives, emetics, or diaphoretics. And although pure crystalline alkaloids were often available, conservative American physicians preferred the old botanical "purges, pukes, and sweats" of the old school of medical treatment. When the quality of botanical supplies began to fall, physicians soon noticed that their prescriptions were not working as well.

The decline in the quality of imported drugs led to the passage of the Drug Importation Act of 1848. This early federal law governing drug quality was initially a success and thousands of pounds of drugs were rejected at major ports. However, a change in administrations in 1849 brought in a group of political

cronies as drug inspectors. The situation became worse than it had been before
the passage of the law and so physicians and pharmacists called for more precise
standards.

Most botanical drugs had no recognized standard of potency. For example,
crude opium was generally expected to be at least 8 percent morphine, but this
was only an informal standard. To facilitate the enforcement of drug purity laws,
the College of Pharmacy of the City of New York called in 1851 for a national
convention of pharmacists to draw up standards for the most popular imported
drugs.

Summary of Period   Proto-professionalism
1820-1850

This call for a national convention of pharmaceutists marks the end of the proto-
professional period. Pharmacy had at last achieved sufficient professional identity
to allow for an assembly of apothecaries, pharmaceutists, and druggists to meet
a national need. And while a wide variety of social, economic, political, and
scientific forces had molded the American drugstore during the proto-professional
period, by the end of the 1840s it had developed the form and function that it
would hold for the next century. When they met in New York in 1851, pharmacists
stood on the verge of a new era.

First Period of Professionalization (1850 to 1910): The Drugstore Era

A key figure in the professionalization of American pharmacy was William
Procter, Jr. Space does not permit a long discourse on his achievements, but no
one has challenged his title as Father of American Pharmacy. This chapter will
focus on a few of his accomplishments which serve as important markers of
pharmacy's progress.

In 1846, Procter became the first professor of practical pharmacy at the Philadelphia College of Pharmacy. The College had been teaching young pharmacists
for a generation, but had never had a professor of pharmacy. Students had been
taught the subjects of Materia Medica (natural history of drugs) and chemistry
by two physician-professors. Pharmacy was not deemed to be an academic subject
and was relegated to the apprenticeship experience. Procter and a few of his young
colleagues petitioned the college's board, which agreed with their arguments that
pharmacy had progressed to the stature of a scientific discipline and appointed
Procter to the professorship.

The professorship enabled Procter to enter the inner circle at the College.
Most significantly, he joined the publishing committee of the College's periodical,
the *American Journal of Pharmacy*. As the only journal of pharmacy in the
United States, it exerted a great deal of influence over the young profession.
Procter rose through the ranks, becoming editor in 1850. Proctor's emergence
as the first permanent pharmacist-editor was indicative of the control pharmacists

were taking over their occupation. They no longer needed physicians to run their schools and journals.

Founding of the American Pharmaceutical Association

When the New York College of Pharmacy called for its national convention in 1851, Procter and his Philadelphia friend and colleague Edward Parrish decided to go to New York to pursue a novel idea. They wanted the convention to achieve its original goal—the establishment of standards for imported drugs—but they also wanted the convention to go further and form a national pharmaceutical organization.

Procter and Porter's call for a national organization was well received in New York, and a second national convention was called for Philadelphia in 1852. Using his position as editor of the *American Journal of Pharmacy,* Procter encouraged participation from all parts of the young nation. The time was ripe for such an organization. Rail and telegraph lines reached out across the countryside and on an intellectual and scientific level, if not a political one, the United States were becoming one nation.

The 1852 convention established a national organization, the American Pharmaceutical Association (APhA). For most of its history, the APhA has counted only a small minority of pharmacists in its membership, but has exerted great influence on professional development. The founding of the APhA came at an opportune time, when pharmacy needed a voice of leadership.

United States Census figures for druggists and apothecaries show that as the 1850s progressed, the growth of American pharmacy accelerated. From 1850 to 1860, the number of physicians per capita did not change significantly, rising from 1:572 to 1:576, while the number of druggists rose from 1:3778 to 1:2850 an increase of nearly 25 percent. This trend continued, at a slightly lower rate, through the rest of the 19th century.

A major cause of this trend was the entry of large-scale manufacturing into pharmacy in the late 1850s. With large firms doing much of the complicated work, less skilled men, who had recently been "mere shopkeepers," entered the ranks of pharmacists. Physicians, already disturbed by counter prescribing, saw pharmacy declining. As one physician put it in 1860, "It is an admitted and lamentable fact that many of those *now* practicing pharmacy are totally incompetent to fulfill the responsibilities of the true apothecary. They know nothing of the science of preparing medicines." The late 1850s also was a time of great economic strife, which increased the tension between physicians and pharmacists.

With the beginning of the Civil War, American pharmacy and medicine communities ceased their battles and called a truce. Business in the cities slowed to a crawl during the war and many pharmacists lost their stores. The war, of course, greatly helped the manufacturers of medicines, who sold huge quantities to the armed forces. Some of the far-sighted firms like Squibb reinvested their profits into new equipment and expansion during the post-war period.

The Classic Drugstore (and Soda Fountain)

The years following the Civil War were witness to the redesign of the American drugstore into its classic form. The work table, which had always been near the front of the shop to benefit from natural light through the front window and to attract customer attention, was moved to the rear of the store, where the laboratory had been previously, and hidden behind a screen. The preparations necessary for compounding prescriptions were now made outside the pharmacy, so an extensive laboratory was no longer needed.

In part, these changes mirrored a trend followed by all retail specialty shops that had at one time featured in-shop manufacturing. Remote manufacturing—which took advantage of economies of scale and sweatshop labor—replaced the out-front style of the antebellum stores. The new arrangement was thought to be more elegant. In the case of pharmacy, it also added a bit of mystery to what the pharmacist did. However, the actual work of the pharmacist was becoming simpler as large manufacturers started to put out finished dosage forms in addition to ingredients for prescriptions.

Of course, moving the prescription department to the back of the store opened up the front for the sale of tobacco, fancy goods, and, best of all, soda fountain specialties. Nothing attracted more business to a pharmacy than a soda fountain. Soda water first entered American pharmacies early in the century, but became popular in the post-Civil War years. Pharmacists possessed the chemical knowledge necessary to handle the early carbonated water generators, which were cranky at best. They also had the knack for making fresh flavorings and mixing up complicated confections. Another factor in the success of the soda fountain was the rise of the temperance and prohibition movements. Pharmacists were seen as solid members of the middle class and their promotion of carbonated beverages was viewed as a support for the major "family values" cause of that era. By 1929, almost 60 percent of American drugstores had a soda fountain. Along with the soda fountain, drugstores of the 1870s added tobacco, candy, and magazines to their offerings. The corner druggist, the man who could mix up a chocolate soda or a good cough syrup, was now established as part of American life.

Physician and Public Outcry

After the Civil War, relations between physicians and pharmacists were bumpy. The truce that existed during the war held briefly, but soon physicians discovered that pharmacists made excellent scapegoats for the failings of their therapeutics. This was particularly true in cases of poisoning. And while many problems could be traced back to physicians, the low level of general competency among pharmacists had indeed led to cases of patients dying from poisonous prescriptions. Additionally, accidental poisonings, usually from rat bait, had been a problem in pharmacies for decades. To cope with these problems, journalists and some physician groups called for poison-control laws, which usually included some serious regulation of pharmacy practices.

A Professional Response

In response to the drive for regulation of pharmacy practice, the American Pharmaceutical Association empowered a committee, headed by John Maisch, to draw up a model state pharmacy act. In acquiescence to the ambivalent attitude of many pharmacists toward legal regulation, the Association published and distributed the model act to all state legislatures without endorsement. As small businessmen, most pharmacists did not want outside restriction of their trade.

During the 1870s, state legislatures began considering in earnest pharmacy bills sponsored by non-pharmacists. In response to this trend, pharmacists in many states organized state-wide associations to coordinate support for their own bills, which were usually versions of the APhA model. Although not enthusiastic about regulation of their businesses, pharmacists wanted a voice in the process.

Most of the laws that were finally enacted called for the establishment of state boards of pharmacy, composed of leading pharmacists appointed by a state authority, to judge which pharmacists were competent to practice. These boards mailed elegant licenses to established practitioners and set up examinations to test newcomers. Laws usually called for three to four years of apprenticeship before licensure. No states required any formal pharmaceutical education.

The more ambitious state associations followed up their work for the passage of a state act and establishment of a board of pharmacy with efforts to get state support for a school of pharmacy. If a state university existed, legislatures would often set up a school simply by authorizing a professor of pharmacy. This one-man department would draw on other university faculty members to provide instruction in a full range of subjects—chemistry, botany, geology, and physics.

Paper Credentials and Models of Professionalism

Despite their humble beginnings, these state schools of pharmacy played an important role in the development of pharmacy as a recognized profession. Before the Civil War, perhaps only one in twenty American pharmacists had finished formal schooling in pharmacy, and that consisted of night courses to supplement apprenticeship training. However, by the 1870s professional credentialing was becoming quite popular in the United States and pharmacists saw clear advantages to basing their claims of status on diplomas and licenses. Even though state laws did not require a pharmacy school diploma for licensure until the early 20th century, the prestige attached to the sheepskin and growing public expectations attracted students to the burgeoning number of schools much earlier.

This new model of professionalism called for the rejection of the old, individualistic model of personal achievement in favor of the modern idea of a "community of the competent" based on paper credentials. For professions like engineering and accounting, this new approach proved successful. Pharmacy, on the other hand, had problems adopting this model completely. Pharmacists were generally extremely conservative and supportive of free enterprise. This new approach was anti-market and so did not gain complete support. Instead, pharmacy adopted the new professionalism in a half-way fashion.

Disagreement over the new professionalism lead to the split which developed within the ranks of the APhA. Near the end of the 19th century, the APhA became dominated by academics, scientists, and the elite of practitioners. They welcomed the new professionalism as a route to greater status within American society. Some of the ordinary members of the Association were concerned that the organization was ignoring the great commercial changes going on around them.

The 1890s were hard times for pharmacists, despite the gay nineties stereotype. Department stores were infringing on pharmacy's traditional turf and the first true chain drugstores were popping up. The Commercial Section of APhA grew restless and broke off to form the National Association of Retail Druggists (NARD) in 1898. Relations between the two groups were cordial at first but quickly deteriorated. The members of NARD had retained the old approach to professional advancement—individual achievement—and worked to resist the movement toward more education, more examinations and more regulation of pharmacy practice. They opposed it both for commercial reasons and out of a deeply held belief in the individual and his own drugstore.

This split within pharmacy and the subsequent contentiousness was indicative of the tension between these parallel paths to professional recognition. For most of the next century this division hindered the profession's climb toward full professional status.

The Drugstore Era in Retrospect

Pharmacy's place in American culture is strongly tied to the vision of the pharmacist as the proprietor of a drugstore. The drugstore itself, that special combination of soda shop, prescription department and general emporium is something of a cultural icon. The proprietors of drugstores were called by the public "druggists," although they preferred the term "pharmacist." "Apothecary" was still retained by a few pretentious shop owners or those who operated a prescription laboratory only.

By the turn of the century, the position of the pharmacist in the American health care system was firmly established. Physicians had agreed to dispense

Summary

medicines only rarely and pharmacists reciprocated by limiting their diagnosing and prescribing to cases of minor ills and emergencies. The pharmacist was known to be the compounder of prescriptions, although this was not a common occurrence. During the drugstore era, pharmacists no longer needed their laboratories and moved the prescription departments to the back of the stores. There they compounded prescriptions when necessary, although compounding got simpler and less costly as the 19th century progressed. For most pharmacists, the prescription department provided only a small fraction of their income and served more as a device to separate them from other retailers.

Although pharmacists gave up their role as primary medical practitioners, they continued to act as secondary providers through the sale of over-the-counter remedies and first-aid items. As general stores and travelling salesmen declined in number, the pharmacist became identified with his role as medical provider.

The drugstore era saw the beginnings of modern professionalism in the passage of state pharmacy laws mandating examinations and licensing. Modern schools of pharmacy, starting with the University of Michigan in 1876, set the stage for scientific advancement and professional development. The path, however, was long, with road blocks set up both by the profession itself and by those within colleges and universities who opposed pharmacy schools.

At the end of the drugstore era, the seeds of great change were already sprouting. Department stores began adding pharmacies in the late 1800s—an experiment that had mixed success, but foreshadowed pharmacies in mass-merchandisers. The 1890s were actually difficult times, but when the new century brought on chain stores, deep price-cutting, and severe competition, the pleasant myth of the gay nineties drugstore, dressed up in all of its finery, became part of the mythos of American pharmacy.

Second Period of Professionalization (1910 to 1965): Educational Reform

During the next half century, pharmacists concentrated on educational reform as the vehicle for professional improvement. The pursuit of professional status charged forward with the pharmacy curriculum as its standard. Just as the old model of the drugstore has lingered on through tremendous changes in science and technology, the belief in increased education as the panacea for all the ills of the American pharmaceutical profession has persisted as well.

New York Law Brings Educational Requirements

In 1905, the State of New York started an important trend by passing a law stating that after 1910, all new registrants in that state would be required to possess a diploma from a recognized school of pharmacy. The minimum course was two years of study. By and large, pharmacists opposed the idea of mandatory formal education. The apprenticeship system, when checked by the state board examinations, seemed to guarantee basic competency. A wide variety of schools were available to those who wanted more education. For example, in 1905 there were over 50 schools offering B.Pharm., Ph.G. or Ph.C. degrees after two years of study; 20 schools offering M.Pharm. and D.Pharm. degrees after three years of study; about a dozen schools offering B.Sc. degrees after four years of study; and four schools offering M.Sc. degrees after five years of study. (Mrtek 1996, 341) But since most pharmacists in 1910 had no degree of any sort, this requirement seemed to be just one more example of too much government.

Pharmacy Leadership Seeks Extended Training

In 1915, two events took place which changed many pharmacists' minds about educational requirements and spurred their leaders into action. First, Abraham Flexner, the respected reformer of medical education, declared that pharmacy was *not* a profession. He argued that although pharmacists did contribute to society through their specialized skill, *physicians* bore the responsibility for the medicines ordered. Soon after Flexner's shocking assertion, the War Department decided that registered pharmacists, even those who had received bachelor's degrees, would not routinely receive commissions because their professional education was so minimal (Mrtek 1976, 342). Perhaps the War Department had a good point. After the turn of the century, the compounding of prescriptions started its great slide and the work of a pharmacist required less specialized skill than it once did.

To help strengthen their position as professionals, pharmacists turned to the best schools and colleges of pharmacy. This is ironic because it was the efforts of the faculties of these schools that permitted mass manufacturers to take over the art and science of pharmacy. Since the 1850s, a handful of pharmaceutical investigators, such as William Procter, applied science to manufacturing problems. Procter, for instance, spent much of his time perfecting new techniques for extracting active constituents from crude drugs. He developed the process of percolation for the preparation of fluid extracts and similar products. His motivation? To popularize a technique whereby a pharmacist could manufacture his own fluid extracts and eliminate the need to purchase those made by large firms. What happened was just the opposite. Big firms copied Procter's technique on a large scale and eliminated almost any need for the pharmacist to continue doing his own percolating. This pattern would be duplicated again and again for the next 100 years.

The irony here is that as pharmacy professors developed new techniques they insisted that their students learn them. This pattern became even more apparent by the middle of this century. Pharmacy professors asked for more classroom hours to teach their students about the science and technology manufacturers were using to take away the main rationale for the profession's being—the making of medicines.

Major changes occurred in pharmacy in the years around 1900 with the emergence of effective synthetic drugs. Out of laboratories in Germany and France came drugs like aspirin and Salvarsan. Aspirin and other anti-inflammatories had an immense impact on medicine, giving physicians safe drugs to use against fever, the dominant symptom of acute infectious diseases. The advances in pharmacology had influenced therapeutics by the turn of the century. Physicians stopped writing prescriptions containing many ingredients hoping one would work. Instead, they usually called for simple mixtures of one or two ingredients. Moreover, the new drugs were usually potent crystalline chemicals that were well suited for tabletting, a finished dosage form perfect for mass production (Gathercoal 1933).

Prohibition and Soda Fountains

Even if pharmacists in the 1920s spent less time compounding prescriptions, they had plenty to do. In 1919, the 18th Amendment to the Constitution prohibited the sale of alcoholic beverages in the United States. The corrupting influences of this failed social experiment are well known, and they extended to pharmacy.

Since beverage alcohols such as whiskey were officially recognized as drugs in the *United States Pharmacopoeia,* pharmacies could legally sell them on prescription. This practice, was abused and strict regulations using special prescription blanks were imposed. However, even the most honest pharmacists, were tainted by this business and pharmacists became the butt of numerous jokes and the subject of many tall tales about liquor.

With taverns closed, the soda fountain business boomed. Many drugstores became little more than soda shops with some old dusty bottles in the back filled with tinctures and fluid extracts. The popularity of druggists may have hit an all time high during the Prohibition years, but it is doubtful that they gained any respect.

During the fabulous growth of the 1920s, educators worked hard to repair the damage inflicted on their profession by Flexner and the War Department. In meetings of the American Conference of Pharmaceutical Faculties, later called the American Association of Colleges of Pharmacy (AACP), educators decided to seek more stringent educational requirements for pharmacists. In 1923, a requirement of four years of high school study was imposed for admission to AACP member schools. In 1925, the two-year Ph.G. courses were eliminated and a three-year minimum installed. Ohio State University required the four-year bachelor's degree in 1925 and was followed by Minnesota and a few other brave institutions in 1927. In 1928, the Association adopted the four-year Bachelor of Science degree as the minimum course of study, although this requirement did not go into effect until 1932.

The objective of this effort was to convince the public (and physicians) that pharmacists were well educated, cultured, professional men. This change came

at a fortunate time. In contrast with the 1890s, the 1920s were years of unprece-
dented prosperity. Times were good in pharmacy, which encouraged educational
reform.

The Great Depression and Repeal

Those who rushed into pharmacy schools in the late 1920s to beat the B.Sc.
requirement came out to find no jobs as the Great Depression deepened. For
those who had established stores, however, the Depression was less trying than
it was for many other shopkeepers. People still got sick and needed medicines,
the soda fountain attracted those with some money, and, no matter how bad
things got, people still bought cigarettes.

In 1933, during the darkest days of the Depression, the 21st amendment to
the Constitution was passed and Prohibition was repealed. People headed to the
bars and the soda fountain business started to decline. However, something made
up for the loss of soda sales. When Prohibition ended, pharmacies had cases of
liquor and the licenses to sell it. For better or worse, alcohol sales became a

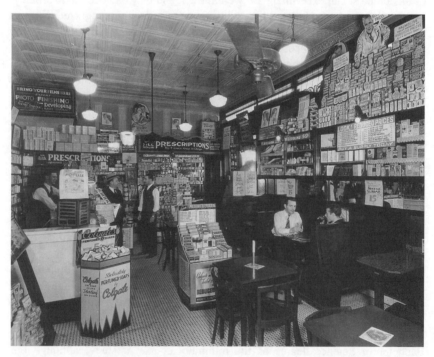

Figure 2.3. Magee Pharmacy, Pittsburgh, PA. c1930. Drug Topics Collection, American
Institute for the History of Pharmacy.

boon to drugstores in the 1930s as the public connected liquor with the place where it was dispensed legally during Prohibition. It is depressing indeed to report that many drugstores in the 1930s survived by selling booze, cigarettes, and chocolate sodas.

The 1930s also brought changes to the store itself. The gradual trend toward self service, which had begun in earnest in the 1920s, continued in the 1930s. By the late 1930s, when the economy had improved, drugstores carried more costly goods—expensive perfumes and, as mentioned, liquor. Store owners opened up the design of their shops so that they could see the entire floor easily from the prescription department in back. The basic store layout featured an elevated prescription department. From a step up, the pharmacist could look down with authority on the customer. In spite of this "elevation", the special art of the pharmacist—compounding medicines—was rapidly disappearing as prefabricated dosage forms flooded the market (Mrtek 1976, 346).

Status of Pharmacists in World War II

As the nation stood on the verge of World War II, the leaders among pharmacists were confident. For nearly ten years, the bachelor's degree requirement had been in effect, raising the standards of the profession. Internally, the profession was undergoing dynamic growth. New organizations—the American College of Apothecaries, the American Institute of the History of Pharmacy, and the American Society of Hospital Pharmacists—were founded during this time of optimism and high ideals.

Again, however, the United States government decided that pharmacists were not to be routinely given commissions in the military. The decision was especially galling since nurses were being commissioned as second lieutenants by the thousands, even though they had less training. Even freshman medical students were commissioned as ensigns in the Navy. However, the Division of Scientific and Technical Personnel of the War Emergency Advisory Committee had concluded that pharmacists were not generally recognized as professionals. The commercialism connected with pharmacy practice seemed to make their expanded training and education secondary.

Moreover, there was no reason to offer pharmacists a special incentive to join the military. All the pharmacists needed could be obtained through the draft because the nation had an overabundance of pharmacists. In 1940, the nation had a population of about 130 million and about 115,000 registered pharmacists working in some 58,000 stores. Today, about 170,000 pharmacists and about the same number of community pharmacies serve a population of 250 million, nearly double the population in 1940. Physicians and dentists, who were needed in much greater numbers in the war effort, continued to receive commissions (Mrtek 1976, 352).

Pharmaceutical Survey and the Five-year Program

Stimulated by the decision of the Advisory Committee and opinion surveys that indicated a low regard for pharmacists, the pharmacy profession decided that a major self-study was in order. On 15 April 1946, the Pharmaceutical Survey was inaugurated. This joint effort of all major pharmacy organizations and the American Council on Education was the most complete study of an occupation ever undertaken. Nearly every aspect of pharmacy was scrutinized, including education, legal controls, organizations, student recruitment, the content of prescriptions, state boards, licensing, and postgraduate education.

Looking back over the results of the survey in 1951, Director Edward C. Elliott commented on pharmacy's uncertain future:

> Whether pharmacy is to be able to have and to hold a real professional status, or whether it is to become stabilized, in most of its practice, as one of the subordinate technological occupations of modern civilization, may be considered debatable questions. The developments of the past generation have tended to make pharmacy a dependent enterprise.
>
> Mass manufacture of medicinals has caused the practicing pharmacist to serve more and more as a mere distributor. Furthermore, and for the most part, pharmacy endeavors to fulfill its traditional, as well as its ever-broadening, responsibilities amidst an expanding jungle of commerce. . . . Here are problems of fundamental importance. Unsolved, they are hazards to any future good fortune of the profession (Mrtek 1976, 353).

The survey made recommendations for change in eleven different areas but the most substantial and controversial changes were those suggested for the pharmacy curriculum. In the words of the General Report of 1949, "It is recommended that the American Association of Colleges of Pharmacy and the American Council on Pharmaceutical Education take the necessary initial steps for the development and establishment of a six-year program of education and training leading to the professional degree of Doctor of Pharmacy, this program to include two or more years of general education and basic science training (Elliott 1950)."

The General Report also encouraged improvements in the four-year program. In 1950, the University of Southern California started the first 2–4 Pharm.D. program, but outside of California this seemed too radical. With the four-year program appearing too conservative, the five-year compromise, already in place at Ohio State in 1948, seemed attractive. In 1954, the AACP recommended the general adoption of the five-year program, beginning with the entering class of 1960.

It is important to realize that when the Pharm.D. debate began in the 1950s it occurred in the context of broadening the education of the future pharmacist. Much of the attraction of the professional doctorate was the added opportunity for more general or liberal education. Pharmacists who followed this new course of study would be well educated and thereby worthy of the respect of other professionals and of the public.

Economic Growth and the Changing Marketplace

While educators debated about the future of the profession, great changes were taking place among practicing pharmacists. The 1950s were boom times, with new, effective drugs on the market. New antibiotics such as tetracycline (1950) and erythromycin (1952) joined the penicillins. Other new drugs of note included warfarin (1954), brompheniramine (1957), chlorpromazine (1954), methotrexate (1955), reserpine (1953), dextromethorphan (1954), tolbutamide (1957), hydrochlorothiazide (1959), hydrocortisone (1952), imipramine (1959), and griseofulvin (1959). Post-war pharmacists were dispensing tablets and capsules which actually cured diseases, rather than just ameliorating symptoms.

The number of prescriptions filled went up over 50 percent, during the 1950s, transforming the prescription department into the economic engine of the drugstore. A relatively stable number of pharmacists worked harder and faster. In the post-war era, suburbia boomed and so did the chains. By concentrating their stores in newer, growing areas of population, chains came to dominate community pharmacy in both urban and suburban areas.

This was the era of "count and pour" pharmacy. Pharmacists were restricted to machine-like tasks. The 1952 Durham-Humphrey amendment to the Food, Drug, and Cosmetic Act had removed much of the pharmacist's autonomy in practice and the APhA Code of Ethics made the pharmacist's limited role quite clear.

> The pharmacist does not discuss the therapeutic effects or composition of a prescription with a patient. When such questions are asked, he suggests that the qualified practitioner [that is, a physician or dentist] is the proper person with whom such matters should be discussed (Elliott 1950).

Pharmacists gained respect from their connection with the new, effective drugs coming on the market, but their new reputation came at the cost of being considered over-educated for a diminished professional function. The pharmacy curriculum had continued to emphasize the physical sciences that underlie the making of medicines even though compounding was disappearing from practice (Higby 1990, 16). The prevalence of this conservative approach to pharmacy education is illustrated by the first sentence of *Remington's Practice of Pharmacy*—"Pharmacy is the science which treats of medicinal substances"—which had not changed in two-thirds of a century (Martin and Cook 1956, 1). The description of the profession's scope in the 1956 edition indicated no significant expansion from the mid-1800s and did not mention the loss of some responsibilities.

Failure of Academic Reform Movement

In retrospect, it is clear that the period of academic reform solidified the place of pharmacy within academia without greatly elevating the position of the pharmacist within the health-care system or society at large. The argument has been made that pharmacists of the 1950s were too concerned with products and not enough with patients. Instead, it may be more useful to view the supposed "product orientation" of the post-war era as a result of the overall calcification of the role of pharmacists. Professional leaders sought peace with physicians and educators strived for recognition from their peers. Practitioners of pharmacy, a majority of whom were independent store owners, concentrated on the business side of their practice in the face of the chain store threat. The professional opportunities available to pharmacists were extremely limited by state and federal laws and by the customs of the physician-pharmacist-patient relationship that had evolved over the previous 100 years. Pharmacists concentrated on overall service to the customer because their other opportunities were so limited.

Attempts to use a more extensive pharmacy school curriculum to elevate the stature of pharmacy failed because in spite of the increased amount of time students spent in school, students were too busy studying advances in industry to get a well-rounded education. It was general education that was to transform pharmacists into "educated men." The irony is that pharmacy students of the 1950s and 1960s spent longer and longer hours learning the scientific basis of the techniques industry used to eliminate compounding, a large part of the traditional *raison d'être* of pharmacy practice.

The end result was that educational reform did not raise the stature of pharmacists within the structure of the health care system or within society at large. Pharmacists learned all the steps necessary for manufacturing medicines but found their practice reduced to counting and pouring. They came out of pharmacy schools tired, with their heads full of unusable information, and with no more general education than graduates of technical schools.

Third Period of Professionalization (1965 to 1990): Changing Practitioners

The decade of the 1960s was a period of turmoil for American society. The civil rights and anti-war movements shook the social order and new rules of thinking and behavior replaced the old. So it went for pharmacy as well. "Clinical pharmacy" was the rallying cry for pharmacy's revolutionaries, who were just as uncertain of what their revolution's results would be as the marchers in the streets.

Rather than a revolution, the clinical pharmacy era (1965–1990) is better seen as a transitional period in professional development. Pharmacists steeped in knowledge about drugs stepped out of the shackles of "count and pour" practice and asserted themselves as "drug information experts." As much as any other 60s movement, clinical pharmacy grew out of the actions of the grass roots (i.e., practicing pharmacists).

The major clinical pharmacy concepts and innovations came from institutional pharmacists. From the 19th century up into the mid-20th century, hospital pharmacists had low status within pharmacy. In the 1800s, they were viewed as marginally competent individuals who did not have the strength of character to run a store. During the first decades of the 20th century, they were still on the fringe of pharmacy.

The special nature of their practice, however, caused hospital pharmacists to band together in organizations from the 1920s on. They practiced manufacturing and compounding pharmacy long after it disappeared from drugstores. As their group identity solidified and organizational numbers reached a critical mass, these groups began to work together. In Denver in 1942 the American Society of Hospital Pharmacists was founded.

In the unique setting of the hospital, pharmacists in the 1940s and 1950s gained more control over the rising number of new drugs and products. Pharmacy and Therapeutics (P & T) Committees and hospital formularies brought pharmacists into the therapeutic side of practice. By the mid-1960s, this involvement increased to the point where Donald Brodie could state:

> The ultimate goal of the services of pharmacy must be the safe use of drugs by the public. In this context, the mainstream function of pharmacy is clinical in nature, one that may be identified accurately as drug-use control (Brodie and Benson 1976).

By "drug-use control" Brodie meant "the sum total of knowledge, understanding, judgements, procedures, skills, controls, and ethics that assures optimal safety in the distribution and use of medication (Brodie and Benson 1976)."

This approach was adopted by programs like the famous ninth floor project of the University of California-San Francisco Medical Center. This project, initiated in 1966, utilized several of the basic components of later practice, including unit doses, pharmacy technicians, a drug information center, and patient drug profiles. As clinical pharmacy demonstrated its utility, hospitals added more staff pharmacists to facilitate greater drug-use control. During the 1970s and 1980s, the number of pharmacists in institutional practice more than doubled to about 40,000, or nearly one-quarter of all practitioners (Pharmacy Manpower Project 1993).

In community pharmacy, the shift to clinical practice started about the same time, but the burdens of business and the distance from the clinical milieu made the transition slower and more difficult. In 1960, Eugene V. White of Berryville, Virginia, started using patient profile cards. Soon afterward he totally remodelled his store into an office-style practice. While few community pharmacists followed White's example completely, many did see a new avenue for professional growth.

A great and gradual paradigm shift had begun in community pharmacy. The person who stood across the counter from the pharmacist was undergoing a transformation from "the customer" into "the patient." After 150 years of caring about the *wants* of *customers,* pharmacists were caring about the *needs* of *patients*.

A few progressive schools of pharmacy quickly adapted to the new concept, adding a few courses in clinical therapeutics to their already full curricula. The 1970s was a difficult decade for pharmacy education as schools opened their doors to hundreds of part-time practitioner instructors who put more and more time demands on the tight five-year curriculum. Some schools opted for six-year Pharm.D. programs, while others cut back some on laboratory courses and all but eliminated general education to include clerkship experience in their five-year programs.

The rapid change at the leadership level of pharmacy is also demonstrated in the 1969 revision of the APhA Code of Ethics. The old 1952 code admonished pharmacists not to inform patients about their drugs. The new code began, "A pharmacist should hold the health and safety of patients to be of first consideration; he should render to each patient the full measure of his ability as an essential health practitioner (The Challeng of Ethics in Pharmacy Practice 1985, 62)."

During the 1970s, graduates of pharmacy schools entered a health care environment relatively hostile to clinical pharmacy. Clinical pharmacy was dismissed as too expensive and time consuming, but the need for clinical skills was manifest. The huge therapeutic advances and the burgeoning drug industry of the 1960s forced pharmacists more and more into decision-making roles. As a profession, pharmacy moved slowly into providing drug information and counselling to patients.

Transition occurred in the 1970s and 1980s, in large part because pharmacy educators, who initially lagged behind practitioners as advocates of clinical practice, saw the prospects for the future. Clinical pharmacy restored meaning to their teaching. Rather than just supporting their own scientific disciplines, professors turned their teaching toward contemporary practice issues and the challenges of the future.

Other Transitions

Other great transitional changes in pharmacy practice also occurred during the period from the mid-1960s to the 1990s. Health insurance developments in the 1950s and the passage of Medicare and Medicaid legislation in 1965, created a complicated yet incomplete system of third-party payment for pharmacy services. Today, the nation stands ready to advance to a new health care system.

Pharmacy is prepared for advances in many ways. The provision of sufficient clinical pharmacy "manpower" remains an issue, but the situation is far less critical than it once appeared because of the great increase of "womanpower" within the profession. In 1950, only five percent of active pharmacists were women. Today the number is approaching one-third of all practitioners, and women may hold the majority of pharmacist positions by the year 2020. It is perhaps too early to gauge the impact of this gender shift on pharmacy—the most rapid in the history of any major American profession (Seventh Report to the President and Congress on the Status of Health Personnell in the United States 1990).

Pharmacy embraced computerization well in advance of other health professions because of its utility in handling and processing insurance claims. Computers were quickly adapted, to provide a wide variety of information services necessary for the provision of patient care. Meeting the drug utilization review regulations of the Omnibus Budget Reconciliation Act of 1990 (OBRA '90) on a national basis would be impossible without the computerization of pharmacies across the country.

At the beginning of the 1960s, pharmacy was truly a "profession in search of a role." Pharmacists had gained a monopoly over the dispensing of prescription drugs but lost much autonomy in their practices after the passage of the Durham-Humphrey Amendment and state anti-substitution laws. Because of the academic reform movement of the early to mid-20th century, pharmacy graduates received a long and rigorous training. They were prepared to take on the new challenges of the clinical pharmacy ideal.

The clinical pharmacy era is best characterized as a transitional period between the years of "count and pour" practice and the dawning era of pharmaceutical care. What changed during this time was not so much what pharmacists knew as how they applied their knowledge. Above all else, pharmacists shared their drug expertise with physicians and with patients. As a movement, clinical pharmacy has its primary roots in institutional practice, ironically the traditional backwater of the profession. In the community setting, "customers" became "patients" and pharmacists began to accept, albeit reluctantly, some responsibility for the proper use of drugs. In both settings, pharmacists had begun to care *about* their patients, even if they were not caring *for* them.

Fourth Period of Professionalization: Full Responsibility and Societal Recognition

If the futurists in American pharmacy are right, we are at the beginning of a new period in our history, the era of pharmaceutical care. The concept, which grew out of Donald Brodie's drug-use control, may complete the move away from "count and pour" practice in ways that clinical pharmacy could not. Pharmacy educators and leaders, who at first lagged behind practitioners, arrived at this concept after a decade or so of speculation on pharmacy's future.

Several general definitions of pharmaceutical care exist. Because this phase of professional development is just beginning, these definitions tend to be a bit vague and idealistic. Still, when one reads that "pharmaceutical care is the responsible provision of drug therapy for the purpose of achieving definite outcomes that improve a patient's quality of life," the challenge is stimulating (Hepler and Strand 1989).

For the historian, the most significant aspect of the pharmaceutical care movement is its voluntary assumption of responsibility without substantial compensation. Motivated by professional pride and the understanding of the problems associated with drug use, pharmacists are adopting the goals set out by the pharmaceutical care model. It may well be that by taking on the responsibility for the proper use of medicines, pharmacists will achieve the societal recognition as full professionals that they have sought for over 150 years. If so, society will confer this status on pharmacists because of what they accomplish in practice, not because of extended curricula or grandiose titles. The individual achievement approach to professional recognition, set aside for a century, may fulfill the dream that paper credentials could not accomplish alone.

In a sense, pharmacy is returning to a high level of professional responsibility after decades of settling for a secondary role. At the beginning of the 1800s, pharmacists became common in American cities and towns. Their major professional function was to provide drugs and medicines of reliable strength and purity. They utilized their specialized knowledge of botany, chemistry, and pharmacy in the selection and processing of crude drugs that became the ingredients of the medicines they compounded. In addition, these pharmacists invented the drugstore, that unique part of American culture where health care and retail intermingled. A century and a half later, American pharmacists invented clinical pharmacy. This new approach to practice that has brought the profession to the threshold of a new era and, after a century, pharmacists' search for a role has come to the beginning of its end.

References

Brodie D. C., and R. A. Benson. 1976. The Evolution of the Clinical Pharmacy Concept. *Drug Intelligence Clinical Pharmacy* 10: 507.

The Challenge of Ethics in Pharmacy Practice. 1985. Madison: American Institute of the History of Pharmacy.

Elliott E. C. 1950. *The General Report of the Pharmaceutical Survey: 1946–49*. Washington: American Council on Education.

Gathercoal, E. N. 1933. *The Prescription Ingredient Survery*. Washington, DC: American Pharmaceutical Association.

Hepler, C. D., and L. M. Strand. 1989. Opportunities and Responsibilities in Pharmaceutical Care. *American Journal of Pharmacy Education*. 53: 12S.

Higby G. J. 1990. Evolution of Pharmacy. In *Remington's Pharmaceutical Sciences*, ed. A. R. Gennaro. Easton, PA: Mack.

Kremers, E., and Urdang, J. *History of Pharmacy*. 4th ed. 1976. Philadelphia, PA: Lippincott.

Martin E., and E. F. Cook. eds. 1956. *Remington's Practice of Pharmacy*. Easton, PA: Mack Publishing.

Mrtek R. G. 1976. Pharmaceutical Education in These United States—An Interpretive Historical Essay of the Twentieth Century. *American Journal of Pharmacy Education* 40: 341.

Pharmacopoeia of the United States of America. 2nd ed. 1928. Boston.

Pharmacy Manpower Project. 1993. Ann Arbor: Vector Research.

Seventh Report to the President and Congress on the Status of Health Personnel in the United States. 1990. Washington, DC: U.S. Government Printing Office.

Society of the New-York Hospital. 1804 A Brief Account of the New-York Hospital. New York: Isaac Collins and Son.

Society of the New-York Hospital. 1811. An Account of the New-York Hospital. New-York: Collins & Co.

Society of the New-York Hospital. 1820. By-laws and Regulations Ordained and Established by the Governors of the New-York Hospital. New-York: Mahlon Day.

3

Health Care in the United States

Earle W. Lingle, Ph.D., R.Ph.

As promising as the concept of pharmaceutical care is, pharmacy is not practiced in a vacuum. Various factors, such as the organization of health care delivery systems, reimbursement methods, laws regulating the practice of pharmacy and medicine, and many others, influence pharmaceutical care. This chapter is intended to discuss the U.S. health care system—a system which is currently in turmoil. By reviewing the structure, financing, problems, and potential for reform of the U.S. health care system, we can better understand how pharmaceutical care can best meet the needs of our growing, aging, and heterogeneous population.

Structure of the U.S. Health Care System

There are many different ways to define the organization of our health care system. First, it might be argued that the term *health care system* is actually a misnomer and what we currently have is a *sickness care system* because of the lack of an emphasis on maintaining health. Another argument might be made that the system is actually a non-system because of the lack of coordination between the different actors. It may also be maintained that the system consists of a group of sub-systems, each with different objectives, members, providers, and services. We will return to this point later in this section.

One method of defining the health care system is by determining who is reimbursing health care providers for their services—the patient or a third party. When a patient reimburses the provider of the care directly, the payment is referred to as the patient's out-of-pocket expense. In health care, a *third party* is defined as an entity that provides reimbursement to a health care provider for services rendered to a patient affiliated with the third party. A third party may either be privately owned or publicly administered. Because of their influence in today's health care system, third-party organizations need to be more closely examined.

Private Health Insurance

Evolution

Private health insurance has not always existed in the form we know it today. In the early 1900's, health insurance policies were similar to accident and disability insurance. They were loss-of-income policies and provided cash payments during certain specific illnesses, such as typhoid, smallpox, and diphtheria. They did not provide payment for health care services but were meant to replace income lost during the disease episode (Health Insurance Association of America 1992).

The Great Depression was a catalyst for the establishment of private health insurance which would reimburse health care providers. In 1929, a group of teachers paid 50 cents per month to Baylor Hospital in Dallas to provide each teacher with up to 21 days of hospital care annually. This was the first of what became known as Blue Cross plans. These plans were followed by the establishment of Blue Shield insurance programs which were similar but reimbursed physicians instead of hospitals. Premiums were usually determined by *community rating*. Under this system, health care costs for a community were averaged and the same premium was offered to each person within that community (Jonas 1986).

The evolution of private health insurance continued during World War II. Because workers were scarce and the government had imposed wage controls, employers offered health insurance as a fringe benefit to attract employees. As more businesses sought health insurance benefit packages the number of insurance companies offering them rapidly increased. These companies determined premium payments by *experience rating*—pricing premiums based on an individual's or a group's medical claims history.

A more recent development in private health insurance is the decision by major employers to self-insure. Instead of paying premiums to an insurance company, self-insured businesses, which are usually quite large, predict the health care expenses for their employees and assume the risks for these costs. The advantages for businesses are such that the number of self-insuring employers has grown rapidly. However, some self-insured businesses have either reduced or dropped their employees' coverage for cancer and AIDS, as well as other diseases which may prove costly (Mariner 1992).

Types

Private health insurance companies offer a multitude of types of policies as a result of their attempts to carve out niches in different markets. In addition, they combine coverages to meet the needs of individual employers or employee groups. The following are the major categories of health insurance as defined by the Health Insurance Association of America (1992).

Hospital/Medical Insurance. This type of insurance provides coverage for specific benefits related to hospital room, board, services, and supplies during a hospital stay. It may also be combined with payment for a doctor's hospital visits and surgical services.

Major Medical Expense Insurance. This insurance usually covers a wide range of medical charges and provides protection for large medical expenses.

Medicare Supplemental Policy. This is often referred to as a "Medigap" insurance policy and provides additional coverage for those persons covered by Medicare, the government-sponsored program for the elderly.

Disability Income Protection. This type of policy provides income for a worker who has become disabled as a result of an accident or illness. The benefit is usually related to the beneficiary's earnings.

Coverage

Approximately 74 percent of the U.S. population is covered by some form of private health insurance, whether they receive it through their employers (61 percent) or purchase it directly (13 percent) (Levit, Olin, and Letsch 1992). Workers in smaller companies, and those who are in retail trade, service industries, or self-employed, are less likely to have employer-sponsored health insurance.

Provision of health insurance by employers has been stimulated by tax policy. Even though health insurance benefits may be considered a substitute for wages, employers can deduct their share of the premiums as operating expenses. Also, health insurance benefits are not subject to the employee's personal income or Social Security taxes (De Lew, Greenberg, and Kinchen 1992). In 1991, health insurance companies collected $244 billion in premiums and paid out $209.3 billion in benefits. The difference, $35.1 billion, was used for administration of the plans, taxes, and profits.

Public Insurance Programs

Federal, state, and local governments have become involved in health care in various ways. Most frequently, their involvement has served one of three purposes: to provide services or to mandate the provision of services by others for the public good; to purchase services for the public good; or to redistribute income. Some health care services cannot be provided in a normal market setting because there is little desire by the public to purchase them or the profit incentives for companies to provide them are too small. The government may either provide these services directly or pass regulations to mandate their purchase or provision.

Examples of government providing or mandating services include the regulation of pharmaceuticals by the Food and Drug Administration and requirements for immunization. The government purchases goods and services to serve the public good when it provides medical research grants through the National Institutes of Health and when it purchases health care services for members of certain segments of society. The government affects income distribution by taxing citizens with higher incomes to pay for health care for persons who are considered poor. This is the basis for the Medicaid program.

It is not possible to survey government's involvement in all aspects of health care, but because of the current interest in health insurance coverage it is important to examine the evolution of public health insurance and examine the two largest programs, Medicaid and Medicare.

Evolution

Not until the early 1900s did industrialization and some social reform begin in this country. The Great Depression and the resulting high unemployment served as important motivating factors, for society to began to change its view of government's role in helping citizens. In 1932, the Committee on Costs of Medical Care reported that a form of national health insurance was needed for this country. However, the politically powerful interest group of organized medicine vehemently opposed. In an editorial of its journal, the American Medical Association wrote, "The alignment is clear—on the one side the forces representing the great foundations, public health officialdom, social theory—even socialism and communism—inciting to revolution; on the other side, the organized medical profession urging principles of sound practice of medicine" (Journal of the American Medical Association 1932). For the next 30 years, the mention of increased government involvement in health care raised the same concerns about socialism and communism expressed by the AMA and their supporters in 1932.

Although President Franklin D. Roosevelt believed there was a need for publicly financed health care for certain segments of the population, he knew the odds were against such a program and instead he opted for Social Security. The passage of the Social Security Act of 1935 was important because the act was to become the basis for future public health insurance plans. In addition to providing a payroll deduction plan for retirement, Social Security provides payments to assist people in paying for essentials such as food, shelter, and medical care. People are eligible if they are both poor and either blind, disabled, elderly, or head of a single-parent family with dependent children. People who fit into these categories are sometimes referred to as the *categorically needy*.

Over the next 25 years, different proposals for public health insurance were put forward, most notably by President Truman, yet no other major legislation was passed until 1960. In that year, the Kerr-Mills Medical Assistance for the Aged Act, which provided medical assistance for the indigent elderly, was successfully steered through Congress by Congressman Wilbur Mills and Senator Robert Kerr. Their reasoning in proposing the act was that since medical expenses consumed such a large part of many elderly people's incomes, public assistance should be provided to those who were not poor enough to be eligible for the welfare payments discussed above.

Buoyed by the support of then-Senator John F. Kennedy and Congressman Lyndon B. Johnson, comprehensive public health insurance for the elderly gained momentum. In 1965, after the assassination of President Kennedy and President Johnson's election, Congress enacted legislation with three primary sections: a federally-administered hospital insurance program for persons of age 65 and older, the disabled, and people with end-stage renal disease (Medicare Part A); a federally-administered supplemental health insurance program that the elderly, disabled, and people with end-stage renal disease could purchase (Medicare Part B); and a state-administered health insurance program for the "categorically needy" and some other poor people (Medicaid).

Medicare

Medicare is the single largest health insurer in the U.S. It covers approximately thirteen percent of the population—31 million elderly people and 3 million people who are under 65 and have disabilities or renal disease (Board of Trustees of the Federal Hospital Insurance Trust Fund 1992). Medicare is administered by the federal government and provides a uniform package of medical care benefits to all recipients regardless of income. Medicare does not pay all medical expenses for its beneficiaries—it does not cover all services and there are certain cost-sharing responsibilities for each eligible person. In fact it is estimated that Medicare covers less than one-half of the medical expenses of the elderly (Waldo, Sonnefeld, and McKusick 1989). Medicare is funded by a combination of payroll taxes, general tax revenue, and premiums.

In general, Medicare does not cover medical care that is not reasonable and necessary for the treatment of a specific illness or injury. Medicare Part A is also known as the Hospital Insurance Plan. It pays part of the cost of inpatient hospital care and related care that is provided by skilled nursing facilities, home health agencies, and hospices. The major items covered by Medicare Part B, also known as Supplementary Medical Insurance, are services and supplies provided by physicians and outpatient hospital facilities. In addition, Medicare Part B covers some home health care, vision care, physical therapy, and mental health services. Pharmaceutical benefits are limited to inpatient hospital coverage, hospice care, and some specific medications on an outpatient basis. A more comprehensive outpatient drug benefit has been considered by Congress and will continue to be debated. People entitled to Part A coverage can enroll in Part B by paying a monthly premium.

A major concern about Medicare is that expenditures are increasing faster than revenue. The aging of the population and decrease in average family size mean fewer workers per Medicare beneficiary. In 1960, there were five workers for each beneficiary. It is estimated that this number will decrease to three by the year 2000 and 1.9 by 2030 (U.S. House of Representatives 1991). Medicare Part A is currently financed by a 2.90 percent payroll tax, but estimates are that Part A costs will equal 3.76 percent of payroll in the year 2000 and 8.62 percent in 2030. Medicare Part B expenditures have increased from $10 billion in 1980 to $40 billion in 1990 and are expected to reach $150 billion (in 1995 dollars) by the year 2030 (Burner, Waldo, and McKusick 1992).

Medicaid

In 1965, there was a major debate over Medicare. Medicaid was given little consideration and passed as a political compromise. Opponents of Medicaid were assured that expenditures would remain relatively small. By 1991, Medicaid covered 24 million people, approximately 10 percent of the U.S. population (Levit, Olin and Letsch 1992), and expenditures had reached $96.5 billion, an increase of 34.4 percent from 1990 (Letsch et al. 1992).

Medicaid is jointly administered by state and federal governments. Although a state can choose whether or not to take part in the program, all 50 states plus the District of Columbia participate in Medicaid. Once a state decides to provide services under Medicaid, federal regulations require that certain services be offered, the population groups eligible for benefits be identified, and reimbursement be specified. Medicaid is financed with a combination of state and federal funds. The federal government's share varies by state and is based on the state's per capita income as compared to the national average. The federal share may range from 50 to 83 percent.

In order to qualify for Medicaid benefits, applicants must meet certain eligibility criteria. Each state sets income and asset limits for qualification. A beneficiary must meet criteria for being *categorically needy*—poor and either blind, elderly, disabled, or a single parent with dependent children (some states include two-parent families if the principal wage earner is unemployed). In addition, some states have programs for people who are considered *medically needy*. The medically needy are the blind, elderly, and disabled, and also single-parent families with dependent children, whose resources are above the income limit, but whose medical expenses exceed their excess income. It is estimated that because of the eligibility categories and differing state income limits, approximately 60 percent of the population below the federal poverty level are not eligible for Medicaid (Swartz and Lipson 1989).

Federal regulations require states that participate in Medicaid provide a basic set of services including inpatient and outpatient hospital services, physician services, laboratory and x-ray services, skilled-nursing facility care, home health care, and some other services. States may also elect to provide optional services which include outpatient prescription drugs, dental services, vision care, and services provided by intermediate-care facilities. All states and the District of Columbia offer outpatient prescription drugs as a benefit, although the programs vary from state to state.

One particular problem in the Medicaid program is expenditure for long-term nursing home care. Medicaid is the only public health-insurance program that pays for such care. In order to become eligible for Medicaid and to receive reimbursement for nursing home care, some elderly people transfer their assets to their children and spend their remaining income on their care. Approximately 43 percent of Medicaid expenditures are used to pay for nursing home care, and as the average age population increases costs can be expected. (De Lew, Green-berg, and Kinchen 1992) Addition of Medicare coverage of nursing home care continues to be considered, but the potential costs of the program makes it politically difficult to enact.

Some people who are elderly, blind or disabled may be eligible for both Medicare and Medicaid. These people are said to be *dually eligible*. In such cases, Medicare provides the primary coverage for hospital insurance (Part A) and states pay the premiums for supplemental medical insurance (Part B) so that Medicare will also cover those services. In addition, state Medicaid programs pay the patient cost-sharing expenses and provide services Medicare does not, such as outpatient prescription drugs and long-term nursing home care.

Summary

Medicare and Medicaid play a major role in the delivery of health care in this country. Approximately one person in four in the U.S. is covered by a public insurance program. Medicare and Medicaid paid approximately 34 percent of all personal health care costs in 1991 and it is estimated that by the year 2000 this will increase to 43 percent (Burner, Waldo, and McKusick 1992). If these programs go unchanged and present trends continue, Medicare and Medicaid will place significant pressures on state and federal budgets.

Managed Care Programs

As health care expenditures increased in the 1970s and 1980s, new health care delivery systems developed to change the incentives for providing care. These new systems are based on three principles: managing the care of patients, using a select group of health care providers, and placing providers at risk financially (Wallack 1992). Because of the way they managed patient care, these new groups became known as *managed care organizations*. The traditional fee-for-service system encourages the use of services that may not be the most appropriate or the most likely to produce the preferred outcome. Theoretically, managed care systems provide incentives to use medical services more efficiently.

Types of Managed Care

Different types of managed care programs have evolved. The two major categories are health maintenance organizations and preferred provider organizations. There are also different models within each of these categories.

Health maintenance organizations (HMOs) are health care organizations that provide a comprehensive set of medical care services to a voluntarily enrolled group of patients. The enrollee pays a fixed amount per month regardless of the amount of services used. This places the HMO at financial risk if total costs are greater than aggregate premiums, but it yields a financial gain if costs are lower than the premium revenue. This system provides incentives to patients and health care providers to minimize utilization and therefore costs.

There are several different models of managed care systems that are considered HMOs. Probably the best known is the *staff model,* in which salaried physicians work in clinical facilities owned by the HMO. In a *group model,* the HMO contracts with one or more physician groups to provide care and usually reimburses them on a capitated basis. Capitation is a reimbursement system in which the medical group or individual practitioner receives a fixed payment per patient over a defined time period regardless of the patient's utilization. Similar to the group model is the *network model.* In the network model, physician providers contract with the HMO to provide services for enrollees. The principal difference between the group and network models is that HMO enrollees usually comprise a small part of a network physician's practice while a group physician sees only enrollees. The fourth model is known as an *individual practice association (IPA).* In this model, the IPA contracts with various individual physicians or associations of independent physicians to provide services for their enrollees. These doctors may be paid on a capitated or a fee-for-service basis.

Preferred provider organizations (PPO) are the second main type of managed care program. These organizations contract with a network of doctors, hospitals, and other providers who provide services to enrollees for a discounted reimbursement. Enrollees in PPOs usually have lower cost-sharing if they go to a health care provider in the network; however, they do have the option to go to a physician or other health care provider outside of the network and pay a greater share of the costs. In an *exclusive provider organization (EPO),* an enrollee who goes to a non-network provider must pay that provider's fee out-of-pocket.

A more recent development in HMOs is the *point-of-service (POS) plan.* This plan may be thought of as a combination of the HMO and PPO models because it integrates characteristics of both. The POS organization contracts with a network of providers and each enrollee has a primary care physician who acts as a "gatekeeper" to control the use of specialists. Physicians may be paid via fee-for-service or capitation reimbursement and enrollees who use health care providers not contracting with the POS share a greater percentage of the costs.

Managed care can be practiced in settings other than those described above.

Managed care techniques are being adopted increasingly by insurers and present a variety of decisions which must be made before services are provided. Cost control methods in use include prior authorization for hospital admissions, second opinions for surgical procedures, provider utilization review, patient case workers, and others.

The differences between these types of managed care organizations are becoming less distinct as each borrows options from the others in an attempt to make their plan more attractive for potential enrollees. Even now it is difficult to determine which of these categories many managed care plans fall into.

Trends

The number of HMOs has decreased since peaking in 1987. In 1992, it was estimated that there were 562 HMOs in the U.S. This is a decrease from 707 in 1987. This decrease in number may be due to the consolidation of different HMOs and attrition of smaller plans. Most of the HMOs in existence today are IPA plans (65 percent). There are only 59 staff model plans remaining (See Table 3-1.). However, enrollment in HMOs has increased. Approximately 43.7 million people were enrolled in a HMO in 1992, a 41 percent increase from 1987. This growth is expected to continue with the offering of POS options. IPA plans have the most enrollees, approximately 21 million in 1992 (see Table 3-1.). Staff model HMOs have shown the smallest growth (Marion Merrell Dow, 1993).

Although PPOs did not become popular until the early 1980s, the number of enrollees has risen quickly. Estimates vary because of differing definitions, but it is thought that in 1992 more than 66 million people were enrolled in some type of PPO plan (Abramowitz 1993).

Effects of Managed Care

There is some disagreement as to the current effectiveness and the future promise of managed care in decreasing health care costs. A recent study estimated that there would be an approximate ten percent reduction in national health care spending if all services were delivered through staff or group model HMOs. However, this would be a one-time drop that would have no effect on the rate of increase of spending (Staines 1993). Some suggest that managed care produces cost savings because of adverse selection. That is, it serves a younger, healthier population. Others suggest that managed care has had little impact on health care spending because enrollment growth in staff and group HMOs—the most effective managed care plans for reducing costs—has been stagnant (Langwell 1992). There is also concern that for-profit HMOs may underserve their enrollees in order to increase profits.

Enrollment in managed care plans will probably continue to increase as employ-

Table 3-1. HMO Enrollment by Type of Plan

	1992		1991		1990		1989	
	Plans	Enrollment (×1000)	Plans	Enrollment (×1000)	Plans	Enrollment (×1000)	Plans	Enrollment (×1000)
Group	71	11,320.1	73	11,190.3	77	10,806.0	85	9,844.8
IPA	363	20,818.6	365	18,171.1	371	16,526.2	386	15,428.0
Network	72	6,858.7	84	6,419.9	98	6,698.3	86	5,431.5
Staff	56	4,743.7	59	4,606.9	64	3,507.7	66	4,326.9
TOTAL	562	43,741.1	581	40,388.2	610	37,538.2	623	35,031.2

Source: Marion Merrell Dow Managed Care Digest, HMO Edition 1993.

ers and insurers realize that uncoordinated care and fee-for-service plans do not adequately contain costs. Managed care is also attractive to patients because it offers comprehensive benefits (including pharmaceuticals) and lower cost-sharing. Add to this the number of government programs, such as Medicaid, turning to managed care for relief from increasing costs, and continued growth for managed care programs should be assured.

Financing Health Care

National health expenditures increased to approximately $752 billion in 1991 (Letsch et al. 1992). In other words, health care costs equaled $2.1 billion per day or $1.43 million per minute in 1991. Americans will spend more on health care this year than on gasoline, cars, trucks, and their parts **plus** the entire military. And the future is even more alarming. It is estimated that if our current laws and medical practices remain unchanged, medical care costs will more than double to $1.7 trillion by the year 2000 (see Figure 3-1.) (Burner, Waldo, and McKusick 1992).

Another important health care cost statistic is the percent of the U.S. gross domestic product (GDP) that is spent on medical care (Figure 3-1). The GDP is the value of all goods and services produced in this country, and the greater the percentage of the GDP we spend on health care, the smaller the amount of

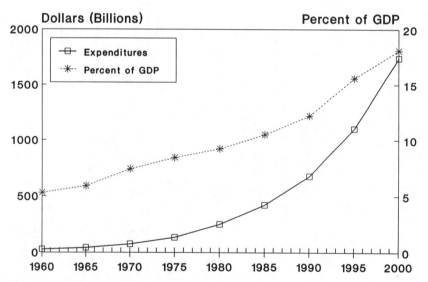

Figure 3.1. U.S. Health Care Expenditures, 1960–2000. *Source:* Burner, S. T., D. R. Waldo, and D. R. McKusick. 1992. National Health Expenditures Projections Through 2030. *Health Care Financing Review.* 14(1):1–29.

money available to purchase other goods and services, such as education and housing. Health care expenditures were 9.2 percent of the GDP in 1980, grew to 13.0 percent in 1991, and are expected to increase to 18.1 percent by the year 2000 (Burner, Waldo, and McKusick 1992).

Use of Funds

National health expenditures are usually divided into two categories: research and construction, and health services and supplies. Research and construction expenditures reached $23.1 billion in 1991, only three percent of the total. Health services and supplies can be divided into personal health care, administration of public programs and the net cost of health insurance, and government public health programs. Because personal health care is responsible for approximately 88 percent of national health expenditures, this area deserves special attention.

Personal health care (PHC) includes all services provided and associated with individual health care. In 1991, per capita PHC costs in the U.S. were $2,518 (Letsch et al. 1992). Hospital care, both inpatient and outpatient, was responsible for 44 percent of PHC expenditures (see Figure 3-2.). This is an increase from 1960, when hospitals represented 38 percent of the costs. Hospital costs also include expenditures for pharmaceuticals used in this setting and physician fees and salaries paid by hospitals. Some of this increase is due to the passage of Medicare in 1965 and its provision of public funding for the elderly's hospital costs. Expenditures for physician services were approximately $142 billion in

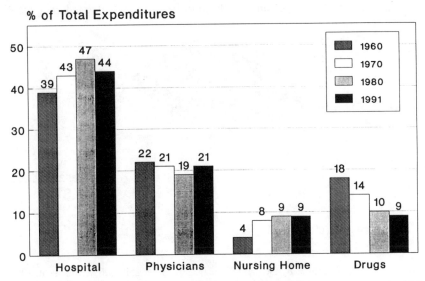

Figure 3.2. Expenditures by Service, 1960–1991. *Source*: Letsch, S. W., et al. 1992. National Health Expenditures, 1991. *Health Care Financing Review*. 14(2):1–30.

1991. This amounts to 21.5 percent of PHC costs and compares to 28 percent in 1960. Nursing home expenditures have increased from about four percent of total PHC costs in 1960 to 9 percent in 1991. This increase may not only be due to Medicaid coverage for the poor elderly but also to the growth of the elderly population.

As a percentage of personal health care expenditures, the cost of pharmaceuticals has decreased, from 17.6 percent in 1960 to 9.2 percent in 1991 (see Figure 3-2.). Although pharmaceutical prices increased at a greater rate than inflation in the 1980s, expenditures for pharmaceuticals still increased at a lower rate than that of expenditures for physician services or nursing home care, and increased at approximately the same rate as hospital services.

Source of Funds

Payment for personal health care (PHC) usually comes from one of four sources: private insurance companies, the federal government, state and local governments, or the patient, who makes out-of-pocket payments directly to the provider. The first three sources of payment are called *third parties* because they become the third player in the patient/health care provider relationship. The source of personal health care payments vary with the service provided.

Overall, third parties were responsible for paying approximately 75 percent of all PHC expenditures in 1991 (Figure 3-3) (Letsch et al. 1992). The tremendous growth in third parties is evident from the fact that only 42 percent of PHC costs were paid by third parties in 1960. Again, most of this increase is due to the implementation of Medicare and Medicaid in 1965. In 1991, the federal govern-

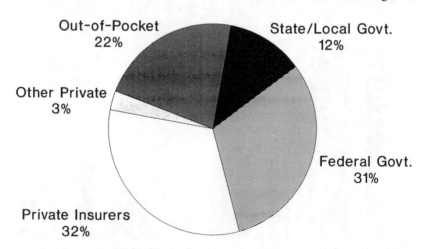

Figure 3.3. Expenditures by Payment Source, 1991. *Source*: Letsch, S. W., et al. 1992. National Health Expenditures, 1991. *Health Care Financing Review*. 14(2):1–30.

ment paid 31 percent of PHC costs while state and local governments paid 12 percent. Therefore, governments are already paying for 43 percent of their citizens' personal health care. Private health insurance paid another 32 percent of PHC costs. Out-of-pocket payments decreased from 56 percent in 1960 to only 22 percent in 1991.

Private insurance and government programs vary in the extent to which they cover different health care services. Out-of-pocket payments concern most consumers because they are direct payments to the provider. Only three percent of hospital expenses are paid out-of-pocket, whereas 55 percent of prescription drug costs are paid directly by patients (see Figure 3-4.). As will be discussed, decreasing out-of-pocket payments insulates the patient from the prices of services. Therefore, consumers are more price conscious with regard to pharmaceuticals than hospital care because a greater percentage of them pay these costs directly. This has direct implications for the pharmacist in providing pharmaceutical care.

Finally, it must be understood that even though we say governments or insurance companies pay for medical care, these payments are derived from individuals. When they pay increased health insurance premiums; federal, state, and local taxes; increased prices for goods and services provided by companies whose health insurance costs have increased; or when their salary drops to help pay for their employer-sponsored health insurance, individuals shoulder the responsibility of paying for health care costs.

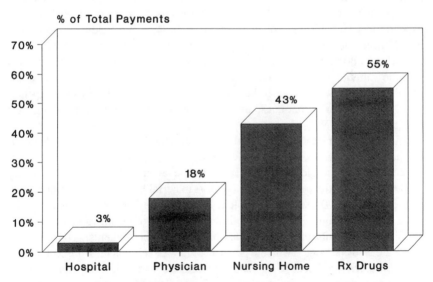

Figure 3.4. Out-of-Pocket Payments by Service, 1991. *Source*: Letsch, S. W., et al. 1992. National Health Expenditures, 1991. *Health Care Financing Review*. 14(2):1–30.

Problems in the U.S. Health Care System

The problems within our health care system are inter-related and attempts to change one area influence the others. However, these problems may be divided into three major categories: costs, access to care, and health status of the population.

Health Care Costs

The previous discussion of health care financing points out the current and potential problems with increasing health care costs. Increasing costs not only have ramifications for health care delivery but also is a foreboding sign for the soundness of the economy. In order to formulate successful strategies to contain rising costs, it is important to understand the underlying causes of the problem.

The greatest factor increasing health care expenditures is *economy-wide inflation*. From 1980 to 1990, general inflation was estimated to account for almost 50 percent of the annual growth of expenditure (Levit et al. 1991). Because inflation is affected by factors such as Federal Reserve Board policies and the world price of oil, economy-wide inflation is difficult to control and is likely to continue to be a factor in increasing costs.

Another cause of rising health care costs is the *increase in the elderly population*. About 12 percent of the U.S. population is 65 years of age or older, and this segment is responsible for approximately 30 percent of medical care expenditures (U.S. Bureau of the Census 1989; Rice and Feldman 1983). The elderly use more services on average than the non-elderly, and the intensity of their care is often much greater and, therefore, more expensive. It is estimated that the number of elderly will increase to approximately 22 percent of the population by the year 2030. If the current ratio of elderly to health care expenditures for the elderly continues, the elderly will use 55 percent of health care services in 2030. Will society accept this?

Another major factor in rising health care costs has been the cost of *technological advancements*. Consider the development of non-ionic contrast material, which replaced radiological dye. The dye had a mortality rate of 1 in every 30,000 uses, and the new non-ionic contrast material has a mortality rate of only 1 in every 250,000 uses. The problem is that the new technology is ten times more expensive and could add $1 billion to the cost of health care. These costs are passed along not only to the users but also to other patients.

We are also confronted with the prospect of new developments from biotechnology laboratories which have tremendous promise for treating many of mankind's ills but are quite expensive to develop. Technological advancements over the past 20 years will probably only be surpassed by developments in the next 20 years, but someone will have to pay for these advancements. Attempts to control the utilization of these technologies have already met and will continue to be met with ethical concerns about rationing health care.

A fourth cause of increasing health care costs is what could be know as the *health insurance effect.* Health insurance effectively insulates consumers from their health care costs and diminishes the effect that increasing the price of products and services has on reducing their utilization. In one study, 34 percent of adults with health insurance did not know the amount of their family's most recent hospital bill, and 78 percent of the respondents did not know what contribution their employer made for their insurance (Anderson 1991). Therefore, there is little financial incentive for patients to question the ordering of tests or procedures. In addition, prices increase because there is little incentive for suppliers or providers to lower prices to gain in market share.

Health care providers sometimes shift costs to private insurance because of the restrictions placed on government payment for Medicaid and Medicare. The resulting costs for insurance providers are evident. Consider these examples: in 1990, General Motors paid out $3.2 billion in health insurance premiums, more than it paid for steel (Castro 1991); Chrysler says health insurance for its employees adds $800 to price of each car it makes; and corporations' spending on health care services and supplies for employees as a proportion of after-tax profits increased from 12.4 percent in 1965 to 41.2 percent in 1980 and to 97.5 percent in 1991 (Cowan and McDonnell 1993). These statistics illustrate why corporate America has become a leader in the call for health care reform.

As the number of lawsuits and amount of liability awards increase, so do the liability insurance premiums for health care providers. These increased costs are passed along to patients or insurers. The threat of such lawsuits encourages practitioners to practice "defensive medicine." The AMA estimated that $21 billion worth of medical care is being utilized each year because of physicians concerns about potential lawsuits (Castro 1991).

Of course there are many other reasons for increased health care costs. These include a lack of information to aid patients in making educated decisions about their medical care; administration costs of private health insurance; duplication of services and competition for patients in many areas; fraud and unnecessary care; and the relatively new added costs for treating AIDS patients. To be effective, any attempt to contain costs must address the factors above.

Access to Care

Access to care is usually measured in terms of the number of Americans who are uninsured. Estimates vary, but between 31 and 36 million people do not have insurance benefits on any given day. This means that approximately 12 to 14 percent of the U.S. population is uninsured. Other estimates suggest that anywhere from 48 million to 63 million people are uninsured for some part of the year (Friedman 1991). These figures do not include the many Americans who have little insurance against catastrophic medical expenses.

It is often assumed that the uninsured are people who are unemployed and ineligible for public funds. However, often this is not the case (see Figure 3-5.). Only about 18 percent of the uninsured are members of a family in which no one is employed (Employee Benefits Research Institute 1992). The ramifications of this statistic are that a combination of two programs, one giving employers incentive to provide benefits and the other providing insurance for the unemployed and their families, could provide access to health insurance for almost everyone in our current system. However, adapting our present health care system, which has greatly contributed to the current crisis, is controversial.

A final point regarding access is that the question should be "access to what?" A person who has access to insurance does not necessarily have access to medical care. As an example, consider pregnant Medicaid recipients. Even though they have publicly financed insurance there is a problem with low birth-weight babies in this population. There may not be transportation available for those who need to travel to reach a health care provider to receive prenatal care. Others may not seek prenatal care at all. Where a person has access to care, what can or should be done to assure the care is given? Whose role is it to provide these assurances?

Quality and Effectiveness of Care

There is little doubt that, overall, the present quality of health care in the U.S. is the highest it has ever been. But it is also apparent that this high-quality care is not available to all. Aggregate measures of the population's health status, such as infant mortality rates and life expectancy, are no better in this country than in other countries that spend less per capita on health care.

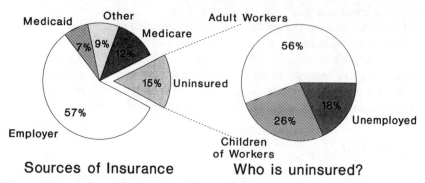

Figure 3.5. Health Insurance Coverage of U.S. Population, 1991. *Sources*: Employee Benefits Research Institute. 1992. *Sources of Health Insurance and Characteristics of the Uninsured.* Washington: Employee Benefits Research Institute. Levit, K. R., G. L. Olin, and S. W. Letsch. 1992. Americans' Health Insurance Coverage, 1980–1991. *Health Care Financing Review.* 14(1):31–57.

In general, the main concerns over the quality of medical care in the U.S. have developed from an excessive or inappropriate use of services. Sources of concern include the variable rates of hospitalization across the country, the overuse or underuse of various diagnostic tests, excessive or inappropriate surgery (such as tonsillectomies and caesarean sections), early discharge from hospitals because of DRG's, variable results of surgeries, and the excessive or inappropriate use of prescription drugs.

One of the problems with ensuring quality of care is that quality has different meanings to different people. To consumers, quality may mean the opportunity to choose a provider or insurer, to an insurer it may suggest the appropriateness of care, and to a clinician it may mean the effectiveness of therapy. However, implicit in the concept of quality medical care is the idea that services should be cost-efficient and cost-effective because unnecessary, excessive, or inappropriate services do not help the patient and may be harmful or waste the patient's resources (Lohr, Yordy, and Thier 1988).

There is little doubt that quality and effectiveness of medical care are inseparable from access to and funding for care. When planning improvements to our health care system, considering the three separately would not only be imprudent but also counter-productive. An example of this policy problem is the provision of pharmaceuticals. Most policy makers understand the importance of access to drug benefits, which are necessary for complete medical care, but are concerned about the costs, direct and indirect, of the benefit and how such a benefit could be financed. In addition, the quality of the benefit must be assured. Pharmaceutical care may be useful in assuring quality, but it raises questions about the provision and documentation of services and about reimbursement.

Representatives of insurers, corporations, the government and consumers have generally come to agree that some changes must occur which will affect the access to, costs of, and quality of health care as provided by the current U.S. health care system. Without such reform we will continue to spend an increasing portion of our resources on health care instead of other pressing social needs, and it will be increasingly difficult to ensure access to effective health care for all Americans.

Reforming a Disjointed Health Care System

Proposals to address the problems regarding access, costs, and quality of medical care vary widely. They represent the diversity of political, economic, and social philosophies found in U.S. society.

Basic Questions for Reform Proposals

In general, when considering different methods by which to change the incentives within our health care system, several questions need to be asked to clarify the proposal.

1) What are the objectives of the plan? Does it attempt to affect costs, access, and/or quality?

2) Will there be a set of basic benefits which all receive?

3) If there is a set of basic benefits, what services are included and who decides what these will be?

4) How much are we, as a society, willing to spend for health care? How will this be measured—aggregate expenditures, per capita expenditures, or percent of GDP?

5) How will these expenditures be financed?

6) Who will administer the program—private insurers, the federal government, state governments, or a combination of these?

7) How will quality of care be measured, monitored, and assured?

8) How much autonomy will patients be allowed regarding their choice of insurance plans, health care providers, and specific medical decisions?

Probably the most difficult issues to address are those related to the financing of the plan and the cost controls utilized. In determining the financing, policymakers must assess the fairness of the proposed funding of the plan. Funding mechanisms may produce economic disincentives, which must be considered, and the political ramifications of any funding mechanism will most certainly be measured by lawmakers. Decisions must also be made regarding the proper cost controls. Some degree of freedom may be taken from the beneficiary in the choice of a health care provider, but this has already been found to be a politically unpopular approach. Also, policies limiting reimbursement for health care providers have to be defined. This, again, may bring political fallout and unwelcome disincentives regarding access to care for beneficiaries.

Prospects for Health Care Reform

Proposals to reform our health care system lie on an ideological spectrum. On one end are those proposals that are egalitarian in nature and consider health care to be a social good, which should be available to all at the same level. An example of this type of proposal is the single-payer system, under which comprehensive medical care benefits would be extended to the entire population and all payments for these services would be made by the federal government. At the other end are those proposals that maintain that health care is a basic good which should be regulated and distributed through a free market. Proposals at this end of the spectrum would remove restrictions that supporters maintain do not allow the free market to work. Most proposals are somewhere between these two and provide a basic set of benefits to all or to a needy portion of the population.

If health care reform follows the same path as other reforms in this country's modern history, a series of incremental changes is likely. Social policy in the U.S. tends to evolve slowly, taking calculated steps but not giant leaps. Most of the U.S. population is satisfied with their health care. Although they believe some changes are needed, most people are concerned about extending the welfare state. In addition, the complexity of both our health care system's problems and the proposed solutions make it difficult to develop a public consensus around any proposal. The perceived effects of reform on individuals' personal health care and the increased funding needed to implement reforms result in a citizenry supportive of more prolonged and methodical change.

This incremental change might result in health insurance reform whereby small businesses and individuals share their risks through health share purchasing cooperatives; regulations prohibiting "preexisting condition" clauses in policies to prevent health insurance companies from refusing to insure persons with health problems; and/or insurance premiums based on a "community rating" of all persons in a geographical area and not based on "experience rating" of an individual's or a business's past medical care. Also, tax system reform may be proposed in order to help individuals or groups purchase health insurance. Another change in the tax system may attempt to lessen the health insurance effect by providing incentives for employers to offer and employees to accept less comprehensive health insurance plans. Finally, malpractice reform could reduce malpractice premiums for health care providers and decrease the practice of "defensive medicine."

Pharmaceutical Care in a Reformed Health Care System

The need for a reduction in health care costs, better access to medical care, and commitments to improved quality and more effective health care all point to the need for pharmaceutical care, and the future looks bright for those who practice it. As health care organizations become more integrated, pharmacists will have better access to clinical information needed to perform their responsibilities. This will be enhanced by the development of new information systems. These systems should also provide a more effective method of determining patient outcomes. In addition, more people will have health insurance benefits and be less affected by financial barriers to care.

Reform will also bring about challenges for pharmaceutical care providers. Managed care networks may exclude some providers unless they can document the effectiveness of the services they provide. Price controls will decrease the margins on ingredient costs and will necessitate better management skills and reimbursement for services provided. Again, documentation of effectiveness may be required. Payers will also try to share their risks with pharmaceutical care providers through capitated payments instead of fee-for-service reimbursement.

The calculation of the appropriate reimbursement levels will be critical for both the payer and the provider of care.

Summary

The U.S. health care system provides the best medical care in the world for those who have access to it. But it is also beset with problems—dilemmas which are interrelated and worsening. The resolution of these problems will not be easy, quick, or perfect.

Pharmacists, as well as other health professionals, are at a crossroads where some will be winners and others will be losers. Only through the provision of care which recognizes the patient as the paramount concern will the profession progress. The health care system offers pharmacy many challenges, but also many opportunities.

References

Abramowitz, K. S. 1993. *The Future of Health Care Delivery in America*. New York: Bernstein Research, Sanford C. Bernstein and Company.

Anderson, K. 1991. Why Health Care Costs are Tough to Cure. *USA Today*. March 11:3B.

Board of Trustees of the Federal Hospital Insurance Trust Fund. 1992. *1992 Annual Report of the Board of Trustees*. Washington: U.S. Government Printing Office.

Burner, S. T., D. R. Waldo, and D. R. McKusick. 1992. National Health Expenditures Projections Through 2030. *Health Care Financing Review*. 14 (1):1–29.

Castro J. 1991. Condition: Critical. *Time*. November 25 (138):34.

Cowan, C. A., and P. McDonnell. 1993. Business, Households, and Governments: Health Spending, 1991. *Health Care Financing Review*. 14 (3):227–48.

De Lew, N., G. Greenberg, and K. Kinchen. 1992. A Layman's Guide to the U.S. Health Care System. *Health Care Financing Review*. 14 (1):151–69.

Employee Benefits Research Institute. 1992. *Sources of Health Insurance and Characteristics of the Uninsured*. Washington: Employee Benefits Research Institute.

Friedman, E. 1991. The Uninsured: From Dilemma to Crisis. *JAMA* 265:2491.

Health Insurance Association of America. 1992. *Source Book of Health Insurance Data 1991*. Washington: HIAA.

Jonas, Steven. 1986. *Health Care Delivery in the United States*. New York: Springer Publishing Company.

Journal of the American Medical Association. 1932. The Committee on the Costs of Medical Care [Editorial]. 99 (23):1950–2.

Langwell, K. 1992. *The Effect of Managed Care on Use and Costs of Health Services* [Staff Memorandum, Congressional Budget Office]. Washington: U.S. Government Printing Office.

Letsch, S. W., et al. 1992. National Health Expenditures, 1991. *Health Care Financing Review*. 14 (2):1–30.

Levit, K. R., et al. 1991. National Health Expenditures, 1990. *Health Care Financing Review*. 13 (1):29–54.

Levit, K. R., G. L. Olin, and S. W. Letsch. 1992. Americans' Health Insurance Coverage, 1980–91. *Health Care Financing Review*. 14 (1):31–57.

Lohr, K. N., K. D. Yordy, and S. O. Thier. 1988. Current Issues in Quality of Care. *Health Affairs*. 7 (1):5–18.

Mariner, W. K. 1992. Problems with Employer-provided Health Insurance—The Employee Retirement Income Security Act and Health Care Reform. *New England Journal of Medicine*. 327 (23):1682–5.

Marion Merrell Dow. 1993. *Managed Care Digest, HMO Edition*. Kansas City: Marion Merrell Dow.

Rice, D. P., and J. J. Feldman. 1983. Living Longer in the United States: Demographic Changes and Health Needs of the Elderly. *Health and Society*. 61:364.

Staines, V. S. 1993. Potential Impact of Managed Care on National Health Care Spending. *Health Affairs*. Supplement 1993:248–57.

Swartz, K., and D. Lipson. 1989. *Strategies for Assisting the Medically Uninsured*. Washington: The Urban Institute and the Intergovernmental Health Policy Project.

U.S. Bureau of the Census, Dept. of Commerce. 1989. Projections of the Population of the United States, by Age, Sex, and Race: 1988 to 2080. *Current Population Reports*. January 1989, Series P–25.

U.S. House of Representatives, Committee on Ways and Means. 1991. *Overview of Entitlement Programs, 1991 Green Book*. Washington: U.S. Government Printing Office.

Waldo, D. R., S. T. Sonnefeld, and D. R. McKusick. 1989. Health Expenditures by Age Group, 1977 and 1987. *Health Care Financing Review*. 10 (4):111–20.

Wallack, S. S. 1992. Managed Care: Practice, Pitfalls, and Potential. *Health Care Financing Review*. 1991 Annual Supplement:27–34.

4

Drug Use and the Health Care System

Hind T. Hatoum, Ph.D.
Robert J. Valuck, Ph.D.

> "Traditionally, all of the health disciplines have been involved to some degree with drugs, but no particular discipline operating at the clinical level has exercised a broad responsibility for the total drug use process. Typically, the drug prescribing, dispensing, and administering functions have occurred independently, with no effective coordination. This situation has resulted in drug misuse, overuse, abuse, and serious untoward effects. The problems in drug therapy management, resulting from the isolation of these functions, led to the thinking that there was a need for one discipline to assume broad leadership and responsibility for the safe and appropriate use of drugs in society (Miller 1983, 14)."

Introduction

The expansion of the pharmaceutical industry since the late 1950s and the resultant plethora of drug products have increased the potential for and concern with iatrogenic diseases associated with drug use. Repeatedly, the call for ensuring rational drug therapy has been made (Rucker 1989). In more recent years, with the increasing emphasis on the need for cost containment in health care expenditures, the economic consequences associated with irrational drug therapy have been of particular interest.

In 1969, President Johnson's Task Force on Prescription Drugs formally documented an array of problems with the use of prescription drugs in the United States health care system (Task Force on Prescription Drugs 1969). The task force went on to propose a series of system improvements, including enhanced physician education in clinical pharmacology and experimentation with various drug utilization review (DUR) methods. It has taken more than twenty years for some of the solutions proposed by the Task Force to be implemented. Most notably, formal DUR programs were required for Medicaid recipients by the OBRA 1990 legislation (Brushwood, Catizone and Coster 1992). However, many problems noted by the Task Force remain unresolved.

Manasse has suggested the label "drug misadventuring" as a broad term inclusive of any iatrogenic disease or complication of drug therapy (Manasse 1989a, 1989b). The author notes that the extensive use of pharmaceuticals in the U.S., as well as the dangers inherent in their distribution, handling, and consumption, has increased the risk of misadventuring. Manasse cites estimates that drug misadventures contribute tens of billions of dollars annually to this country's spiraling health care costs; such estimates are even more troubling in light of expert opinion that these problems are, if anything, under-reported and undervalued in terms of their impact. Manasse advocates the development of a public policy dealing with this problem.

Indeed, some attention over the past twenty-five years has been centered on the identification, documentation, and to some extent the prevention of various forms of drug misadventuring. Strand et al. (1990) have proposed a useful descriptive typology for dealing with and preventing drug-related problems (See Table 4-1). However, just as drug-related problems were the result of a lack of a coordinated system of drug use, so were the efforts to address them fragmented. We contend that the concept of rational drug therapy needs to be expanded beyond the prevention of drug misadventuring and should be conceptually founded upon a thorough understanding of the entire drug use process as it exists in the United States today. Such an understanding will provide a unifying framework for both system reforms designed to foster optimal drug use and the development of a patient-centered philosophy of practice.

This chapter is based on the premise that the drug use *process* in the health care system is suboptimal and therefore is not conductive for the delivery of pharmaceutical care. In addition there are several forces, both internal and external to pharmacy, that create major obstacles to the delivery of pharmaceutical care. Therefore, the profession of pharmacy must endeavor to transform the existing process into a drug use *system* designed to promote the rational prescribing, preparation, distribution, use, monitoring, and evaluation of drugs and drug therapy.

The following sections provide descriptions of and elaborations on the steps comprising the drug use process, as well as illustrative empirical evidence of the potential negative consequences to patient care associated with inconsistencies or problems arising at each step of the process. Forces precipitating change in

Table 4-1.   Major Types of Drug-Related Problems

A patient is experiencing (or has the potential to experience) an undesirable event (medical problem, complaint, symptoms, diagnosis, or syndrome) that is of psychological, physiological, social, emotional, or economic origin, and is a function of the patient's

1. needing pharmacotherapy but not receiving it (a drug indication),
2. taking or receiving the wrong drug,
3. taking or receiving too little of the correct drug,
4. taking or receiving too much of the correct drug,
5. experiencing an adverse drug reaction,
6. experiencing a drug-drug, drug-food, or drug-laboratory interaction,
7. not taking or receiving the drug prescribed, or
8. taking or receiving a drug for which there is no valid medical indication.

Source: Strand, L. M., R. J. Cipolle, and P. C. Morley. 1992. *Pharmaceutical Care: An Introduction,* p. 11. Kalamazoo, MI: The Upjohn Company).

the drug use process are reviewed, including demographic, epidemiological, technological, social, economic, and political factors. These factors are both divergent and convergent in nature, creating a "push-pull" demand for optimal drug therapy. Pharmacy practitioners, adopting the care model when delivering pharmaceutical services, are in a position to help their public realize optimal drug therapy by turning challenges and obstacles into opportunities. Pharmacists must assume the lead role in guiding the drug use process in a positive direction, towards a coordinated, multidisciplinary drug use system with a united approach.

The Drug Use Process in the United States Health Care System

In the mid-1960s, Brodie was the first to advocate the notion of drug-use control as "the keystone to pharmaceutical service . . . the mainstream function of pharmacy (Brodie 1967, 63)." Brodie defined drug-use control as the system of knowledge, understanding, judgments, procedures, skills, controls, and ethics that assures optimal safety in the distribution and use of medication. He further stated, "Drug-use control provides a purpose, it gives a direction, it recognizes need and fulfillment in the patient-pharmacist relationship, it is the basic ingredient which underlies the essentiality of pharmacy and its service (Brodie 1967, 65)." Brodie suggested that drug-use control encompasses the chain of events from the development of a drug to the completion of the drug's task in the patient's body. The term applies to community, institutional, and industrial pharmacy practice, as well as pharmacy education. Brodie's article represents the first major attempt to view drug use as a *process* and to relate the role of the pharmacist to steps within that process.

Evolution of the Drug Use Process Concept

As the fundamental nature of pharmacy practice has evolved over the past 100 years, so has our conceptualization and understanding of the complexities of the drug use process. Briefly, the profession of pharmacy has seen three major stages of development in its recent past: the traditional, or drug-distribution stage; the transitional, or clinical-pharmacy stage; and the patient-focused, or pharmaceutical-care stage. These stages are described in considerably more detail by Higby in Chapter 2. Across these stages, the focus of pharmacy practice has expanded to include the drug products, the specialized clinical services, and, most recently, the professional responsibility for outcomes associated with drug therapy in individual patients.

Parallelling this "professional role evolution" has been an expansion and a revision of what has or should have constituted the drug use process. In an era when pharmacists were primarily the compounders and the dispensers of medicines, the drug use process might have been described as beginning with the discovery, extraction, or synthesis of raw drugs and ending with the sale of the finished, compounded prescription to the patient (Mrtek 1982). During the era of expansion of clinical pharmacy, the scope of practice grew to include the delivery of several pharmaceutical services, e.g. pharmacokinetic dosing, therapeutic monitoring, provision of drug information, nutritional support, and the compilation of medication histories. The notion of the drug use process had shifted to place much less emphasis on compounding and considerably more emphasis on clinical service delivery.

Since the mid-1970s, many experts have argued that pharmacy should be defined as a system which renders a health service by concerning itself with knowledge about drugs and the application of this knowledge to man and animals (American Association of Colleges of Pharmacy 1975). More recently it has been advocated that this knowledge about drugs should constitute the theoretical base of pharmacy practice in the 1990s and well into the twenty-first century (Brodie, McGhan, and Lindon 1991). For this assertion to hold true, the drug use process must be viewed in terms of the application of specialized knowledge to any and all aspects of drug use. Pharmacists' unique education and skills represent an enabling mechanism by which they may affect many aspects of drug use. Tools the pharmacist has available include consultation with physicians on therapies of choice, monitoring the ability of drugs to achieve therapeutic objectives in patients, and, ultimately, making recommendations accordingly.

We believe that, to assume the clinical role engrained in a patient-centered philosophy of practice, pharmacists must develop a keen understanding and appreciation of the fact that their role revolves around the drug use process. Using the model of the drug use process as described in the next section, pharmacists will have a frame of reference to link their pharmacotherapy expertise to the needs of their patients.

The Drug Use Process Model

The concept of coordinated efforts to achieve the optimal use of drugs is encompassed in the multi-stage model referred to as the "Drug Use Process (DUP)" (Knapp et al. 1974; Hutchinson and Witte 1983; Kirking 1986). As we suggested earlier, an expansion of focus beyond problem identification and prevention to one of fostering rational drug therapy is needed. This expansion, however, requires patients as well as all health professionals to play a role in the drug use process and to consider that all actions related to drug therapy represent a continuum. The "systems perspective" espoused here (and depicted in Figure 4-1) necessitates interrelated and coordinated decisions with a focus on patient problems and the means to achieve the desired therapeutic endpoints.

Presently, the drug use process is disjointed and inefficient in manpower use and resource consumption. Physicians, pharmacists, and nurses spend significant amounts of time carrying out technical tasks in isolation and without adding professional value, and many professional activities are poorly coordinated

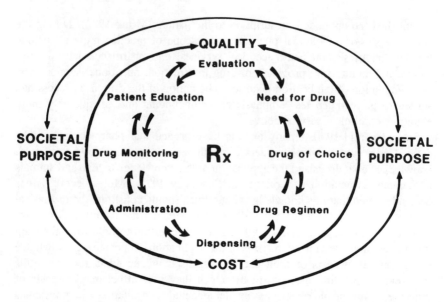

Figure 4.1. A Systems approach to rational drug therapy: A model of the drug use process. (*Source*: Hutchinson, R. A., R. K. Lewis, and H. T. Hatoum. 1990. *DICP Ann Pharmacother* 24 (June):634).

(Hutchinson, Lewis, and Hatoum 1990). As a result, patients may be placed at risk and unnecessary costs in terms of morbidity, mortality, and wasted resources may be added.

The following sections describe each of the eight steps of the drug use process. Along with the descriptions are discussions of reported incidents documenting suboptimal drug therapy and identifying opportunities for pharmacists to improve therapeutic outcomes.[1] It should be kept in mind that errors and failures may occur at any point in the DUP and that for the process to function optimally, each step must be completed without problems. For example, if a drug is not administered properly, it matters little that tasks such as selection and dispensing have been carried out properly (Hutchinson, Lewis, and Hatoum 1990).

Step One: Perception of the Need for a Drug

The high cost of drugs and potential risk of undesirable consequences from the misuse of drugs require health care professionals and patients to be circumspect in their decisions to seek and to use drug therapy. Patient needs and alternative therapies (including no therapy) must be considered before either prescription

---

[1]This section of the chapter borrows heavily from an article by Hutchinson, Lewis, and Hatoum (*DICP Ann Pharmacother* 1990; 24:633–6). Readers are referred to this citation for further details.

or over-the-counter drug therapy is initiated. However, evidence shows that physicians are inclined to use pharmacologic forms of treatment even when non-pharmacologic modes of therapy are more advantageous, and that physicians frequently prescribe medications for durations far exceeding the recommended length of therapy (Manning et al. 1986).

A classic example of unnecessary and nonindicated use of drug therapy is the prescription of antibiotics to treat the common cold (Meyer 1988). This unnecessary use of antibiotics may lead to clinical complications, including the development of resistant strains of bacteria and a multitude of untoward health consequences, and to an unnecessary increase in the cost of drug therapy (Hutchinson, Lewis, and Hatoum 1990).

The need for drug therapy must be carefully evaluated and weighed against the alternatives for every patient in each situation of possible utilization. Both health professionals and patients must realize that all illnesses do not necessitate drug therapy. Because of the cost of drugs and the potential for adverse effects, drugs should be used only when indicated. Pharmacists should monitor drug utilization in all practice settings and assist in establishing guidelines to discourage unnecessary drug use. Given that two-thirds of all patient visits to physicians result in a prescription (Koch 1982), pharmacists should also become directly involved in the decision to use drug therapy. Pharmacists can become involved by documenting important drug-related information in patient profiles or medical charts, establishing consultative arrangements with physicians in all practice settings, and providing inservices and other forms of education for medical staff, area physicians or group practices, and patients.

Step Two: Selection of Drug of Choice

The second step in the drug use process is the selection of the most appropriate drug. This decision should be based on therapeutic goals, patient variables, and costs. Any deviation from this practice is less than optimal (Hutchinson, Lewis, and Hatoum 1990). One dilemma for the physician at this step can be summarized as follows:

> The basic motivations behind a physician's choice of drug therapy must be considered to be rational. [S]/He would be expected to select the product that would do the most good with the least possible side effects, and perhaps the lowest cost. In most cases of drug [of choice] selection, however, physicians try to make a rational decision under conditions of uncertainty (Avorn and Soumerai 1983).

A number of factors that foster suboptimal prescribing have been identified. Hutchinson, Lewis, and Hatoum (1990) noted that some of the most common factors are the rapid rate of new drug introductions to the market, the profusion of promotional product information, failure to keep abreast of current drug topics, careless evaluation of drug information, and the underestimation of the true cost and toxicity of drugs. A review of the literature by Valuck (1992) also identified medical practice "fads," office or clinic location (e.g., urban versus rural), and a variety of physician demographic variables as being correlated with irrational prescribing. A high frequency of suboptimal prescribing practices has been reported in the literature (Davis and Cohen 1981; Avorn and Soumerai 1983; Baum et al. 1985).

One plausible explanation for the frequency of suboptimal prescribing, pointed out by Hutchinson, Lewis, and Hatoum, is that, while a significant amount of time and effort is required to understand drugs and their actions, physicians have limited time available for reading and understanding the medical and pharmaceutical literature. The American College of Physicians reported that continuing education in pharmacology for physicians is largely random, incomplete, and subject to bias (Meyer 1988). New information on available drug therapy is reported at an unbelievably rapid pace. It is quite optimistic to suggest that health care professionals in general and physicians in particular have the time to keep up with this information. Moreover, skepticism has been voiced regarding the validity of published literature—be it in professional journals or materials sponsored by pharmaceutical firms (Smith 1977; Brink 1986).

When given the opportunity to influence selection of drugs of choice, through physician education, consultation, or service on pharmacy and therapeutics committees, pharmacists have demonstrated their ability to improve drug prescribing. Pharmacists have targeted specific drugs that were subject to suboptimal prescribing with success. For example, direct contact between pharmacists and physicians is believed to have generated important changes in the nature and cost of drug use and to have decreased the average cost per course of therapy (Avorn and Soumerai 1983).

In an age of rapid technological advancement, maintaining expert knowledge of every aspect of health care is beyond the scope of any single profession, let alone individual practitioners. One societal solution to the exponential growth in drug-related information may be to sanction experts in each field and to follow a professional team approach in assuring optimal health care delivery (Hutchinson, Lewis, and Hatoum 1990). Empirical evidence supports the contentions that pharmacists make sound therapeutic recommendations when given therapeutic objectives, and that physicians are willing to accept such recommendations (Lobas, Lepinski, and Abramowitz 1992; Hatoum and Akhras 1993).

Step Three: Selection of Drug Regimen

The third step of the drug use process is the selection of a specific drug regimen. A drug regimen includes the dose, dosage form, route, frequency of administration, and duration of drug therapy. In this step, the most appropriate regimen should be selected for accomplishing the desired goals based on patient-specific variables. Potential problems to be averted include underdosing, overdosing, drug interaction, inappropriate routing, and inappropriate dosage form (Hutchinson, Lewis, and Hatoum 1990).

Problems in this step exist and deviations from acceptable standards have been cited. In one study, nearly 90 percent of 87 patients monitored received theophylline doses that exceeded recommended guidelines, and more than 81 percent of these patients experienced toxicity (Burkle and Gwizdala 1981). In another study, 52 percent of a 42-patient study group received intravenous cimetidine when oral therapy was indicated (Kimelblatt et al. 1982).

The pharmacist's role in the selection of drug regimen has great potential for reducing costs and increasing the proper and safe use of medications. In a 1979 study, pharmacists employed in a newborn intensive care unit demonstrated that they could not only achieve cost savings but could also prevent unwanted clinical outcomes. In this study, calculation errors made by pediatricians and nurses were 10 times greater or smaller than the correct dose, but the errors made by pharmacists were all within 1 percent of the correct dose. Pediatricians and nurses made these calculation errors respectively 40 and 56 percent of the time. Moreover, the pediatricians and nurses were incorrect in their judgment of the appropriate dose in 19 and 59 percent of the cases, respectively (Perlstein et al. 1979).

Other studies have shown that pharmacists are able to adjust aniticoagulant therapy as well as experienced physicians (Chenella et al. 1983); that they are able to avert dose-related toxicities from digoxin therapy (Lewis, Cooper, and McKercher 1976); and that they are able to apply their knowledge of pharmacokinetics to customize aminoglycoside antibiotic dosage regimens in hospitalized patients (Schloemer and Zagozen 1984). Ample opportunities exist in a wide variety of practice settings for pharmacists to have a positive impact on patient care within this step in the drug use process.

Step Four: Provision of Drug Product

The fourth step of the drug use process is the preparation and dispensing of the drug product. Historically, pharmacists have spent the majority of their time compounding and dispensing prescriptions. Today, the need for compounding has decreased, while the need for effective and efficient drug distribution systems has increased (Hutchinson, Lewis, and Hatoum 1990).

This step of the drug use process has received the most attention in the pharmacy literature since Barker and McConnell (1962) reported that one dose in six was given in error at a large university hospital. In fact, in terms of systems improvement, one can safely say that the unit-dose method of distributing pharmaceuticals, now in place in over 90 percent of U.S. hospitals, has been successful in decreasing both medication errors and the total cost of drug distribution and administration (Black 1984).

Improving the system of drug distribution without implementing changes in the overall drug use process does not necessarily ensure optimal drug therapy. If this were the case, one would not expect problems with drug therapy in hospitals using the unit-dose system. In the unit-dose system, pharmacists dispense medications as ordered, in unit dose packaging. However, while this system ensures correct dispensing, it does not necessarily ensure that the medication selected is appropriate or that nurses administer the dispensed dose to the patient on time or at all. The system employed by most hospitals for dispensing and administering medications allows neither the pharmacists nor the nurses to assume full control for coordinating these two steps. Hence, medication errors continue to be reported (Davis and Cohen 1981; Barker et al. 1984).

In the community, drug administration is in the hands of patients, their family members and their caregivers, and correct administration becomes a function of the individual's education about and understanding of the need for drug therapy, as well as the patient's willingness to abide by the instructions given. Because of these variables, any drug distribution system, regardless of setting, must have supportive clinical services to ensure proper drug use.

As we approach the 21st century, pharmacists need to understand technological advances and incorporate them into their daily practices. Not only can technologies such as robotics help minimize nonprofessional tasks, it can also offer the opportunity to develop distribution systems that will provide continuous care to patients when they move from one setting to another (e.g., inpatient to outpatient). This is of particular concern given the existing financial pressure for the early discharge of patients from hospitals. Once discharged, patients are expected to seek services from community pharmacies. Community pharmacists are in most cases faced with assessing these patients' needs based on incomplete information. Existing technology can be applied to this problem in useful ways. For example, "smart cards" may be able to provide the community pharmacist with a patient's medical history, including any recent hospitalizations, thus enhancing the pharmacist's ability to provide comprehensive patient care and optimal drug therapy.

At least one newly contemplated health care program for the nation is, in fact, centered around the use of "smart cards" to link services with patient demographic and clinical data. It remains, however, the responsibility of pharmacists to define the information needed to ensure appropriate care and be the conduit for the delivery of patient-oriented pharmaceutical care.

Step Five: Consumption or Administration

The fifth step of the drug use process is the consumption (in the community) or administration (in the inpatient setting) of medication, i.e., the administration of the right drug, to the right patient, by the right route, at the right time, in the right amount, and for the right duration. Problems in drug administration exist due to the lack of effective coordination between those responsible for prescription, distribution, and administration—normally three different health professionals.

Recently reported medication administration errors are no different from those reported in the early 1960s (Barker and McConnell 1962; Koren, Barzilay, and Greenwald 1986).

In hospital settings, medication errors are often linked to nursing services regardless of the origin of the error. Moreover, nurses, as professionals, are questioning the wisdom of continuing to assume responsibility for non-nursing tasks (Nichols 1981). Nursing time devoted to drug administration has not been thoroughly studied (Hatoum 1990). However, it seems reasonable that it is not cost-effective for these highly trained health care professionals to continue to perform technical tasks.

Some institutions have approached the identified problems in this step with a pharmacy-coordinated drug dispensing and administering system. Pharmacy-coordinated drug administration teams were shown to have a positive impact by decreasing the amount of error and human suffering, as well as by decreasing the direct and indirect costs associated with medication administration (Jozefczyk, Schneider, and Pathak 1986). However, this positive impact does not necessarily ensure the continuation of such a program, as both pharmacy and nursing staff continue to think of steps four and five in the drug use process as independent processes in terms of both cost to their departments and consequences on patient care.

Consumption of drugs in the outpatient or community setting is complicated by patient non-compliance as well as the apparent lack of formal systems or processes to ensure that drugs are consumed appropriately.

Step Six: Monitoring Effects of Drug

In the sixth step of the drug use process, drug therapy is monitored for effectiveness and/or adverse effects. This step is crucial, given that inappropriate medication monitoring may lead to prolonged illness and to increased resource consumption.

There are many established methods and parameters for monitoring the effectiveness of drug therapy, especially in inpatient settings (Elenbaas 1986). Pharmacokinetic monitoring of drug therapy has been an important advancement and is especially valuable with drugs that have narrow therapeutic indices and are sensitive to patient-specific variables. However, determinations of serum drug concentrations represent additional health care resource consumption and must be used efficiently and effectively. Moreover, some physicians may not possess the pharmacokinetic training necessary to use serum assays properly, leading to waste of health care resources (Guernsey et al. 1984). Pharmacists have repeatedly been shown to be the most effective health care professionals in providing pharmacokinetic services in hospitals (Winter, Herfindal, and Bernstein 1986; Smith et al. 1987).

Opportunities for application of pharmacokinetic skills to patient care are present for pharmacists outside institutional settings as well. Guidelines for drug therapy monitoring, which were developed in collaboration with physicians, provide pharmacists practicing in home health care, nursing homes, community care, and other settings with the chance to positively impact therapeutic outcomes in this step of the drug use process. Measuring blood pressure and, more importantly, monitoring patient compliance are two examples of tasks pharmacists can take on and thereby play a key role in improving drug-therapy monitoring in a community setting.

Proper monitoring of drug therapy also entails the prevention (or early detection) of adverse drug reactions (ADRs). An ADR is generally defined as "any response to a drug which is noxious and unintended in doses used for prophylaxis, diagnosis, or therapy (World Health Organization 1975)." Although some ADRs are severe and may result in death, the literature has emphasized morbidity, drug-related hospital admissions, increased hospital stays, and related costs (Manasse 1989a, 1989b). In addition to their impact upon patients' quality of life, ADRs needlessly increase resource consumption. In one study, patients with one or more ADRs stayed in hospital an average of 13.7 days more than patients with no ADRs (Spino, Sellers, and Kaplan 1978).

Appropriate monitoring is pivotal and of most concern for medications that are potent and possess narrow therapeutic indices. Clozapine, warfarin and digoxin are examples of powerful drug therapies that require careful therapeutic monitoring. We anticipate introduction of additional therapeutic agents requiring strict monitoring systems like the closed system of distribution and monitoring required for clozapine.

Monitoring for drug-related complications or adverse events is rather complicated since drugs are not frequently identified as the cause of patients' problems. In this regard, pharmacists appear more apt to suspect drugs as the source of problems than physicians or nurses (Garnett 1983). Pharmacists have both an opportunity and a responsibility to minimize the incidence of ADRs, regardless of practice setting.

Step Seven: Patient Education

The seventh step in the drug use process is patient education. In this step patients are educated about their drugs to assist in compliance with the prescribed regimen and the early detection and reporting of drug-related adverse events. This stage of the drug use process is becoming one of the most important, as evidenced by the formal congressional recognition of this professional function in the OBRA 1990 legislation.

A recent investigation by the Office of the Inspector General (OIG) for Health and Human Services, which described the effects of patient noncompliance, placed particular emphasis on the ambulatory elderly population. In this population, 55 percent of patients do not follow their prescribed regimens (Office of the Inspector General 1990a). The OIG report concludes that noncompliance with medication regimens increases the use of resources such as hospitals, nursing homes, and clinics and results in unnecessary treatments. Noncompliance can also lead to therapeutic failure, which in some instances results in serious complications or death. Moreover, the report points out that educating patients is the best way to improve compliance with drug therapy and emphasizes that patient education should not be construed to mean simply repeating directions or handing out printed materials. Rather, patient education is a process entailing gathering data, individualizing instructions, prompting and supporting the patient, and following up on and evaluating the patient's response to therapy to determine the success of the treatment in improving patient outcomes (Hatoum, Hutchinson, and Lambert 1993). Opportunities abound for pharmacists to overcome traditional obstacles; to use their knowledge and expertise to improve patient understanding, compliance, and clinical outcomes through counseling and education; and to enhance their professional standing as they conform with the OBRA 1990 mandates.

Step Eight: Evaluation and Follow-up

The eighth and final step of the drug use process is the evaluation of drug therapy effectiveness in light of therapeutic objectives and observed patient outcome. As with any process where goals and objectives have been set, it is important to monitor the patient's reponse as compared to desired endpoints. Having such information in hand will facilitate the pharmacists achieving their profesional responsibility.

Summary

Rational drug therapy has traditionally been viewed as the right drug, in the right dose, at the right time, for the right patient. Today, the emphasis on cost containment has added an extra dimension: cost-effectiveness of therapeutic regimens.

Most steps of the drug use process have not been extensively studied. Evidence to date shows duplication of efforts and suboptimal decisions, with little concerted effort to identify means for improvements that may have a favorable impact on costs and patient outcomes. The increasing cost and complexity of drugs, along with the inconsistencies that exist in drug use, demonstrate a need for a complete review of the drug use process.

The drug use process, as it currently operates in the United States, is not conducive to the provision of a systematic approach to therapy. The steps in this process are often carried out independent of each other and poorly performed by a variety of health professionals (Hutchinson, Lewis, and Hatoum 1990).

The development of strategies for increased provision of optimal drug therapy through the use of pharmacists as drug therapy experts is both relevant and possible. The profession of pharmacy is in a prime position. Expanded clinical services, coupled with a patient-centered philosophy of practice, could allow for a better coordination of the entire drug use process. The needs are apparent, the skills of pharmacists are well documented, and the opportunity awaits.

Perspectives on the Drug Use Process

The use of drugs in the United States is strongly influenced by a variety of factors that define our society, its culture, and its norms. These factors include, but are not limited to, trends in demography, epidemiology, technology, social structure and function, economics, and politics. As Manasse notes:

> In our pluralistic, individualistic, and competitive society, our collective drug use behavior reflects a phenomenon that is unique to the United States but parallels pharmaceutical consumption trends in other parts of the developed world. In short, we are a drug-taking society whose outlook centers on the general view that every malady has a treatment solution and that this solution lies mainly in the use of medicinal agents (Manasse 1989b).

Within this set of broader forces, a variety of collective "actors," each with unique interests, strengths and limitations, bring differing demands and expectations to the drug use process. The Task Force on Prescription Drugs suggested that at the very least, the interests of the following groups be considered (Task Force on Prescription Drugs 1969):

1. The drug users (patients using legitimate drugs)
2. The drug makers (manufacturers of prescription and nonprescription, and generic and brand name products)
3. The drug distributors (dispensing physicians, pharmacies, pharmacists, and the "applying" professions)
4. The drug prescribers (the prescribing professions)
5. The payers (government, private insurance, and managed-care plans)
6. The regulators (local, state, and federal government agencies)
7. The policymakers (local, state, and federal legislative bodies)

Given this variety of forces and actors, drug use must be viewed as a dynamic rather than a static process; the ways in which the process is invoked and implemented must change to meet the evolving needs of American society. The remainder of this chapter is devoted to a discussion of some of the more prominent forces and interests shaping the present-day drug use process.

Forces Precipitating Change

Planning for the future requires a realistic assessment of the major trends that are influencing and will continue to influence health care, including pharmacy practice. Each trend holds within it threats and opportunities for the profession of pharmacy in general and for its practitioners in particular.

Demographic Factors

Demographic data clearly show that the population of the U.S. is growing older. By the year 2000, the median age in the United States will be 36 years, compared to 29 years in 1975; the 35 million people over age 65 will represent about 13 percent of the population, in contrast to 8 percent in 1950; and the population of the "oldest old"—those over age 85—will have increased by about 30 percent to a total of 4.6 million (Spencer 1989). The influence of the aging population in shaping national health policy was recently demonstrated by the repeal of the Medicare Catastrophic Coverage Act of 1988 (repealed in 1989 under pressure from Medicare beneficiaries). Few pharmacists would argue that the elderly offer challenging opportunities for pharmaceutical services, but few have been successful in devising practice models that meet the needs of the elderly population and satisfy the professional goals in economically efficient ways. The profession's greatest success in this field to date lies is the provision of pharmaceutical services to institutionalized elderly in long-term care facilities (Penna 1991).

Further, by the year 2000, the racial and ethnic composition of the American population will be different than it is today. Caucasians other than Hispanics will represent a smaller proportion of the total population, only 72 percent compared with 76 percent today. In contrast, Hispanics are a fast-growing population group. Some estimate a rise from 8 to 11.3 percent of the population, to more than 31 million Hispanics by the year 2000. Blacks will increase their proportion of the population from 12.4 to 13.1 percent. Other racial groups, including Native Americans, Asians, and Pacific Islanders, will increase from 3.5 to 4.3 percent of the total population (Spencer 1989).

These demographic changes are important for pharmacists to consider, given the growing literature base that demonstrates the existence of ethnic and racial differences in pharmacologic response to medicines (Levy 1993). For example, black patients may respond very differently than white patients to anti-hypertensive drug therapy (Saunders 1988; Hall 1990); Chinese patients may require lower doses of and be more sensitive to the sedative effects of benzodiazepines than whites (Wood and Zhou 1991); and Hispanic patients may experience a greater incidence of side effects than whites with tricyclic antidepressant medications (Kalow 1982). Pharmacists should endeavor to be cognizant of the ethnic and racial composition of their patient populations in order to provide optimal pharmaceutical care.

Also of concern to pharmacists are the issues of access to care and provision of care in economically impoverished, inner city neighborhoods. Some researchers have noted problems and obstacles to providing pharmaceutical services in poor and underserved urban areas (Reutzel et al. 1993), but their conclusions tend to support our contention that pharmacists possess sufficient skills, resources, and formal role legitimation (e.g., under OBRA 1990) to provide pharmaceutical care regardless of location.

Epidemiological Factors

A gradual but definite change has occurred in the nature of the illnesses afflicting the U.S. population. Partly because of public health practices (Public Health Service 1979), partly because of advances in drug therapy, and partly because of the aging of the population, we have eliminated most serious acute illnesses as major public health concerns. The vast majority of patients cared for today have chronic illness or the acute manifestations of chronic disorders. Hypertension, arthritis, congestive heart failure, asthma, diabetes, glaucoma, alcoholism, cancers, and AIDS have supplanted polio, chicken pox, colds, and middle ear infections as the maladies which consume most of our health care resources (Public Health Service 1990). Yet our health care system is still oriented toward treating acute illness. As Penna (1991) notes:

> We train our physicians, nurses, and pharmacists in the acure care setting; the management of chronic illness is patient-initiated; and our compensation practices are based on the fee-for-service model developed for the care of the acutely ill. Pharmaceutical services are especially episodic: we wait until chronically ill patients determine that they are out of their medications before they seek renewals; we do a perfunctory evaluation of therapy at the time of new or renewal prescription orders rather than conduct comprehensive examinations of patients' medication regimens, desired outcomes and compliance assessments.

Given the shift from acute to chronic illness in the United States, the importance of an understanding of the entire drug use process is even more apparent. In order for long-term drug therapy regimens to remain optimal, or to be modified as necessary, constant and careful monitoring of all steps of the drug use process must be maintained.

Technological Factors

Today's pharmaceutical industry is producing drugs that are potent, effective, target-specific, and precise in their action, but great in their risks and high in their costs as well. Biotechnology has produced (and will continue to produce) drugs to treat illnesses that have evaded successful treatment, and some of these drugs require special storage and new administration techniques and procedures. Pressures to control the costs of these agents will continue; issues and debate with regard to cost-effectiveness of these drugs will continue to emerge; and the potential for serious harm to patients from the inappropriate use of these agents will continue to grow. There will likely be mounting pressure to restrict such potent drugs to special status—to be prescribed and/or dispensed either by specifically qualified practitioners or in special settings, facilities, or distribution systems (Penna 1991). Pharmacist monitoring of the use of these powerful compounds throughout the drug use process will be increasingly important in years to come.

Information technology is changing the way we access, store, and use information. It is expanding our access to new sources, types, and amounts of information as well. In the not too distant future, pharmacists practicing in community pharmacies may no longer face the lack of access to patient medical information which, has limited their ability to make clinically significant decisions. Indeed, the development of centralized health care databases (whether at the local, state, or regional level) is the key to the creation of a more rational, systematic, and cost-effective health care delivery systems (Rucker 1992). Such databases are an integral part of recently proposed national health care reforms.

Robotics is revolutionizing the drug distribution process. Large volume prescription distributors, such as mail order pharmacies, are using robots to pick, count, pour, label, and record prescription orders. Pharmacists must understand the impact of such technological advancements on their present and future practices, roles, and opportunities. On one hand, technological advances appear to decrease the social need for pharmacists. On the other hand, there is a well-documented need for drug *knowledge* experts, and the adoption of robotics to assist in distributive tasks may actually help future pharmacists to assume the more clinical role that pharmaceutical care requires.

Social Factors

Pharmacy, as a profession and as an integral part of the health care system, is experiencing a restructuring that closely mirrors trends in American society. John Naisbitt, in his best-selling book, Megatrends—Ten New Directions Transforming Our Lives, articulated several dimensions along which our society is experiencing change. They include the following shifts (Naisbitt 1982):

1. From an industrial to an information society
2. From forced technology to high tech/high touch
3. From a national economy to a world economy
4. From short term to long term
5. From centralization to decentralization
6. From institutional help to self help
7. From representative democracy to participatory democracy
8. From hierarchies to networking
9. From north to south
10. From either/or to multiple option

Several of these trends are particularly relevant for pharmacy practitioners (Hatoum 1990). Already discussed in this chapter have been shifts from an industrial to an information society; from short term to long term; and from either/or to multiple option (in terms of the vast number of drug therapy and product choices existing today).

Two of the remaining megatrends merit discussion here as well. One is the shift from forced technology to high tech/high touch. Naisbitt contends that each time a new technology is introduced, a counterbalancing human reponse is needed or else the new technology may be rejected. With regard to pharmacy practice, clinical services such as therapeutic monitoring and evaluation must accompany the utilization of potent new pharmaceuticals. If not, there indeed may be a societal backlash when an unacceptable level of adverse effects and costs is reached without improvement in health status.

The other megatrend of particular relevance to pharmacy practice is the shift from institutional help to self help. An increasingly sophisticated public with higher education has a growing interest in its own health care. The availability of convenient, inexpensive diagnostics (e.g., pregnancy tests and blood glucose monitoring kits); health and medical information; and effective and safe medication provide fertile ground for the growth of this movement in the United States. While people desire the freedom to self-diagnose and self-medicate (that is, to make their own health care decisions), they also demand accurate, personal, and available information resources (Penna 1991). Pharmacists are in a unique position to meet this demand and should strive to maintain their respected status by applying pharmaceutical care principles to the use of nonprescription as well as prescription medications by their patients.

Arnold Relman, former editor of the *New England Journal of Medicine,* presented another perspective when he described and discussed what he considers to be three "revolutions" which have occurred in the U.S. health care system since World War II (Relman 1988). According to Relman, the first revolution was the "Era of Expansion" which ran from the late 1940s through the 1960s. This period saw all aspects of the United States health care system grow at a rapid pace, along with most sectors of the U.S. economy. The number of hospitals, physicians, and commercial health insurance carriers climbed. Blue Cross and Blue Shield plans became dominant payers for health care services. Medical schools produced larger numbers of highly trained physicians geared towards specialized practice, and technological advances reached into all aspects of medical care—diagnostic, medical, surgical, pharmacological, and others. Medicare and Medicaid were added to Title XIX of the Social Security Act in 1966, putting government in the business of paying for health care services directly. Finally, this era saw the birth of investor-owned health care enterprises, mostly in the form of hospital chains. These businesses arose in response to a very favorable system of insurance (third party) payment based on billed charges and the prospect for continued growth and market penetration.

The second revolution Relman labeled the "Revolt of the Payers" or the "Era of Cost Containment," and it occurred in the 1970s and early 1980s. Growth in the health care sector, fueled by rapid expansion in the capacity for service provision and a payment system based on charges, began to concern those responsible for paying the cost of insurance premiums or program administration—largely employers and the federal government. As health care expenditures rose from four percent of the U.S. Gross Domestic Product (GDP) in 1965 to over 11 percent in the early 1980s (today the figure approaches 14 percent of GDP), cost containment became the goal. This goal was pursued by various means, including prospective payment for Medicare services (based on diagnosis-related groups, or DRGs), global budgeting at the local and state levels, and the evolution of managed care arrangements (e.g., HMOs, PPOs, and EPOs). Cost-containment efforts were directed at the use and provision of pharmaceuticals as well. From the early 1970s to the present day, third-party payment for prescription drugs has steadily increased (Myers 1987); with this increase have come the many faces of pharmacy-related managed care arrangements (Burns and Cordero 1991).

Relman concludes that we have now entered the "Era of Assessment and Accountability" (the third revolution in medical care). While the third-party payers have put forth their best efforts to curb rising costs, many observers have noticed that, for the most part, the quality and outcomes of the medical services purchased (including pharmaceuticals) are either poorly understood or virtually unknown. As Relman puts it:

> It is bad enough, the payers say, to be confronted with uncontrollable medical costs, but the situation becomes intolerable if in addition no one knows what benefits accrue from the services we pay for or the quality of those services. To control costs, without arbitrarily reducing access to care or lowering the quality of care, we will have to know a lot more about the safety, appropriateness, and effectiveness of drugs [and other services] (Relman 1988).

It is difficult to predict the outcome of the vigorously debate on health care reform in the United States as changes are occurring at a rapid pace and issues are in a state of flux. What is certain, regardless of the outcome of the debate, is that pharmacists can play a pivotal role in determining and increasing the cost-effectiveness of drug therapies. The application of drug utilization review methods (both at the clinical and aggregate levels) provides one means by which pharmacy may meet the mandate of assessment and accountability.

Economic Factors

As noted in previous sections, the rapid escalation in total health care expenditures in the United States over the past 20 to 30 years has caused concern among patients, providers, and payers alike. The economic costs associated with the overuse, underuse, or inappropriate use of pharmaceuticals in particular have not been fully identified (Hatoum 1991). Among the many economic forces to consider in examining this problem are the nature and role of the U.S. pharmaceutical industry and its impact on health care delivery; the existing patterns of health care spending in the final years of patients' lives; and the trend towards "value for money" in the delivery of health services.

The pharmaceutical industry is under scrutiny as the health care policy debate continues. Growth of the pharmaceutical industry depends upon further innovation, as well as creation and maintenance of demand for these new products. Growth in the sales of some products may be achieved through switches from prescription to non-prescription status. In either case, it is important to achieve a balance between apropriate drug therapy use and marketing and promotional activities of pharmaceutical firms—that is, promotion of pharmaceutical agents while simultaneously minimizing the rate of inappropriate drug use and drug-related problems. Pharmacists have an important role to play as providers of objective information to physicians, patients, and payers regarding the use, monitoring, and cost-effectiveness of drugs and drug therapy.

Also of relevance to pharmacy is the issue of health care spending in the last year of life. Twenty years ago, Victor Fuchs highlighted the difficult decisions which must be made regarding the allocation of scarce resources to the care of the elderly or terminally ill patients (Fuchs 1975). Regardless of the outcome of this social debate, we should expect drug therapy to continue to play a prominent role in sustaining human lives.

Finally, in the "Era of Assessment and Accountability," the costs and benefits of drugs and drug therapy to individual patients and to society will be under increased scrutiny from those who produce, purchase and consume them. The rapidly growing field of pharmacoeconomics is gaining the interest of everyone from government policy makers to medical staff and administrators in hospitals and other managed care settings (McGhan 1993), and represents one avenue by which pharmacy can help to meet the public mandate of assessment and accountability.

Political Factors

As mentioned earlier, there are a number of relevant "actors" in the drug use process (i.e., drug consumers, makers, distributors, prescribers, payers, regulators, and policy makers). Each of these groups of actors has a unique set of interests, demands, and resources that they bring to bear on issues relating to drugs and public policy. It is, therefore, inevitable that the interests of such a wide variety of actors conflict at times and converge at others. A discussion of some of the divergent perspectives on drug use follows in the next section of the chapter.

With respect to pharmaceuticals and their use in American society, Manasse noted several issues that have inherent political implications (Manasse 1989b). They are:

1. Drug approval, surveillance, and regulatory processes
2. Manufacturer image, influence, and impact
3. Professional group stature and credibility
4. Credibility, impact, and influence of professional organizations

Each of these areas directly influences the political agenda, political decision-making, and public policy. The interplay of economic, social, and institutional forces affects the political domain and vice versa. Ultimately, then, the success or failure of drug-use-related political decision-making is largely determined by the confluence of social, political, and economic forces (Manasse 1989b).

Given that many debates relevant to the profession of pharmacy are settled in the political arena, an understanding of policy-making within the U.S. political system would be useful to pharmacists (e.g., to fully understand both the nature and impact of the OBRA 1990 legislation). Not only are the *provisions* of particular public policies or decisions relevant, but the genesis, formulation, implementation, and evaluation of those policies are crucial for those towards whom the policies are directed. In the case of OBRA 1990, issues relating to the implementation of the mandatory patient counseling provisions have been of particular concern to practicing pharmacists, state pharmacy licensure boards, and Medicaid program administrators, (Hatoum, Hutchinson, and Lambert 1993; Brushwood, Catizone, and Coster 1992).

Finally, within health care reform and the role of the pharmacist in a newly-reformed health care system, there are political issues of concern to the public at large. Pharmacists have the responsibility to make both the public and policymakers aware of their role and their contributions to optimal pharmaceutical care. This role is based upon the extensive training that pharmacists receive, their accessability in most communities, and their patient-centered philosophy of practice. Toward this end, a number of pharmacy-related professional organizations recently joined with the National Consumers League and more than 45 other state and regional groups to form the Coalition for Consumer Access to Pharmaceutical Care (CCAPC). The coalition has sent representatives to congressional hearings, trade and press briefings, and meetings with groups of legislators to stress the benefits to the health care system that can occur through better use of pharmacists' services and proper management of medications (American Pharmaceutical Association 1993). Ultimately, it is hoped that these efforts will result in further congressional recognition of the value of pharmaceutical care, building on that which was established by OBRA 1990. Pharmacists need to actively participate, both at the public as well as the professional pharmacy association levels, in policy issues impacting their role in the delivery of pharmaceutical care to the public.

Divergent Perspectives on Drug Use

As described above, the wide range of actors involved in the drug use process all have particular interests and perspectives regarding what constitutes the rational use of prescription medications in our society.

For example, patients have a right to expect safe and effective drug therapy when it is indicated, and also have a right to safe and appropriate handling and dispensing of prescribed medicines. Patients do, however, contribute to suboptimal drug therapy outcomes by not getting prescriptions filled, by not getting prescriptions refilled when extended use is indicated, by combining the use of prescription medications with other substances or foods which are contraindicated, by storing medications improperly, and by using medications intended for use by other persons (Manasse 1989b).

From another perspective, physicians have broad cultural, social, and legal authority to prescribe as they see fit for any patient in any context. Professional organizations representing prescribers defend this broad authority through legal and professional means (Manasse 1989b).

Providers of "alternative" medical therapies also affect the drug use process. For example, homeopaths, herbalists, and advocates of megavitamin therapy or macrobiotic diets are gaining popularity in the United States; it has been estimated that approximately 10 percent of the U.S. population used one of these forms of alternative medical therapy in 1990 (Wood and Zhou, 1991). This statistic has implications for pharmacists relating to the role of "traditional" prescription drugs vis-a-vis these medicines, herbs, vitamins, or foods; the role of the pharmacist vis-a-vis alternative medical providers; and the effects of increasing utilization of different types and numbers of providers on the health care delivery system.

Pharmaceutical manufacturers have a somewhat different orientation. As Manasse notes:

> Although an inherent "social good" undergirds the reason for being in pharmaceutical manufacturing, the industry exists mainly as a business and behaves, for the most part, as a business. The ultimate aim of the industry, therefore, rests on minimal regulation and oversight, highest sales, highest profitability, highest return on investment, and shortest delay in recovering investment expenses (Manasse 1989b).

Pharmaceutical manufacturers are affected by the policies and actions of health professionals. Thus, it is in the manufacturers' best interests to involve themselves in profesional policy development (e.g., therapeutic interchange, prescribing privileges). Drug manufacturers have lobbied extensively at the state and federal levels to inhibit certain professional practices or regulatory mandates that impinge upon their market definitions (Victor 1987).

The distribution of prescription drugs takes place in a number of ways. Most commonly, community pharmacies, hospitals, ambulatory care centers, correctional facilities, military installations, home health care agencies, and nursing homes are the source of prescribed medicines for patients. Other outlets for prescription drugs include mail order pharmacies and dispensing physicians. Each of these distributors has an interest in retaining and expanding market share, creating debates over the most appropriate channels for distributing prescribed drugs to the U.S. population. Similar debates take place over the control of over-the-counter (OTC) medicines, or those drugs which have the potential for switching from prescription to OTC status. In most cases, such debates are settled by the political interaction of lobbyists, scientists, regulators, and policy makers.

Finally, third-party payers have an interest in minimizing expenditures and maximizing the health status of their subscriber populations. As a result, many third-party payers incorporate the concepts of cost-sharing (deductibles, copayments, etc.) into their prescription drug benefit plans, along with an array of more complex administrative mechanisms such as generic or therapeutic interchange, drug utilization review, and the use of drug formularies.

Convergent Perspectives on Drug Use

Despite the number of interested actors and the differences in their perspectives on the drug use process, there exists a growing body of support from a variety of sources for an increased role for pharmacists in preventing drug misadventures:

- The U.S. Office of the Inspector General (OIG) has concluded that clinical pharmacy services add value to patient care and reduce health care utilization costs (Office of the Inspector General 1990b). The OIG recommended that the Health Care Financing Administration (HCFA) facilitate the process of providing pharmaceutical care.

- The Public Health Service's *Healthy People 2000* objectives endorse the role of pharmacotherapy in primary and secondary prevention of disease (i.e., primary prevention via vaccination, and secondary prevention via management of chronic conditions) (Public Health Service 1990). The Public Health Service further recommended that, by the year 2000, 75 percent of pharmacies establish linked systems to provide drug reaction or interaction alerts for medications dispensed from different sources.

- Food and Drug Administration Commissioner David Kessler has stated that the primary responsibility for the proper use of drugs lies with physicians and pharmacists (Kessler 1991).

- The Joint Commission on the Accreditation of Healthcare Organizations (JCAHO) has incorporated the concept of pharmaceutical care into its hospital and home care pharmacy standards, thus recognizing the value of pharmacists in the provision of quality health care (Joint Commission 1991a; Joint Commission 1991b).

- Third-party payers have begun to notice the value of pharmacists in achieving cost-containment objectives, thus providing economic justification for the expansion of pharmaceutical care in managed care settings (Myers 1987).

- The National Consumers League has joined with a number of professional pharmacy associations to form the Consumer Coalition for Access to Pharmaceutical Care, whose function is to lobby Congress in the area of health care reform (see previous sections).

These examples are only a fraction of the growing base of evidence that the concept of pharmaceutical care is receiving support from providers, consumers, regulators, and payers across the United States.

Pharmaceutical Care: A Model to Optimize the Drug Use Process

We believe that, as a result of a myriad of forces and actors impacting the drug use process, there exists no single professional group or strategy sufficient for the optimization of the drug use process. As a result, patient care is often influenced by competing interests. These intrests disagree about what constitutes optimal drug therapy and who should be in control, thus increasing the risk of drug misadventuring.

We further contend that there is a significant degree of agreement from a wide variety of sources that pharmacy practitioners, adopting the care model for delivering pharmaceutical services, are in a unique position to help their public realize optimal drug therapy by turning challenges and obstacles into opportunities. Pharmacists should assume the lead role in guiding the drug use process in the positive direction, that is, towards a coordinated, multidisciplinary drug use system aimed at achieving optimal drug therapy for the public.

References

American Association of Colleges of Pharmacy. 1975. *Pharmacists for the Future. The Report of the Study Commission on Pharmacy*. Ann Arbor: Health Administration Press.

American Pharmaceutical Association. 1993. Coalition Promotes Pharmaceutical Care. *American Pharmacy* NS33 (9):73–4.

Avorn, J., and S. B. Soumerai. 1983. Improving Drug-therapy Decisions Through Educational Outreach: A Randomized Controlled Trial of Academically Based "Detailing." *New England Journal of Medicine* 308:1457–63.

Barker, K. N., et al. 1984. Consultant Evaluation of a Hospital Medication System: Analysis of the Existing System. *American Journal of Hospital Pharmacy* 41:2008–16.

Barker, K. N., and W. E. McConnnell. 1962. The Problems of Detecting Medication Errors in Hospitals. *American Journal of Hospital Pharmacy* 19:360–9.

Baum, C., et al. 1985. Drug Use and Expenditures in 1982. *JAMA* 253:382–6.

Black, H. J. 1984. Unit Dose Drug Distribution: A 20-year Perspective. *American Journal of Hospital Pharmacy* 41:2086–8.

Brink, C. J. 1986. Reading with a Critical Eye (editorial). *American Journal of Hospital Pharmacy* 43:1697.

Brodie, D. C. 1967. Drug-Use Control: Keystone to Pharmaceutical Service. *Drug Intelligence in Clinical Pharmacy* 1:63–5.

Brodie, D. C., W. F. McGhan, and J. Lindon. 1991. The Theoretical Base of Pharmacy. *American Journal of Hospital Pharmacy* 48:536–40.

Brushwood, D. B., C. A. Catizone, and J. M. Coster. 1992. OBRA 90: What It Means to Your Practice. *U.S. Pharmacist* 17 (10):47–52.

Burkle, W. S., and C. J. Gwizdala. 1981. Evaluation of "Toxic" Serum Theophylline Concentrations. *American Journal of Hospital Pharmacy* 38:1164–6.

Burns, J., and C. E. Cordero. 1991. *Business & Health Special Report: Managed Care Comes to Prescription Drugs.* Montvale, NJ: Medical Economics Publishing.

Chenella, F. C., et al. 1983. Comparison of Physician and Pharmacist Management of Anticoagulant Therapy of In-patients. *American Journal of Hospital Pharmacy* 40:1642–5.

Davis, N. M., and M. R. Cohen. 1981. *Medication Errors: Causes and Prevention.* Philadelphia: George F. Stickley.

Elenbaas, R. M. 1986. When to Monitor Blood Drug Levels. *Hospital Therapeutics* (July):27–37.

Fuchs, V. R. 1975. *Who Shall Live? Health, Economics, and Social Choice.* New York: Basic Books.

Garnett, W. R. 1983. Adverse Drug Reactions: Detection, Assessment, Reporting, and Prevention. In *Basic Skills in Clinical Pharmacy Practice*, ed. M. D. Ray, 209–49. Chapel Hill, NC: Universal Printing and Publishing.

Guernsey, B. G., et al. 1984. A Utilization Review of Theophylline Assays: Sampling Patterns and Use. *Drug Intelligence in Clinical Pharmacy* 18:906–12.

Hall, D. H. 1990. Pathophysiology of Hypertension in Blacks. *American Journal Hypertension* 3:366S–371S.

Hatoum, H. T. 1990. Megatrends a la Pharmacy: Potential and Promise. *Hospital Pharmacy* 25:825–8, 36.

Hatoum, H. T. 1991. The Social and Economic Impact of Inappropriate Drug Therapy. Paper read at 3rd Annual Focus on Illinois Clinicians Conference: Pharmaceutical Care as an Issue of Public Policy, 1 October 1991, Chicago, Illinois.

Hatoum, H. T., and K. Akhras. 1993. 1993 Bibliography: A 32-year Literature Review on the Value and Acceptance of Ambulatory Care Provided by Pharmacists. *Annals of Pharmacotherapy* 27:1106–19.

Hatoum, H. T., R. A. Hutchinson, and B. L. Lambert. 1993. OBRA 90: Patient Counseling—Enhancing Patient Outcomes. *U.S. Pharmacist* 18 (1):38–45.

Hutchinson, R. A., R. K. Lewis, and H. T. Hatoum. 1990. Inconsistencies in the Drug Use Process. *DICP Annals of Pharmacotherapy* 24:633–6.

Hutchinson, R. A., and K. Witte. 1983. How to Get Started—Planning Clinical Pharmacy Services. In *Basic Skills in Clinical Pharmacy Practice*, ed. M. D. Ray, 21–46. Chapel Hill, NC: Universal Printing and Publishing.

Joint Commission on Accreditation of Healthcare Organizations. 1991a. *1991 Accreditation Manual for Hospitals*. Chicago: JCAHO Publications.

Joint Commission on Accreditation of Healthcare Organizations. 1991b. *1991 Accreditation Manual for Home Care*. Chicago: JCAHO Publications.

Jozefczyk, K. G., P. J. Schneider, and D. S. Pathak. 1986. Medication Errors in a Pharmacy-coordinated Drug Administration Program. *American Journal of Hospital Pharmacy* 43:2464–7.

Kalow, W. 1982. Ethnic differences in Drug Metabolism. *Clinical Pharmacokinetics* 7:374–400.

Kessler, D. A. 1991. Communicating with Patients about Their Medications. *New England Journal of Medicine* 325:1650–2.

Kimelblatt, et al. 1982. Use Review of Cimetidine Injection. *American Journal of Hospital Pharmacy* 39:311.

Kirking, D. M. 1986. Drug Utilization Review: A Component of Drug Quality Assurance. In *Final Report of the APhA Pharmacy Commission on Third Party Programs*. American Pharmaceutical Association, 81–91. Washington, D.C.

Klein, T. 1983. Detailing and Other Forms of Promotion. In *Principles of Pharmaceutical Marketing*. 3rd ed., ed. M. C. Smith, 400–17. Philadelphia: Lea & Febiger.

Knapp, D. A., et al. 1974. Development and Application of Criteria in Drug Use Review Programs. *American Journal of Hospital Pharmacy* 31:648–56.

Koch, H. 1982. Drug Utilization in Office-based Practice: A Summary of Findings. *National Ambulatory Medical Care Survey; National Health Survey Series* 13 (65):1–9. Hyatsville, MD: National Center for Health Statistics.

Koren, G., Z. Barzilay, and M. Greenwald. 1986. Tenfold Errors in Administration of Drug Doses: A Neglected Iatrogenic Disease in Pediatrics. *Pediatrics* 77:848–9.

Levy, Richard A. 1993. *Ethnic & Racial Differences in Response to Medicines*. Reston, VA: National Pharmaceutical Council.

Lewis, K. P., J. W. Cooper, and P. L. McKercher. 1976. Pharmacists' Effect on Digoxin Use and Toxicity. *American Journal of Hospital Pharmacy* 33:1272–6.

Lobas, N. H., P. W., Lepinski, and P. W. Abramowitz. 1992. Effects of Pharmaceutical Care on Medication Cost and Quality of Patient Care in an Ambulatory-care Clinic. *American Journal of Hospital Pharmacy* 49:1681–8.

Manasse, H. R. 1989a. Medication Use in an Imperfect World: Drug Misadventuring as an Issue of Public Policy, Part I. *American Journal of Hospital Pharmacy* 46:929–44.

Manasse, H. R. 1989b. Medication Use in an Imperfect World: Drug Misadventuring as an Issue of Public Policy, Part II. *American Journal of Hospital Pharmacy* 46:1141–52.

Manning, P. R., et al. 1986. Changing Prescribing Practices Through Individual Continuing Education. *JAMA* 256:230–2.

McGhan, W. F. 1993. Pharmacoeconomics and the Evaluation of Drugs and Services. *Hospital Formulary* 28:365–78.

Meyer, B. R. 1988. Improving Medical Education in Therapeutics. Health and Public Policy Committee, American College of Physicians. *Annals of Internal Medicine* 108:145–7.

Miller, W. 1983. Functional Elements of Clinical Pharmacy Practice. In *Basic Skills in Clinical Pharmacy Practice*, ed. M. D. Ray, 1–20. Chapel Hill, NC: Universal Printing and Publishing.

Mrtek, R. G. 1982. 1940 to 1960: The Rise of Commercialism. *Drug Topics* 126 (8):112–4.

Myers, M. J. 1987. Thirty-party Programs. In *Effective Pharmacy Management*. 4th ed. Kansas City, MO: Marion Labs.

Naisbitt, John. 1982. *Megatrends: Ten New Directions Transforming Our Lives*. New York: Warner Books.

Nichols, B. 1981. Standardized Education for Nursing. *American Journal of Hospital Pharmacy* 38:1455–8.

Office of the Inspector General. 1990a. *Medication Regimens: Causes of Noncompliance*. Washington, DC: U.S. Department of Health and Human Services, Publication OAI–04–89–89121.

Office of the Inspector General. 1990b. *The Clinical Role of the Community Pharmacist*. Washington, DC: U.S. Department of Health and Human Services, Publication OAI–01–89–89020.

Penna, R. P. 1991. Creating Our Futures. Paper read at Indiana Pharmacy Consensus-Building Conference, 31 May 1991 Indianapolis, Indiana.

Perlstein, P. H., et al. 1979. Errors in Drug Computation During Newborn Intensive Care. *American Journal Diseases in Childhood* 133:376–9.

Public Health Service. 1979. *Healthy People: Surgeon General's Report on Health Promotion and Disease Prevention*. Washington, DC: U.S. Department of Health and Human Services.

Public Health Service. 1990. *Healthy People 2000: National Health Promotion and Disease Prevention Objectives*. Washington, DC: U.S. Department of Health and Human Services.

Relman, A. S. 1981. Journals. In *Coping With the Biomedical Literature: A Primer for the Scientist and the Clinician*, ed. K. S. Warren, 67–78. New York: Praeger Publications.

Relman, A. S. 1988. Assessment and Accountability: The Third Revolution in Medical Care. *New England Journal of Medicine* 319 (18):1220–2.

Reutzel, T. J., et al. 1993. Inner-city Pharmacies: Can They Meet the OBRA '90 Mandates? *American Pharmacy* NS33 (5):44–51.

Rucker, T. D. 1989. Pursuing Rational Drug Therapy: A Macro View a la the USA. *Journal of Social Administrative Pharmacology* 5 (3/4):78–86.

Rucker, T. D. 1992. National Health Ensurance: The Lesson of Baseball, Diapers, and Pecan Parlors. *Journal of Clinical Computing* 20 (5&6):176–97.

Saunders, E. 1988. Drug Treatment Considerations for the Hypertensive Black Patient. *Journal of Family Practice* 26 (6):659–64.

Schloemer, J. H., and J. J. Zagozen, 1984. Cost Analysis of an Aminoglycoside Pharmacokinetic Dosing Program. *American Journal of Hospital Pharmacy* 41:2347–51.

Smith, M. C. 1977. Drug Product Advertising and Prescribing: A Review of the Evidence. *American Journal of Hospital Pharmacy* 34:1208–24.

Smith, M., et al. 1987. Aminoglycoside Monitoring: Use of Pharmacokinetic Service Versus Physician Recommendations. *Hospital Formulary* 22:92–102.

Spencer, G. 1989. Projections of the Population of the United States, by Age, Sex, and Race: 1988 to 2080. *Current Population Reports, Population Estimates and Projections*. Series P-25, No. 1018. Washington, DC: U.S. Department of Commerce, Bureau of the Census.

Spino, M., E. M. Sellers, and H. L. Kaplan. 1978. Effect of Adverse Drug Reactions on the Length of Hospitalization. *American Journal of Hospital Pharmacy* 35:1060–4.

Strand, L. M., et al. 1990. Drug-related Problems: Their Structure and Function. *DICP Annals of Pharmacotherapy* 24:1093–7.

Task Force on Prescription Drugs. 1969. *Final Report*. Washington, DC: U.S. Department of Health, Education, and Welfare.

Valuck, R. J. 1992. Macro-level Screening Criteria to Identify Suboptimal Prescribers of Controlled Substances. Master's thesis, University of Illinois at Chicago.

Victor, K. 1987. New Kids on the Block. *National Journal* (Oct 31): 2726–30.

Winter, M. E., E. T. Herfindal, and L. R. Bernstein. 1986. Impact of Decentralized Pharmacokinetics Consultation Service. *Hospital Physician* 43:2178–84.

Wood, A. J. J., H. H. and Zhou. 1991. Ethnic Differences in Drug Disposition and Responsiveness. *Clinical Pharmacokinetics* 20:350–73.

World Health Organization. 1975. *Requirements for Adverse Reaction Reporting*. Geneva: WHO Publications.

5

The Process of Change in Pharmacy
Donald O. Fedder, Dr. P.H., M.P.H.

I hear and I forget,
I see and I remember
I do and I understand
Confucius

Introduction: Concepts of Change

Change has been defined as:

> to make different the form, content, future course—of something, to become
> transformed or converted, and to pass gradually (. . into) as from summer into
> autumn, from youth to adulthood, from student to practitioner (Random House
> College Dictionary 1980)

From Ecclesiastes we learn, "there is no new thing under the sun (Eccles. 1:9)"
and from others that even when we think there is change, little really does change
(Plus ça change, plus c'est le même chose (Karr 1849)) Yet each of us in our
own lives recognizes changes that occur both in ourselves and around us. One
of the objectives of this book is to encourage change in the practice of pharmacy.
In order to achieve this objective we must consider the concept of change as a
constant and then consider the energy needed to overcome resistance to change.
Certainly, practitioners have a need to understand the management of change in
their patients, in their colleagues, and in themselves.

Seasons change, people change, conditions change and we all learn to accommodate to these in some manner. Some changes are beyond individual control
and seem to be spontaneous. Thus clothes styles, cultural norms, sexual conduct
change over time apparently with little direction or predictability. Invention and
discovery (e.g., the airplane, automobile, computers, atomic energy and space
exploration) have led to revolutionary changes with broad cultural implications.
Large segments of society havev redefined "acceptable behavior" to include
couples living together and having children without the benefit of marriage; the
use of language that to some is considered "filthy"; and the acceptance of persons
in communities and work places regardless of race or gender. Many of these

changes seem to have occurred almost randomly, and in many cases there appears to have been little organized societal effort to control or manage the change. In health care, discovery and invention have, over time, led to major changes. These changes present opportunities to manage the profession for the benefit of society, and to improve everyone's quality of life.

Many changes are directly attributable to human behavior, such as smoking and other addictive pursuits, sedentary lifestyle, and violence. Causes of change that are not directly ascribable to human behavior include public policies, poverty rates, and access to health care. Consideration of change must include consideration of the nature of change and analysis of the goal in managing change. As we attempt to define change, we should consider the futurists, who attempt to predict change by examining past history, analyzing trends, and interpreting social needs. We should also consider chaos theorists, who believe that change is not predictable but random.

In any event, change is going on all around us and, in some cases, it would behoove us to intervene to create change. Thus, the focus of this chapter is on determining the need for and the management of change, especially as it relates to the delivery of pharmaceutical care.

Professional Practice

Social scientists define professions as "occupations with special power and prestige granted by society because professions have special competence in esoteric bodies of knowledge linked to central needs and values of the social system, and because professions are devoted to the service of the public, above and beyond material matters (Larson 1977)."

Perspective will affect interpretation of this definition. Three groups, each with a different perspective, interpret this definition with respect to pharmacy: the practitioners who provide services and who generally define the profession, the patients (clients) who are the recipients of services, and society as a whole, which provides the authority and often the resources for the practice. Many practitioners believe that by dint of their education and training, only they have the capacity to make decisions about the profession and their clients. Recipients may agree in principle but are increasingly concerned that their interests are overridden when in conflict with those of the professional. While professionals often feel that they systematically process knowledge in a rational, scientific manner, and that decisions are as free of error as possible, recipients of those services expect near-perfection and tend to tolerate only zero error. Society has similar expectations with regard to error-free practice and further expects an extraordinarily high degree of altruism and good faith from all parties to assure high-quality, low-cost care. The system's imperfections may prove to be the driving force for change in the delivery of health care.

Modes of Behavior

Peter Temin, Professor of Economics at Massachusetts Institute of Technology, described professional behavior in terms of "three distinct 'modes' or ideal types without implying that anyone follows any single mode all the time." He characterized these as "instrumental, customary, and command behaviors (Temin 1980)."

The first mode of behavior, *instrumental* or *rational*, is behavior based on logic, reason and/or science. In economic terms, this is marketplace behavior, in which one is ceaselessly striving to attain profit-maximization. In the context of outcome orientation, "profit" may be interpreted as a predictable therapeutic outcome. This behavior mode connotes consistent behavior "indicating it does not lead to internal contradiction." Those familiar with the Drug Use Evaluation (DUE) literature will understand why Temin speaks of physician prescribing as customary rather than instrumental behavior.

The second mode of behavior, *Customary* or *traditional*, is behavior that continues that which "was done yesterday . . . more or less." Patterns of behavior may be set in training, as in an apprenticeship or mentoring situation. Temin adds "more or less" because behaviors do change, sometimes because of lack of institutional memory or simply by modification—but the changes are consistent with the prior learned behavior. While physician prescribing is best described as customary behavior (i.e., learned and continued based upon a preceptor-student model), organizational behavior is a true representation of customary behavior. Most professionals probably consider their behavior to be rational or instrumental.

The third behavior mode, *Command*, is seen in situations in which one person can order another to perform an action (or not perform an action) with the connotation that a penalty may be imposed for non-compliance. Patient education (i.e., the transmitting of the therapy regimen) is frequently "command behavior," although better results may be achieved by negotiating and contracting with the patient.

The reader should understand that the value of this behavioral topology is not to categorize people (i.e., to label them or put them in boxes) but rather to learn to recognize and understand behaviors that need to be either reinforced or changed. This need to reinforce or change behavior leads us to the next step in our analysis.

The Study and Process of Change

As indicated, change can be either planned or spontaneous. Historians, futurists, and a wide array of social scientists, each with different perspectives and methods for study, all examine unplanned change. For example, a historian records and studies past events and attempts to explain how, when, and why they occurred. We have all heard the sage advice that those who do not study history are condemned to repeat it. Futurists use many strategies to predict the future based on past experiences and trends, and the study of theory. Others use different methods to understand phenomena and perhaps to manage them.

Diffusion

The dissemination of new ideas to a population of interest has been termed the "diffusion of innovation." Everett M. Rogers, who published the seminal texts on diffusion research, defines diffusion as a "process by which an innovation is communicated through certain channels over time among members of a social system (Rogers)." He goes on to describe the innovation-*decision* process, in which "an individual . . . passes from first knowledge . . . , to forming an attitude toward the innovation, to a decision to adopt or reject, to implementation . . . , and to confirmation of this decision (Rogers)." These definitions make clear the concept that communication requires mutual understanding by the communicants, NOT just the transfer of knowledge or information. Only proper communication results in a decision to adopt or reject the new idea.

Rogers and his colleagues identified nine academic disciplines ("research traditions") and listed their major contributions to research. The earliest were the anthropologists, who gathered data from populations often by "participant observation (Rogers, 48)." Although one can garner remarkable insights this way, there are problems of generalizability and time that make this method impractical for the study of many problems. However, as change agents anthropologists have been quite successful in the promotion of a new idea within a society or system (Rogers). They have also provided insights into the consequences of innovations.

Major contributions were also made by rural sociologists, whose early work involved promoting the use of hybrid seed, insecticides, and fertilizers. This work led to the development of the agricultural extension services. Rural sociologists elaborated on the S-shaped adopter distribution curve[1] and made observations of characteristics of the adopters at various stages along this curve, the perceived attributes of innovations, communication channels, and the characteristics of the opinion leaders.

Public health and medical sociologists examined the adoption of such things as pharmaceuticals, vaccinations, and family planning methods. The classic studies in this area were conducted by Columbia University sociologists Elihu Katz, Herbert Menzel, and James Coleman, and were funded in part by a grant from Charles Pfizer and Company in the late 1950s. Their work demonstrated

---

[1]Curve that occurs when number or percentage of adopters is plotted on the ordinate (Y axis) and time is plotted on the abscissa (X axis).

the importance of interpersonal networks of adopters and the important role of opinion leaders in the dissemination of information and the adoption of the product. Although they were entirely ignorant of the prior hybrid corn studies, they were able to add a dimension to these studies. By reviewing pharmacy prescription files to determine who prescribed the specified drug by when, Katz, Menzel, and Coleman gained an objective measure of adoption. Prior studies depended a great deal on recall information, a much more problematic outcome measure.

Other disciplines that contributed to research were marketing, communication, and even geography. Geographers examined diffusion, particularly of technological innovations, and added to their studies the spatial dimension (i.e., the distances between innovator and adopter), that needs to be considered by the change agent. Interestingly, with the proliferation of new ideas, technologies, and products, the time between innovation and adoption has been compressed in many instances. However, time compression is not automatic and cannot be assumed when the change advocated requires significant behavioral change.

Diffusion research has focused on eight broad areas:

1. Earliest awareness of innovation
2. Rate of adoption of different innovations within a social system
3. Characteristics of innovation
4. Characteristics of opinion leaders
5. Interactions of communicants within in diffusion networks
6. Rates of adoption in different social systems
7. Communication channel usage
8. Consequences of innovation

Diffusing innovations has been shown to be a robust method for implementing change. However, the mere transfer of information—for example, the describing the benefit of a recommended behavior—does not automatically translate into adoption of the change by the target population. Returning to Rogers definition, communication between innovator and adopter must result in mutual understanding followed by an adoption or rejection *decision*.

The Innovation-Decision Process

In the innovation-decision process, one initially becomes aware of a new idea or concept and may develop an interest in or an attitude about it. One may then decide to adopt or reject the idea or concept. If the result is positive, implementation and then confirmation occur. This is not an instantaneous process, and the adoption is not necessarily permanent. (See Figure 5-1.) An advocate for change (that is, the change agent) should consider attributes of the target population, the characteristics of the decision-making unit, and the *perceived* characteristics of the innovation when choosing the methods (channels) for communication. For example, early in the adoption curve, one would seek out the opinion leaders, as chances are good they can persuade their colleagues of the need for or usefulness of the innovation. Adoption and endorsements by opinion leaders provide credibility that may be capitalized on by the change agent (e.g., to promote the concept of pharmaceutical care). Late in the process, one would single out those who had not adopted the innovation. Between these two extremes, the majority is the target. One can analyze the pace of adoption by estimating the number of people in the target population and determining the percentage who have adopted the innovation at various points in time. Such analyses have determined that there is a normal distribution of adopters over time that can be plotted. (See Figs. 5-2 and 5-3.)

Note that the curves in Figures 5-2 and 5-3 represent the same data. The S curve in Figure 5-2 represents the cumulative percentage of the population that has adopted the innovention over time, while the normal curve in Figure 5-3 shows the percentage that adopted the innovention in each time segment. The labels in Figure 5-3 refer to the characteristics of the adopters, based on research. So, if we determine that only 16 percent have adopted the procedure, the communication channels need to be broad (e.g., multi-media, community or system wide). If only 16 percent have NOT adopted (i.e., the hard to reach or "laggards"), strategies must be quite selective and well-targeted.

Planned Change: The Scope of Health Promotion and Health Education

Before discussing the process of planned change, a few definitions are in order to explain the context of the change process. The key concepts requiring definition are *health promotion, lifestyle,* and *health education. Health promotion* is defined as "the combination of educational and environmental supports for actions and conditions of living conducive for health" (Green 1991). Environmental supports are all approaches to improving health other than education. Environmental supports may include social, political, economic, organizational (including community activism), legal, and regulatory efforts. Conditions of living include all conditions subsumed in the term "lifestyle," not just those related to health.[2] *Lifestyle* connotes patterns of behavior chosen by an individual that have an impact on the individual's health, even if the individual is unaware of the impact. Patterns of behavior, which generally develop from decisions an individual makes over time, are "a composite expression of the special and cultural circumstances

---

[2]Examples include "housing, eating, playing, working, and just plain loafing." (Temin, 1980).

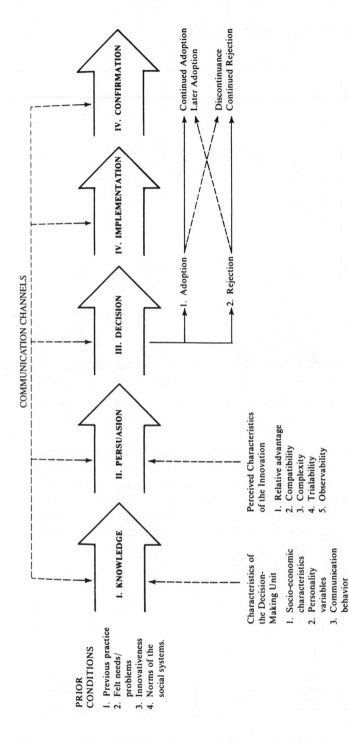

Figure 5.1. A model of stages in the innovation-decision process.

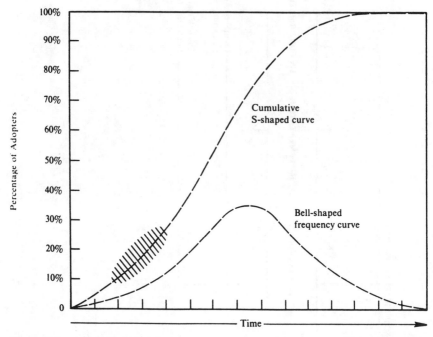

Figure 5.2. The bell-shaped frequency curve and the s-shaped cumulative curve for an adopter distribution.

that condition and constrain" the person (Green, 1991, p.3). Conditions of living expand the lifestyle construct to include "the more complex web of culture, norms, and (the) socio-economic environment". (Green, p.17).

As discussed, many disciplines are involved in planned change, and the changes advocated by clinical and public health practitioners are quite relevant to the practice of pharmacy. In the discussion of diffusion, we spoke of the role of

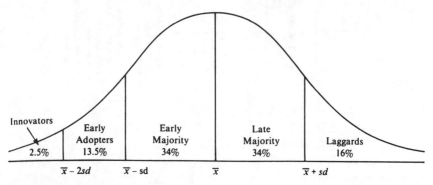

Figure 5.3. Adopter categorization on the basis of innovativeness.

communication in creating an awareness of and interest in the innovation. This process, when characterized as health education, connotes that the subject has received some information (i.e., that knowledge has been transferred from the educator (sender) to the recipient (receiver)) and that the subject has processed or internalized the information for some purpose. The point is that it is not sufficient for the subject to just know something. The preferred result would be an action, and it would help if there was either empirical or theoretical support for predicting the outcome.

Health education is the field of endeavor that uses education to achieve a behavioral change that will result in a health benefit. Steuart explains, "The essence of health education is its scientific concern with the role of human behavior, individual, and societal, in the natural history of health and disease . . . with an operational focus on those planned influence-attempts directed toward maintenance, reinforcement, or modification of behavior in the extent to which this may demonstrably affect curative, rehabilitative and disease preventive processes, and the promotion of health (Steuart 1993)."

Although many disciplines overlap with health education, the essential concept in the definition is an identified relationship (or link) between the educational strategy and the outcome. The field is eclectic in that it draws from many disciplines, and the expectation is that a "behavioral analysis" or assessment precedes any action taken. This analysis revolves around identifying behaviors that contribute in any way to the problem of concern and prioritizing the effects of the behaviors on that problem. One might compare this analysis to a physical assessment of a patient.

Performing this analysis certainly sounds intuitive, but consider the way in which traditional or customary behavior occurs. The reader may find the following example familiar. A patient presents with a set of risk factors including Stage I HBP (152/96 mm Hg), elevated cholesterol (TC 234 mg/dL), and body weight 30 percent above ideal. Past experience may suggest placing the patient on both antihypertensive and cholesterol lowering drugs since patients don't respond well to dietary restrictions. Also, since weight reduction is so difficult, the practitioner may omit a suggestion to lose weight so that the patient will not be confronted with another failure.

Health education concepts suggest other strategies. Since behavioral changes will predictably provide long term benefits, and since even when drug therapy is indicated, behavioral changes are necessary, the practitioner should, when possible, add a behavioral prescription to the drug therapy recommendation. This combination may effect a change that maximizes the effectiveness of the drug therapy while minimizing risks. Although there are professional health educators, some complete with certification, the premise of this chapter is that ALL practitioners, especially pharmacists, need to understand and utilize health education and promotion strategies with patients, their families, and the community to improve the management of disease, prevent the development or exacerbation of disease, and, importantly, to improve the lifestyle of patients and their families. This premise contrasts what Steuart called "the insidious tendency to slant professional (health education) preparation in the direction of those aspects . . . more relevant to . . . preventive and promotive programs with large populations than to curative and rehabilitative programs for smaller groups with special needs (Steuart 1965)."

Health education gave rise to health promotion because of the need to enhance health rather than just prevent disease and also because of the recognition of the need to develop "structural measures" of support (Kickbush 1986). Thus, health promotion targets both the behavioral and environmental determinants of health by combining educational, political, regulatory, and organizational strategies to achieve changes that contribute to the health of the community (Green and Ruchard 1993).

Analyses for Change: The PRECEDE—PROCEED Framework

Although there are many models of health behavior, the PRECEDE-PROCEED model, which was "founded on the disciplines of epidemiology; the social, behavioral, and educational sciences; and health administration," is both strongly grounded in theory and utilitarian in application (Green and Kreuter 1991). A major strength of this model is that its analytical process begins at the top, with the impact of the problem on quality of life or human values (i.e., the analysis begins at the end). In the PRECEDE phase, problems are sorted into behavioral and environmental groups, and factors are classified based or whether they predispose, reinforce, or enable the behavior in question. This organization of the determinants of behaviors is iterative and orders the determinants by importance and feasibility. This PRECEDE phase drives the PROCEED phases (the action or intervention stages) of the model to maintain the link between specific behavioral factors and the health and quality of life issues of interest to the analyst. Therefore, this model increases the likelihood that the advocated behavioral and/ or environmental changes will result in improvement of the identified problems.

The utility of this comprehensive planning process is that it avoids many of the false starts and blind alleys that are common when issues are addressed by trial and error. Designing a program based on the specifics identified in the analyses is much more effective than addressing issues haphazardly. Thus, planners may withhold the urge to set up lectures or seminars, delay the production of another pamphlet, or avoid victim blaming, when the issue may be, for example, accessibility of clinics or availability of transportation.

Green et al. have enumerated five phases in the PRECEDE analysis and three phases in the PROCEED interventions. (See Figure 5-4.) Phase one is a *social* diagnosis, preferably performed in conjunction with representatives of the community at risk, to identify social indicators of quality of life. Phase two examines

PRECEDE

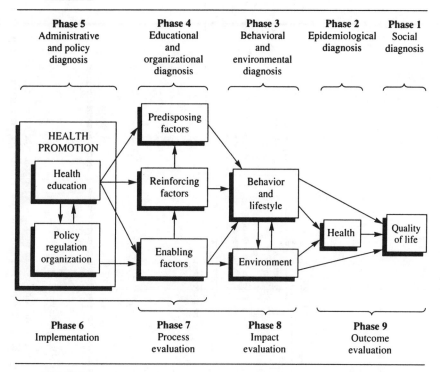

Figure 5.4. The PRECEDE–PROCEED model for health promotion planning and evaluation.

the indicators and dimensions of health by the application of *epidemiological* methods. Phase three then separates the correlates of health into their *behavioral* and *environmental* components. In Phase four, *educational* and *organizational* analyses elicit a set of factors that predispose, reinforce, or enable the identified behaviors or that have an environmental component. *Predisposing factors* are those factors attributed to the individual (i.e., the patient); *reinforcing factors* are those factors attributed to others that either reinforce or discourage the individual's behaviors; and *enabling factors* are those factors external to the individual and his support system. Enabling factors include skills, resources, or barriers that may help or hinder the specified behavior. Phase five is an administrative and policy diagnosis, which uses information gathered in phase four to design of an implementation program. Phases six through nine involve initiation of the implementation program, followed by process, impact and outcome evaluations.

Figure 5.5 is an example of a completed PRECEDE-PROCEED analysis that resulted in a health promotion intervention for an elementary school. The analysis

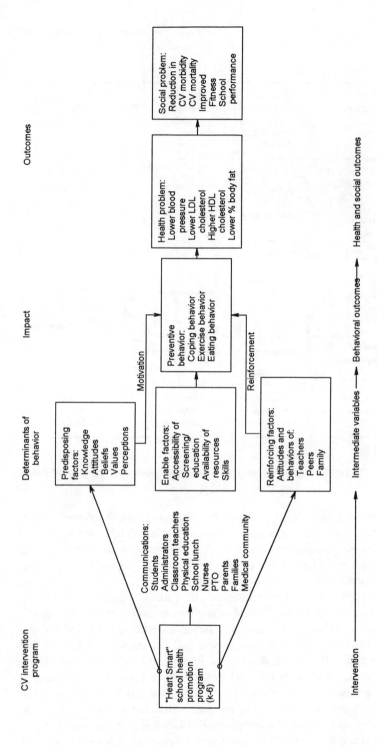

Figure 5.5. Application of the PRECEDE model in a cardiovascular health promotion program for school-age children. [From A. M. Downey, G. C. Frank, L. S. Webber, et al., *Journal of School Health* 57 (1987): 98–104; Printed by permission of the publisher.]

began with the social problems and elicited a series of behaviors that affect that problem. Preventive behaviors were then determined from the literature, and their determinants (factors) were iterated and prioritized. Only then was a program plan developed, tested, and implemented. A typical pharmacy intervention is more likely to deal with patients with chronic disease and would focus on both treatment behaviors (e.g., make a commitment to control the disease, follow the prescribed therapy regimen, keep appointments with physicians) and secondary prevention measures (e.g., coping, exercise, and eating behaviors). For a full discussion of this framework, the reader is referred to Green & Kreuter (1991).

Why Pharmacy?

Patterns of Illness

We have spent much time developing the concepts and analyses of change without addressing the fundamental question of why change is important to the practice of pharmacy and the delivery of pharmaceutical care. Let us step back and examine some changes in the patterns of illness and in the causes of death and disabilities in the U.S. Donald Vickery, in an examination of mortality data in the U.S., divided the 100 year period starting in 1875 into three distinct periods, which he called the Age of Environment, the Age of Medicine, and the Age of Lifestyle. (See Figure 5-6.) The Age of Environment, 1875–1930, was a period in which the U.S. death rate more than halved, largely as a result of public health measures such as immunization, sewer and water purification, the creation of public health departments, improved sanitation, and the development of disinfectants. The Age of Medicine, 1930–1950, saw a further decrease in the death rate as a result of drug and technology development that transformed medical care from symptom control and palliation to cure. The Age of Lifestyle, 1950–1970, began with a slowing of the rate of decrease of the death rate, even though a great number of discoveries and innovations were introduced (e.g., open heart surgery, coronary care units, heart transplants, coronary artery surgery, and innumerable new therapeutic agents). The rate of decrease of the death rate increased again in the early 1970s and has continued almost unabated into the 90s (Vickery 1978). (See Figure 5-6.)

The Centers for Disease Control (CDC) graph (See Figure 5.7) underscores the point that the next major step in lowering our death rate is to change the living conditions of the majority of our population (i.e., to change behaviors that affect health). This step is important because the major causes of mortality in the U.S. today are more amenable to behavioral interventions than to traditional medical interventions. All health practitioners need to understand the importance of this step, if they are to improve the outcomes in their patients. As pharmacists increase their focus on health outcomes, behavioral diagnoses and interventions will increasingly become essential components of pharmaceutical care.

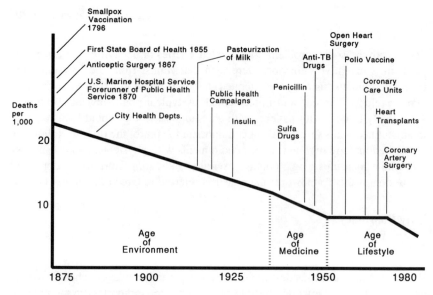

Smallpox
Vaccination
1796

Open Heart
Surgery

First State Board of Health 1855   Pasteurization
                                    of Milk   Anti-TB   Polio Vaccine
Anticeptic Surgery 1867   Drugs

U.S. Marine Hospital Service   Coronary
Forerunner of Public Health   Penicillin   Care Units
Service 1870   Public Health
                      Campaigns

Deaths
per   Heart
1,000   City Health Depts.   Insulin   Transplants
                                                   Sulfa
20   Drugs
                                                             Coronary
                                                             Artery
                                                             Surgery

10

              Age   Age   Age
              of   of   of
              Environment   Medicine   Lifestyle

1875   1900   1925   1950   1980

Adapted From Vickery, Donald M. LifePlan For Your Health,
Addison Wesley Publishing Co., 1978

Figure 5.6. (Source: Vickery, Donald M. LifePlan For Your Health, Addison Wesley Publishing Co., 1978. Reprinted with permission.)

The Patient-Practitioner Behavioral Model

The basis for recommending pharmacists' participation in patient care can be illustrated using the Patient-Practitioner Behavioral Model (See Figure 5.8.) (Fedder 1982, 113–117). The model depicts a patient initiating a visit to a physician, receiving a prescription order, procuring the medication, and taking the medication. The model demonstrates that the patient bears the major responsibility or "burden" in the process. The patient must initiate the physician visit, accept the prescription order and have the order filled, take the medicine according to instructions, renew the prescription, make and keep the follow-up medical appointment, and continue the therapy. Clearly, patients could benefit from a support system that included their physician and pharmacist. Within the traditional Patient-Pharmacist behavior system, there are three opportunities for the pharmacist to provide enhanced patient services each time a prescription is dispensed: upon receipt of the prescription order, when determining its appropriateness, and upon presentation of the prescripted medication to the patient. There are tasks that the pharmacist performs independently, but there are also tasks that require the assistance of others. There are a number of participants (or variables) in the therapeutic equation, only one of which is the pharmacist. The diagnosing of disease and the prescribing of therapy are legally the practice of medicine.[3]

---

[3]This, also, defines the practice of dentistry, osteopathy, and podiatry, but explicitly not pharmacy.

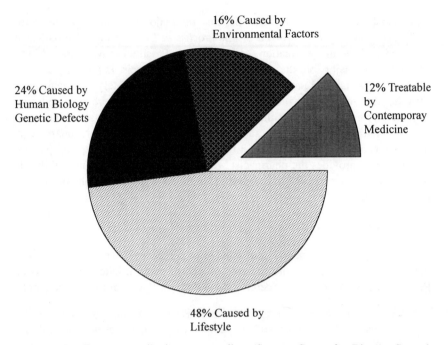

16% Caused by
Environmental Factors

24% Caused by
Human Biology
Genetic Defects

12% Treatable
by
Contemporay
Medicine

48% Caused by
Lifestyle

Figure 5.7. Factors contributing to mortality. (Source: Center for Disease Control, 1979.)

PATIENT–PRACTITIONER BEHAVIOR: AN INTERACTIVE MODEL

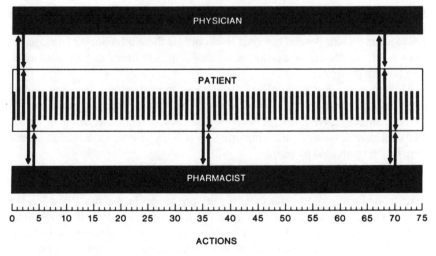

PHYSICIAN

PATIENT

PHARMACIST

0 5 10 15 20 25 30 35 40 45 50 55 60 65 70 75

ACTIONS

Figure 5.8. Patient–practitioner behavioral model.

Pharmacists, especially those who dispense the majority of prescriptions in the U.S., are generally not involved in this process *at its inception*. The patient is a second variable in the equation, and the Patient-Practitioner Behavioral Model illustrates the major role the patient plays. The pharmacist is a third player. If both the physician and patient perform their roles appropriately, the pharmacist **may be able** to assure that results will follow. However, there are conditions beyond pharmacists' control that may limit their capacity to assure outcomes (e.g., the patient may not return, the physician may countermand the pharmacist, the patient may be non-responsive to the drug). The point is that each patient-client contact provides the pharmacist with an opportunity and responsibility to provide service appropriate to the case. That this is a shared responsibility must not be dismissed.

Change: The Mission of Pharmacy and Pharmaceutical Care

In order to place this discussion of change in perspective, we need to examine the mission of pharmacy and the role of pharmaceutical care. The American Pharmaceutical Association recently adopted the following mission statement:

> The mission of pharmacy is to serve society as the profession *responsible for the appropriate use* of medications, devices, and services to achieve optimal therapeutic outcomes.

Pharmaceutical care, as defined by Hepler and Strand and as elaborated over recent years, suggests that the pharmacist has the ability to design, implement, and monitor therapeutic plans that will result in definable outcomes. This process requires the integration of a knowledge base and the use of change strategies that will assist the patient in many ways. Taking medicine, making and keeping appointments, and adjusting diet and exercise patterns are often behaviors essential to achieving the desired outcome. Not only are these behaviors not automatic, but too often patients do not know what specifically needs to be done, much less how to do it.

Therefore, the first principle of patient education should be the provision of explicit directions for drug use and advice regarding any expected manifestation of drug effect (e.g., flushing, increased urinary output, coloration of urine, transient dizziness, or other symptoms). Warnings or contraindications should certainly be provided as well.

Even something as simple as prescription label instructions may be problematic. For example, take the commonly used direction "Tab. i t.i.d." Most pharmacy computer programs translate this to "one tablet three times a day" on the label, but provide no further elaboration. I have often challenged professional audiences, both students and active practitioners, to explicitly state the times of day a dose should be taken based on this direction, and received every possible permutation. Three times a day could mean every 8 hours around the clock, before, with, or after meals, or at 8 AM, 2 PM, and 8 PM, depending upon the drug prescribed and the patient's particular requirements. Yet rarely does someone in the audience ask what drug was prescribed. The point is that a myriad of labels go to patients each day with no further explanation—so how does the patient know when to take the medicine? Obviously, there are many more complex issues that we may assume the patient understands when he does not. The pharmacist should also assess the patient's ability to follow the regimen. Scheduling, opening prescription containers, restrictive diets, and timing of interacting medicines all pose problems for some patients. If it appears that the patient will have difficulty, alternative arrangements may be required. Finally, practitioners need to elicit from the patient an agreement to follow the therapy regimen. Only if these steps have been followed can one begin to consider whether patients are compliant with their regimen.

Pharmacists are not autonomous agents regarding the patient and his or her therapy; the prescriber clearly has a major responsibility. However, there are many roles for pharmacists that rest entirely within their professional domain and require neither permission nor the delegation of prescriptive authority by others to be taken on. These roles include the education, monitoring, counseling, and follow-up of the patient and diagnosing and prescribing non-prescription therapies for primary or self care of clients. The pharmacist remains the most accessible of health professionals, one for whom the public has a great respect and to whom they turn for many of their self-care needs. In the decades before World War Two, that is, before the "Age of Medicine," pharmacists and physicians often found themselves competing for the patient. In a clear effort to diffuse this conflict, a truce was called, which made physicians responsible for diagnosing illnesses and prescribing therapies and pharmacists responsible for dispensing medicines. The passage of the Durham-Humphrey Act reinforced the distinction between those drugs that required prescription from an authorized prescriber and those that did not. With the rapidly increasing numbers of prescription drugs available, many of which have narrow therapeutic indices, pharmacists are positioned and should be expected to help solve problems of patient education and monitoring for unintended events due to drug therapy.

Today, it is clear that the public needs the services of many different professionals if they are to wend their way through the thicket of powerful drugs and devices that are available. Even those items deemed safe when labeled uses are followed can be dangerous when used in combination. Again, shared responsibilities require the intelligent delivery of pharmaceutical care along with other medical care modalities.

Operationalization

This chapter about change would be incomplete without some discussion of how to approach the operationalization of change strategies in a practice. There are a number of skills needed that are NOT subsumed under the rubric of pharmaceutical care. Pharmaceutical care delivery must be economically viable. It should not be surprising that pharmacy school curricula are increasingly including practice management components taught by people trained in business disciplines. Even if their knowledge and skills are limited, pharmacists must develop management strategies for implementation of practice innovations. For example, in the usual high-volume community pharmacy, the dispensing function may take 80 to 90 percent of personnel time. If the pharmacist is so involved in dispensing, how can he or she allocate the time required for in-depth patient education and counseling? Since there are identified patient needs that should be met by pharmacists, pharmacists must plan or redesign their practices to address these needs. Modalities include increased use of well trained technicians, introduction of more technology and robotics, and the use of more unit-of-use packaged products, as well as work-flow analyses and the application of technology to the design of the physical plant (i.e., the pharmacy).

The fiscal implications of any new service need to be assessed and a marketing plan developed (Frederiksen, Solomon, and Brehony 1984). The skills required for this process are not generally resident in the usual accounting firms but must be developed by innovative pharmacists with input from business-discipline trained professionals. Tutorials or business school coursework could be helpful. True change (i.e., large scale implementation of pharmaceutical care) will be inconsistent and ineffectual without a dramatic change in management practices in pharmacies. Facilitating the integration of new services requires the combined wisdom of many. As Allan R. Cohen recently wrote, (O)ne of the dirty little secrets of modern business life is that bosses no longer know answers (Cohen 1993). You may wish to keep this in mind as you go about the process of continually changing your practice. Change may be a constant but it must be managed to be effective.

References

Cohen, A. R. 1993. *The Portable MBA in Management*. New York: John Wiley & Sons.

Fedder, D. O. 1982. Managing Medication and Compliance: Physician, Pharmacist-Patient Interactions. *Journal American Geriatric Society*, 30(11) 113–7.

Frederiksen, L. W., L. J. Solomon, and K. A. Brehony, eds. 1984. *Marketing Health Behavior, Principles, Techniques and Application*. New York: Plenum Press.

L. W. Green, and M. W. Kreuter. 1991. Health Promotion Planning: An Educational and Environmental Approach. Palo Alto, CA: Mayfield Publishing Co.

Green, L. W., and L. Ruchard, 1993. The Need to Combine Health Education and Health Promotion: The Case of Cardiovascular Disease Prevention. *Promotion & Education Quarterly, The International Journal of Health Promotion and Education*, No. 0, Dec. 93, p. 11–7.

Kickbush, I. 1986. World Health Organization, keynote address before Canadian Public Health Association, 1986 as quoted in Green & Kreuter. 1991 Health Promotion Planning: An Educational and Environmental Approach. p. 14. Mayfield Publishing Co.

Larsen, M. S. 1977. *The Rise of Professionalism: a Sociological Analysis*. Berkley and Los Angeles: University of California Press.

The Random House College Dictionary, Revised. 1980. New York: Random House.

Steuart, G. W. 1965. Health Behavior and Planned Change: An Approach to the Professional Preparation of the Health Education Specialist. *Health Education Monographs* 20:3–26.

Temin, P. 1980. *Taking Your Medicine, Drug Regulation in the United States*. Cambridge: 12–7. Cambridge: Harvard University Press.

Vickery, D. M. 1978. *LifePlan for Your Health*. Addison Wesley Publishing Co.

6

Assessment of Health-Related Quality of Life by Health Care Professionals

Kathleen M. Bungay, Pharm.D.
William A. Gouveia, M.S.

Introduction

An important aspect of change, which affects the diffusion of pharmaceutical care, is the simultaneous evaluation and diffusion of quality of life measurements that relate to health. This chapter will introduce the reader to the concept of the quality of life as an essential consideration of all who provide health care.

Traditionally, health has been considered from a medical point of view. Discussions of health have centered on activities associated with repairing injury, alleviating pain, and eliminating illness. As medical science advanced and the conditions under which we live improved, this narrow view of health has become inadequate. Today's health professionals and their patients are faced with decisions that require a broader definition of health, a definition that considers the patient's entire life, not simply the biological manifestations of the chronic or acute condition under treatment. New health-related thinking extends the medical model of care beyond the traditional definition of care by trained health care professionals.

While this more complete view of health has received much attention during the past decade, it is not a new concept. As long ago as 1948, the constitution of the World Health Organization (WHO) defined health as more than freedom from disease; WHO expanded the boundaries of health to include "complete physical, mental, and social well-being (World Health Organization 1948)."

Most contemporary health practitioners and health services researchers have adopted this expanded view of health and now strive to consider the impact a disease and its treatment have on patients' entire lives. The traditional medical approach is still essential. However, patients, payers, and policy makers are increasingly demanding explanations as to how the medical care provided promotes health. These explanations must consist of more than laboratory results, clinical opinions, or diagnoses of diseases. Information about physical and social functioning and mental well-being are also required to answer the questions now being posed.

These "non-clinically" defined components of health are currently the focus of a considerable number of studies. An entire area of research has evolved to capture and evaluate data necessary to provide insights into patient health outcomes. This area of study is known as health-related quality of life and is particularly relevant to pharmacy in the current and future health care environment.

In the new era, information about functional status, well-being, and other important health outcomes will be used by policy analysts and by managers of health care organizations. Policy analysts will compare costs and benefits of competing ways of organizing and financing health care services, and managers of health care organizations will seek to obtain the most value for each health care dollar. The information will also be used by clinician investigators who will evaluate new treatments and technologies and by health care practitioners who will try to achieve the best possible patient outcomes. A primary source of new information on general health outcomes is standardized patient surveys. These tools are currently becoming accepted by clinicians and have been serving health services and social science researchers effectively during the past decade.

Study of health-related quality of life is a specifically focused area of investigation within the larger field of health services research and/or quality of life research. Standardized questionnaires are used to capture health-related quality of life data in a variety of settings, by either self-administration, telephone interview, personal interview, observation, or postal survey. In the jargon of this field of research, these standardized *questionnaires* are often called *instruments, tools, surveys, scales,* or *measures.* These terms are used interchangeably in the literature. *Psychometrics,* the science of designing questionnaires to measure attributes of individuals, is fundamental to the study of health-related quality of life.

While quality of life refers to an evaluation of all aspects of our lives, including such things as where we live, how we live, how we relax, and how we work, health-related quality of life encompasses only those aspects of life that are dominated or significantly influenced by personal health or activities performed to maintain or improve health (Bungay and Ware 1993). Advances in medical science have encouraged this attention to health-related quality of life, because medical care is no longer limited to providing only death- or disease-averting treatments. Today, maintaining or restoring quality of life is an important therapeutic goal for many medical conditions, among them arthritis and diabetes. These conditions having no medical cure, therefore medical treatment is targeted at controlling disease progression and symptoms. Health-related quality of life measures enable the physician to capture appropriate data and thereby monitor disease effects and treatment impacts in terms that are relevant to patients and that reflect the quality of their lives.

Personal Health Services in the U.S.

The first officially recognized dispensing of health services occurred between 1875 and 1930. During this time, hospitals were established mostly by voluntary community boards and church bodies. The church bodies, of course, had a long history of caring for the poor, and this tradition was transformed into the modern hospital. Capital came from the millionaires created by the tremendous industrial development following the Civil War.

Between 1928 and 1933, the first national study of the extent of morbidity and the use of and expenditures for personal health services was conducted. This study was known as the household survey. In 1946, hospitals began to collect data on expenditures for health services and the census bureau served as a source for mortality information. The prevailing assumption was that there was a relationship between mortality, morbidity, and the presence or absence of health services.

From 1965 to the present there has been an intense concern with how to *manage* health services. Federal mandates have required activities such as utilization review of hospital care, and agencies have been created to determine the appropriateness of construction, distribution, and renovation of hospitals. During this period, the Health Maintenance Organizations (HMOs) introduced competition to the medical marketplace.

Medicare and Medicaid legislation in 1966 promised equal access to high-quality health care for the aged and the poor and set a tone for health care policy in the United States. The preamble of the Medicare legislation states that equal access to high-quality health care is a fundamental right of U.S. citizens. Three attributes of care were deemed important in this legislation: access, affordability, and quality. Efforts have since been launched to improve access to health care, such as the efforts to increase medical school enrollment. Efforts to control and contain costs have been attempted during the last two to three decades.

In 1976, a report was published called the Forward Plan. The report stressed the need for a conceptual framework for the evaluation of health care.

> Activities directed toward the development of a more systematic framework for the analysis of the health domain are a very high priority and are designed to increase our power to forecast and to predict the consequences of alternative policies. . . . With respect to our health sector phenomenon, we are a long way from being able to make such predictions with even a minimal degree of certainty. The goal in this Forward Plan is to improve the health of the American

people. The objectives are: to assure equal access to quality care at a reasonable
cost and to prevent illness, disease and accidents. (Bergner, 1976, p. 396).

Achieving quality in the delivery of pharmaceutical care and assessing the outcomes of this care are a more recent focus of the evaluators and managers of
the health care system. Legislation introduced during the last 30 years has deemed
quality care imperative. However, many efforts to evaluate the system of care
have been focused on controlling costs and providing access.

Evaluating the Quality of Care

The best measure of quality is not how well or how frequently a medical service
is given, but how closely the result approaches the fundamental objectives of
prolonging life, relieving distress, restoring functioning and preventing disability (Lembecke 1952).

Before attempting to assess the quality of care, either in general or in particular
site or situation, it is necessary to come to an agreement on what constitutes
quality. To measure quality without a firm agreement on how to define it is to
court disaster (Donabedian 1980). Donnabedian suggests begining to measure
quality by examining the performance of health professionals.

The management, by a health care professional, of a clearly definable episode
of illness in a given patient has been termed the simplest unit of care (Donabedian
1988). It is possible to divide this management into two domains: the technical
and the interpersonal. Technical care is the application of the science and technology of medicine and other health sciences to the management of a personal health
problem. Interpersonal care is the management of the social and psychological
interaction between client and practitioner. Technical care has been called the
science of medicine and interpersonal care its art.

Assessment of the quality of health care has been classified[5] into three categories: structure, process, and outcome. The following section will describe what
each of these categories represents, explain who is involved in each category of
evaluation, describe methods used to monitor each category, and present examples from a pharmacy practice setting.

Approaches to Assessment of Quality Care

The Structure of Care

Structure denotes the attributes of the settings in which care occurs. Evaluations
of structure address the relatively stable characteristics of the providers of care,
the tools and resources providers have at their disposal, and the physical and
organizational settings in which providers work. Structure includes the attributes
of material resources (such as facilities, equipment, and money), human resources

(such as the number and qualifications of personnel), and organizational structure (such as staff organization, methods of peer review, and methods of reimbursement). The concept of structure also includes the human, physical, and financial resources that are needed to provide care. The term embraces the number, distribution, and qualifications of professional personnel and the number size, equipment, and geographic disposition of hospitals and other facilities. But the concept of structure goes beyond the factors of production to include the ways in which the financing and delivery of health services are organized, both formally and informally. Health insurance is an aspect of structure, as are the organization of the medical staff in a hospital, and the presence or absence of a quality review effort. The basic characteristics of structure are its stability, its function as a producer of care or a feature of the "environment" of care, and its influence on the kind of care provided.

Evaluation of the quality of the structure of a health system is completed by inspectors, engineers, architects, national licensing boards, and medical boards. Structure is measured in many different units. For example, units could be the number of licensed practitioners, assurance that all practicing practitioners are licensed, or the assurance that the pharmacy conforms to fire and safety codes.

Farris and Kirking (1993) proposed *examples of structure criteria* by which to evaluate the quality of pharmaceutical care. These include licensing of the pharmacists, presence of appropriate drug information references, sufficient inventory, record-keeping capabilities (e.g., computers), usable pharmacy counter space, trained and/or certified technicians, designated area for compounding, pharmacy business manager, financial stability, private patient counseling area, and proximity of non-prescription medications to pharmacists.

The Process of Care

The process of care is what is actually done in giving and receiving care. Within the process the patient seeks care and carries out instructions and the practitioner makes a diagnosis and recommends or implements treatment. The primary object of evaluation is the development of a set of activities that go on within and between practitioners and patients (Donabedian 1980).

One very good example of how the system monitors the process is the creation of the Peer Review Standard Organizations (PRSOs) for physician peer review. In fact, most evaluations of the process of care have their roots in peer review. Peer professionals have developed, discovered, or set a precedent for some practice standard that has become accepted by the medical community. The evaluation of the process is conducted by health care professionals.

A judgment concerning the quality of the process may be made either by direct observation or, for a less accurate representation, by review of recorded information. Quality of the process of care is defined as normative behavior. The norms are derived either from the science of medicine or the ethics and values of society. Measurements of the process are determined by previous scientific research and discoveries and published literature with accepted standards.

Dispensing the correct medication is one measurement of the process of pharmaceutical care (Katz et al. 1963). In the strategy proposed by Donnabedian there are *technical* and *interpersonal* aspects to the process of care. The *technical* responsibilities of the pharmacist include gathering prescription information, entering the prescription into a computer, reviewing patients' profiles, obtaining medication from stock, labeling medication containers, assessing the appropriateness of the drug and dosage prescribed, checking for drug allergies and interactions (drug-drug or drug-food), monitoring adverse events, and assessing patient compliance. The *interpersonal* skills a pharmacist, or any healthcare professional, require include listening, being sympathetic or empathetic to the patient, being friendly, and showing concern and consideration. Use of interpersonal skills should not be exception to the rule when delivering care.

Outcomes of Care

The outcomes of care are the effects of care on the health status of patients and populations. Improvements in the patient's knowledge and salutary changes in the patients' behavior are included under a broad definition of health status, as is the degree of the patient's satisfaction with care. Although most health professionals agree that quality outcomes are a goal of care, little emphasis has been placed on their evaluation and even less emphasis placed on documenting achievement. Using the definition above, the patient is the best source of information to evaluate the outcome. Information is garnered from patients using scientifically designed and tested surveys which have been proven to be reliable and valid. The surveys may also be interviewer-administered or telephone-administered. The use of patients' assessments of their care and their health to evaluate outcomes has received increased attention over the past few decades. Currently, patient self-administered questionnaires are used in health care policy decisions as well as in clinical practice. However, the methods used to create these questionnaires pre-date the current awareness in the health care community.

Historical View of Patient-Based Health-Related Quality of Life Assessments

The use of standardized surveys to assess functional status and well-being can be traced back over 300 years. Methodologic interest, however, has been greatest during the last half of this century (Katz et al. 1963). The psychometric techniques of scale construction, now widely used in the health care field, have been available for most of the past century (Guttman 1944; Likert 1932; Thurstone and Chave 1929). The study of methods to measure health-related quality of life began with physicians' attempts to measure patient functioning. The Karnofsky Functional Status Assessment (Karnofsky and Burchenal 1949) and the New York Heart Association Classification (Criteria Committee of the New York Heart Association 1979) were among the first instruments developed to capture data about a patient's level of physical activity. The first health-status instruments sought to distinguish among patients' functional states and included symptoms, anatomic findings, occupational status, and activities of daily living. These early instruments were significant because they provided a standardized approach for physicians to document the consequences of the patient care being provided. The early tools found application in inpatient studies designed to evaluate the functional status of patients with severe disabilities.

The first modern health-status questionnaires appeared in the 1970s, when social scientists and clinical experts came together with a common research agenda to answer questions about the consequences of the medical care provided. Most health measures prior to the 1970s were not based on scale construction methods. The early tools were quite long but the data they captured were valid, reproducible, and relevant. Their focus was multi-dimensional, providing assessments of physical, psychological, and social health. The development, refinement, and use of the early instruments helped to establish the foundation for today's studies. (Ware et al. 1993; Patrick and Erickson 1993) Many of these early measures are still popular today and will be familiar to readers. These early measures include Quality of Well-Being Scale (Fanshel and Bush 1970) Sickness Impact Profile (Bergner et al. 1976) the Health Perceptions Questionnaire (Ware 1976) and the OARS (Pfeiffer 1975) Tools of more recent origin include the Duke-UNC Health Profiles (Parkerson et al. 1981), the Notthingham Health Profile (Hunt, McEwen, and McKenna 1985), and the Medical Outcomes Study 36-Item (SF-36) Health Survey (Ware and Sherbourne 1992).

Common to all of these assessment tools is a theoretical framework that views the measurement of biologic functioning as an essential but inadequate component of the comprehensive evaluation of health. Beyond the documentation of organ system functioning, lies the assessment of general well-being and behavioral functioning which is central to the traditional medical view of health. This broader assessment of health is necessary because basic biologic abnormalities can extend into a person's behavioral functioning and sense of well-being, disrupting the person's health-related quality of life (Ware 1991). The impact a disease can have on a person's life can be likened to a rock dropped into the center of a still pond. The rock sends out ripples over the entire surface of the water just as a disease affects or the entirety of a patient's life, not just organ function. All of the circles detailed in Figure 2-1 are affected and must be addressed in a health-related quality of life assessment if a comprehensive understanding of the patient's condition is to be achieved.

Interest in health-related quality of life was expanded greatly in 1989 when the United States Congress passed the Omnibus Reconciliation Act, which in-

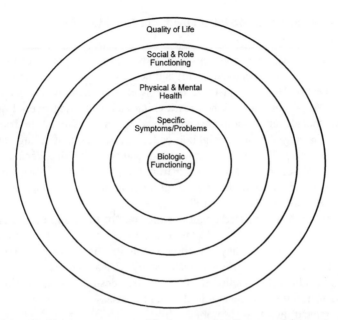

Figure 6.1. Health status concepts. The impact of a disease and its treatment often affects more than the biologic functioning of the patient. Biologic abnormalities and imbalances can impact other important areas of the patient's life such as general well-being and behavioral functioning. The analogy often used to describe this impact is that of a rock hitting the surface of a still pond, sending ripples over the entire surface of the water. Adapted from Ware, J. E. 1991. Conceptualizing and Measuring Generic Health Outcomes. *Cancer*:67(suppl):3.

cluded as part of its mandate patient outcomes research. This legislation required the Secretary of Health and Human Services to establish a broad-based, patient-centered outcomes research program and created the Agency for Health Care Policy and Research. The Agency monitors the effectiveness of specific medical treatments by including assessments of patients' functional status, general well-being, and satisfaction with the medical care provided (Omnibus Reconciliation Act 1989). In addition to research, a major focus of the agency is the promotion of clinical practice guideline development, database development, and information dissemination.

Additionally, both academic and industry researchers interested in evaluating alternative medical, surgical, and pharmacological treatments have shown great interest in including health-related quality of life in their investigations. Researchers in pharmacoeconomics have accepted health-related quality of life assessments as a valid approach to documenting the consequences of using medicines. These specialized researchers look forward to including health-related quality of life findings in their economic assessments of competing therapeutic options.

Components of Health-Related Quality of Life Measures

Health-related quality of life focuses on those aspects of quality of life that are specifically related to personal health and activities to maintain or improve that level of health. Health is just one of the twelve domains of life identified by Campbell to be considered when researching and evaluating overall quality of life. The other eleven domains are community, education, family life, friendships, housing, marriage, nation, neighborhood, self, standard of living, and work (Campbell 1981). The term "health-related quality of life" has been adopted by researchers to set their research apart from the more global concept of quality of life identified by Campbell and to reflect more accurately the scope of their research (Patrick and Erickson 1988).

In assessing health-related quality of life, one of three approaches is usually taken. Researchers can either select tools that focus on *general* (sometimes called generic) health status or they can choose tools that are more narrowly focused on specific aspects of the *disease* under study. For a comprehensive picture of patient's health-related quality of life, it is often desirable to *include both types* of assessment tools, the general health and the disease-specific, in projects with a health-related quality of life objective.

General Health Status Instruments

General health status instruments evaluate aspects of health relevant to all ages, races, sexes, and socio-economic backgrounds. Questions in a general health status questionnaire are not defined by the disease or disorder under study. These questions have historically covered the full range of the state of disease or illness and have therefore emphasized the negative end of the health continuum. Increasingly, this limitation in older general health status instruments is being recognized and outcomes researchers are constructing general health status tools that extend measurements into the well-being end of the health spectrum (Ware 1991). General health status tools are by definition multi-dimensional, generally evaluating at least four key health concepts: physical functioning, social and role functioning, mental health, and general health perceptions (Ware 1994).

Disease-Specific Health Status Instruments

Often it is necessary to focus on the particular impact that a certain disease has on patients. In such cases, general health status tools are inadequate to provide the information needed. To overcome this limitation, condition-specific or disease-specific measures are often used to supplement the general health status instrument. The more narrowly focused disease-specific measures request detailed information about the impact a disease and its treatment has on the patient from his or her perspective. While items in both general health status measures and

Table 6.1. General Health Concepts

Concepts	Definition
Physical	
Physical limitations	Limitations in performance of self-care, mobility, and physical activities
Physical abilities	Ability to perform everyday activities
Days in bed	Confinement to bed due to health problems
Bodily pain	Ratings of the intensity, duration, frequency of bodily pain and limitations in usual activities due to pain
Social and Role	
Interpersonal contacts	Frequency of visits with friends and relatives
	Frequency of telephone contacts with close friends or relatives during a specific period of time
Social resources	Quantity and quality of social network
Role functioning	Freedom from limitations due to health in the performance of usual role activities such as work, housework, school activities.
Mental	
Anxiety/depression	Feelings of anxiety, nervousness, tenseness, depression, moodiness, down heartedness
Psychological well-being	Frequency and intensity of general positive affect
Behavioral/emotional control	Control of behavior, thoughts, and feelings during specific period
Cognitive functioning	Orientation to time and place, memory, attention span, and alertness
General Health Perceptions	
Current health	Self-rating of health at present
Health outlook	Expectations regarding health in the future

Adapted from Ware, J.E. 1987 Standards for Validating Health Measures: Definition and Content. *J Chron Dis.* 40:473–480.

in disease-specific measures may appear to ask the same question, those in the disease-specific tool are phrased to direct patients to think about their specific disease, its symptoms, or its treatment rather than disease or limitations in general. Additionally, using disease-specific measures allows inclusion of domains of specific interest for the disease under study and the patients it afflicts. Some areas previously investigated with disease-specific questionnaires are sexual functioning, nausea and vomiting, pain, cancer, arthritis, epilepsy, HIV infection, anxiety and depression, asthma, and rhinitis (Patrick and Deyo 1989; Wu et al. 1991; Juniper and Guyatt 1991; Juniper et al. 1993; Schipper et al. 1993; Meenan 1982).

Psychometrics

The literature is expanding with reports of general health and disease-specific health-related quality of life research. As with any field of research, the studies being reported in the literature meet various levels of scientific rigor. Readers of these reports must have a basic understanding of psychometrics to draw appropriate conclusions from health-related quality of life study findings.

Psychometrics is the science of developing standardized tests or scales to evaluate attributes of an individual. It is used in the field of health assessment to translate people's behavior, feelings, and personal evaluations into quantifiable data. These data, once captured, need to be both relevant and correct if they are to provide useful insights into health-related quality of life.

There are two psychometric properties that any measurement scale or instrument must possess: reliability and validity. Additionally, useful measuring scales must be sensitive to change and must be accepted by the clinician, investigators, and respondents.

Reliability

When measuring reliability, the scientist is concerned with the relationship between true variation and random error (Selitz, Wrightman, and Cook 1976). Evaluations assess the consistency and repeatability of measurement. Reliability estimates are useful because they allow the researcher to examine the consistency of results from different measures thought to evaluate the same thing (Stewart 1990). These estimates can be obtained by capturing data using the same tool on repeated administrations or by using alternative forms of a measure.

Validity

There are a number of key questions that must be answered if researchers are to have confidence in the data captured using health-related quality of life instruments. All are related to the validity of the assessment. Do the questions in the instrument really measure the concept under study? Do respondents understand the questions being asked? Are the response categories appropriate for the questions? *Validity* is the extent to which differences in test scores reflect the true differences in the individuals under study.

Sensitivity

Perhaps the least studied and documented aspect of health-related quality of life measures at this time is sensitivity (McHorney et al. 1992). Researchers evaluating sensitivity are concerned with detecting the true changes that occur in a health concept over time. It is important, when assessing sensitivity, that measures of change over time cover the entire range of a particular health concept.

Acceptability for Use

Clinicians, investigators, and respondents will have valuable opinions about the acceptability of various health-related quality of life instruments. How easy the measure is to use, to score, and to interpret are all valid concerns. The completion rate, the extent of missing data, and the number and nature of complaints about the tool are all clues about the acceptability of the measure for use in a research or clinical setting. Acceptability is also expressed as respondent burden. Regardless of the administration format (self-administered, telephone interview, personal interview, observation, or postal survey) failure to consider respondent burden can doom any survey project.

Today's researchers strive to achieve a balance between an increase in reliability (achieved by asking more questions) and an increase in respondent burden (achieved by asking fewer questions). Some short-form multi-item scales derived from much longer measures are now in use. These short forms achieve an acceptably high level of precision when compared to their longer parent versions and are much more acceptable to respondents, investigators, and clinicians. The MOS SF-36 (McHorney et al. 1992) and the Duke Health Profile 17-item (Parkerson, Broadhead, and Tse 1991) are two examples of short-form scales recently available.

The Future of Health-Related Quality of Life Research

The agenda for the future of health-related quality of life research is quite full. Health-related quality of life measures appearing today are shorter and more user friendly than earlier versions. These shorter tools are gaining acceptance in clinical practice as well as in industry and academic research. The trend towards shorter, more focused tools is expected to continue. Other methodologic developments are also expected. A parallel research agenda is the application of these tools in clinical practice. Both agendas require interpretation of the patients' scores and amalgamation of data from patient scores with traditional biologic markers of disease. Future research will test the use of these combinations in therapeutic decision-making as well as in monitoring therapy. Only when we know the health-related quality of life of very healthy individuals, very disabled individuals, and all those in-between can findings from health-related quality of life research have meaning and find application. Establishing community norms and characteristic patterns within population segments is also an important research objective for many contemporary scientists.

The future research agenda, as it pertains to pharmacists, has three similar but not identical purposes: to continue to measure and define health states, to assist with monitoring patients' care, and to provide information with which to manage an individual patient's care. Each of these three purposes is illustrated with examples.

Findings from the Medical Outcomes Study have been instrumental to measuring and defining health. Information gained using these tools in clinical drug trials has enabled the exploration of how to use health-related quality of life assessments as monitoring parameters. The clinical application of health-related quality of life research is only just now being realized. The use of this information in routine care and in making decisions about therapy is not yet common practice.

The Medical Outcomes Study

Results from the Medical Outcomes Study (MOS) (Tarlov et al. 1989; Stewart et al. 1989; Wells et al. 1989) have taught researchers and clinicians a great deal about measuring and defining health. In the MOS, a more comprehensive approach to the assessment of health was first embraced. One of the major objectives of the MOS was the development of practical tools for monitoring patient outcomes and their determinants in routine medical practice. In particular, the study was designed to evaluate the impact of chronic disease on patient functioning and well-being and to determine if key features of medical care were associated with more favorable patient outcomes. Today, after 8 years and baseline data on over 22,000 patients, information from approximately 2,500 patients followed over 4 years continues to inform research agendas (McHorney n.d.; Ware et al. n.d.[a]; Ware et al. n.d.[b]; Stewart and Ware 1992).

Quality of life Research in Clinical Trials

Research on furthering the use of health-related quality of life instruments as monitoring tools in clinical practice, has been conducted in the context of clinical drug trials. Clinical trial planning is driven largely by companies' need to develop their products and obtain regulatory approval to market them. Despite great demand in the U.S. and abroad for information about product attributes beyond traditional measures of safety and efficacy, the only practical opportunity to conduct patient-based research on these attributes has been the integration of health-related quality of life components with Phase II, III, or IV studies. The results of this combination have been synergistic. Both clinical practice and the science of psychometrics have benefited from information from these combined studies.

The results of these clinical trials containing health-related quality of life assessments are increasingly present in both the general medical literature and medical specialty journals from which clinicians derive new information for patient care decisions. Another trend that has added relevance to the health-related quality of life data is the shift of the locus of decision making away from individual practitioners and toward provider organizations such as managed-care and managed-pharmacy benefit programs. These organizations systematically seek information on product attributes, including health-related quality of life data, to assist in decisions about products to acquire or to recommend to participating practitioners.

Using Health-Related Quality of Life Assessments in Routine Patient Care

Standardized measures capturing patient perspectives regarding their physical functioning, social and role functioning, mental health, and general health perceptions are likely to appear in routine patient records in the near future. Comparing individual scores with regional or national norms may provide health professionals with clues to hidden health problems. A series of health-related quality of life assessments taken over time can provide the clinician with valuable information.

In a report of experiences using patient-based health-related quality of life assessments to monitor patients' care in a busy dialysis clinic, Meyer et al. (1994) relate that health-related quality of life surveillance has done more than give quantitative expression to the staff's intuition. The surveillance reveals new information, and the information revealed is qualitatively different from that provided by the assessments that are otherwise made in the care of patients. The authors suggest that patient-based assessment can improve the management of individual patients and can contribute to the epidemiology of treatment.

To the individual patient, health-related quality of life assessments provides a language in which to describe experiences that he or she may find difficult to express, or may not think to formulate unless prompted. It also aids the patient in reconstructing experiences that he or she may not remember clearly. By objectifying the patient's subjective experience, health-related quality of life assessment makes the experience more consistently accessible to the staff who share responsibility for his or her care. It puts his experience on the agenda for discussion, whether or not technical aspects of his care currently compete for attention. The authors maintain that clinicians can make meaningful interpretations of individual patients' scores and that these interpretations enhance rather than summarize the collective understanding of a conscientious medical team.

"It is important to note that if one understands responses to health status assessments as a form of speech, then by entering the results of HQL (health-related quality of life) assessment into the medical record, one is asking the patient to make entries in the record. A health status database offers patients who wish to do so the opportunity to share their experiences over the course of illness and treatment with other patients who face similar clinical situations. Such a database could also be a valuable tool for clinicians trying to help patients make decisions."

Pharmacoeconomists will also find increasing use for health-related quality of life research. As the techniques for including patient preferences in economic assessments improve, pharmacoeconomists will be a primary user of health-related quality of life measures.

Regardless of the final shape health care reform takes, patients, who can chose providers or health care programs, and payers, who can restrict or limit coverage, will continue to require answers to their questions about the outcomes of medical care options and will continue to demand high-quality outcomes. Providing these answers will remain a key objective of industry and academic researchers and clinical practitioners. Health-related quality of life will likely remain central to many research agendas and be accepted as a component of clinical practice.

Conclusions

The study of health-related quality of life requires a multi-dimensional, multi-disciplinary approach. Assessments must include components that evaluate, at a minimum, the health concepts of physical functioning, social and role functioning, mental health, and general health perceptions. Additionally, the full continuum of these concepts must be included, from illness-specific to the well-being. Approaches to the capture of health-related quality of life data include the self-administered questionnaire, the personal interview, the telephone interview, observation, and postal survey. The assessment instruments must possess acceptable reliability, validity, and sensitivity, and they must be accepted by clinicians, investigators, and participants. Psychometrics is an essential part of health-related quality of life research, especially in today's research settings which require shorter, more focused measures. The application of health-related quality of life research findings is just now beginning to be realized. However, as cost pressures continue to dominate health care, these research results will most certainly play an important role in documenting the outcomes of treatment and in justifying pharmaceutical care.

References

Bergner, M., et al. 1976. The Sickness Impact Profile: Conceptual Formulation and Methodology for the Development of a Health Status Measure. *International Journal of Health Services* 6:393–415.

Bungay, K. M., and J. E. Ware. 1993. *Measuring and Monitoring Health-Related Quality of Life*. Kalamazo, MI: The Upjohn Company.

Campbell, A. 1981. *The Sense of Well-being in America: Recent Patterns and Trends.* New York: McGraw Hill.

Criteria Committee New York Heart Association. 1979. *Nomenclature and Criteria for Diagnosis of Diseases of the Heart and Great Vessels.* 8th ed. Boston: Little, Brown & Co.

Donabedian, A. 1988. The Quality of Care: How Can It Be Assessed? *JAMA* 260:1743–8.

Donabedian, A. 1980. *The Definition of Quality and Approaches to Its Management.* Vol. 1, *Explorations in Quality Assessment and Monitoring.* Ann Arbor: Health Administration Press.

Fanshel, S., and J. W. Bush. 1970. A Health-status Index and Its Applications to Health-services Outcomes. *Operations Research* 18:1021–66.

Farris, K. B., and D. M. Kirking. 1993. Assessing the Quality of Pharmaceutical Care. II Applications of Concepts of Quality Assessment from Medical Care. *Annals of Pharmacotherapy* 27:215–23.

Guttman, L. A. 1944. A Basis for Scaling Qualitative Data. *American Sociological Review* 9:139–50.

Hunt, S. M., J. McEwen, and S. P. McKenna. 1985. Measuring Health Status: A New Tool for Clinicans and Epidemiologists. *J R Coll General Practice* 19:806–26.

Juniper, E. F., and G. H. Guyatt. 1991. Development and Testing of a New Measure of Health Status for Clinical Trials in Rhinoconjunctivitis. *Clinical and Experimental Allergy* 21:77–83.

Karnofsky, D. A., and J. H. Burchenal. 1949. The Clinical Evaluation of Chemotherapeutic Agents in Cancer. In *Evaluation of Chemotherapeutic Agents*, ed. C. M. Macleod, 191–205. New York: Columbia Press.

Katz, S., et al. 1963. Studies of Illness in the Aged: The Index of ADL: A Standardized Measure of Biological and Psychosocial Function. *JAMA* 185:914–19.

Lembecke, P. A. 1952. Measuring the Quality of Medical Care Through Vital Statistics Based on Hospital Service Areas: 1. Comparitive Study of Appendectomy Rates. *American Journal of Public Health.* 42:276–86.

Likert, R. 1932. A Technique for the Measurement of Attitudes. *Archives of Psychology* 140:5–55.

McHorney, C. A., et al. 1992. The Validity and Relative Precision of MOS Short-and Long-form Health Status Scales and Dartmouth COOP Charts. *Medical Care* 30:MS253–65.

McHorney, C. A., et al. In press. The MOS SF-36 Short Form Health Survey (SF-36): III Tests of Data Quality, Scaling Assumptions, and Reliability Across Diverse Patient Groups. *Medical Care*.

Meenan, R. F. 1982. The AIMS Approach to Health Status Measurement: Conceptual Background and Measurement Properties. *Journal of Reheumatology* 9:785–88.

Meyer, K. B., et al. 1994. Monitoring Dialysis Patients' Health Status. American Journal of Kidney Disease. 24:267–79.

Omnibus Reconcillation Act 1989. Public Law 101–239.

Parkerson, G. R., Jr., et al. 1981. The Duke-UNC Health Profile: An Adult Health Status Instrument for Primary Care. *Medical Care* 19:806–26.

Parkerson, G. R., W. E. Broadhead, and C. K. Tse. 1991. Comparison of the Duke Health Profile and the MOS Short-form in Health Young Adults. *Medical Care.* 29:679–83.

Patrick, D. L., and R. A. Deyo. 1989. Generic and Disease-specific Measures in Assessing Health Status and Quality of Life. *Medical Care* 27(suppl):S217–32.

Patrick, D. L., and P. Erickson. 1988. Assessing Health-related Quality of Life for Clinical Decision Making. In *Quality of Life: Assessments and Application*, eds. S. R. Walker and R. M. Rosser, 9–49. Nancaster, England: MTR Press.

Patrick, D. L., and P. Erickson. 1993. *Health Status and Health Policy. Allocating Resources to Healthcare*. New York: Oxford University Press.

Pfeiffer, E., ed. 1975. *Multidimensional Functional Assessment: The OARS Methodology*. Durham: Duke University Center for the Study of Aging and Human Development.

Schipper, H., et al. 1984. Measuring the Quality of Life of Cancer Patients: The Functional Living Index-cancer: Development and Validation. *Journal of Clinical Oncology* 2:472–83.

Selitiz, C., L. S. Wrightsman, and S. W. Cook. 1976. *Research Methods in Social Relations*. 3rd ed. New York: Holt, Rinehart, and Winston.

Stewart, A. L. 1990. Psychometric Considerations in Functional Status Instruments. In *Functional Status Measurement in Primary Care*, 3–26. New York: Springer Verlag.

Stewart, A. L., and J. E. Ware, eds. 1992. *Measuring Functioning and Well-being: The Medical Outcomes Study Approach*. Durham: Duke University Press.

Stewart, A. L., et al. 1989. Functional Status and Well-being of Patients with Chronic Conditions: results from the Medical Outcomes Study. *JAMA* 262(7):907–13.

Tarlov, A. R., et al. 1989. The Medical Outcomes Study: An Application of Methods for Monitoring the Results of Medical Care. *JAMA* 262(7):925–30.

Thurstone, L. L., and E. J. Chave. 1929. *The Measurement of Attitude*. Chicago: University of Chicago Press.

Ware, J. E., 1991. Conceptualizing and Measuring Generic Health Outcomes. *Cancer* 67(suppl):3.

Ware, J. E., 1994. The Status of Health Status Measurement. *Annual Review of Public Health 16*. Palo Alto: Annual Reviews.

Ware, J. E., et al. 1993. *SR-36 Health Survey, Manual and Interpretation Guide*. Boston: Nimrod Press.

Ware, J. E., et al. In press. Comparison of Methods for the Scoring and Statistical Analysis of the SF-36 Health Profile and Summary Measures: Summary of Results from the Medical Outcomes Study. *Medical Care*.

Ware, J. E., Jr. 1976. Scales for Measuring General Health Perceptions. *Health Services Research* 11:396–415.

Ware, J. E., Jr. 1991. Measuring Functioning, Well-being, and Other Generic Health Concepts. In *Effect of Cancer on Quality of Life*, ed. D. Osoba, ch. 2. Boca Raton: CRC Press.

Ware, J. E., Jr., and C. D. Sherbourne. 1992. The MOS 36-Item Short-Form Health Survey (SF-36). *Medical Care* 30:473–82.

Wells, K. B., et al. 1989. Detection of Depressive Disorder for Patient Receiving Prepaid or Fee-for Service Care: Results from the Medical Outcomes Study. *JAMA* 262(23):3298–302.

World Health Organization. 1948. *Basic Documents: World Health Organization*. Geneva, Switzerland: World Health Organization.

Wu, A. W., et al. 1991. A Health Status Questionnaire Using 30 Items from the Medical Outcomes Study: Preliminary Validation in Persons with Early HIV Infection. *Medical Care* 29:786–9.

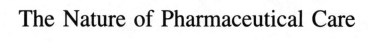

The Nature of Pharmaceutical Care

7

Pharmaceutical Care—An Overview

Lucinda L. Maine, Ph.D.
Richard P. Penna, Pharm.D.

Introduction

The primary purpose of this chapter is to offer an operational definition of pharmaceutical care. To achieve this purpose, the evidence that pharmacy has identified a deficiency or a major public health need, and has made a philosophical commitment to strive to fill that deficiency or meet that need will be reviewed. That evidence is the heart of this chapter's first major section. The remainder of the chapter will draw attention to the significant amount of work that must be done to transform pharmacy into a profession which is committed not only to caring about the outcomes of patients' drug therapies but also to assuming the responsibility for those outcomes. The implications of these commitments will be studied in greater detail in subsequent chapters. This chapter will close with a review of the initial steps that have been taken by both individual practitioners and researchers and professional and regulatory bodies to expedite a paradigm shift that will make pharmaceutical care the model for contemporary pharmacy practice.

Roots of Pharmaceutical Care

Pharmacy: A Profession Familiar with Change

Pharmacy, like all professions, must evolve continuously to meet the needs of society, and is therefore no stranger to change. As with most professions, pockets of resistance within the profession challenge the innovators and slacken the pace of change, which is nonetheless inevitable. Rufus A. Lyman, founding editor of the *American Journal of Pharmaceutical Education,* noted the following with respect to change in pharmacy education:

Some were violently opposed, the majority were indifferent. Support did come from a few farseeing laymen who recognized the importance of the pharmacist and the drugstore in the public health service. It also came from a handful of practicing druggists who were readers of pharmacy's history and who had learned the part the pharmacist has played in the past in science, in industry, in research, in education, and in the art of living, and who had a vision of greater things for the future (Kremers, and Urdang, 1976, 254).

(E. Kremers, J. Urdang History of Pharmacy 4th Ed Lippincott, Phila 1976)

Change Through History

As detailed in Chapter 2, in the pharmacy profession's earliest days its practitioners were primarily involved with the gathering, identification, testing, and purification of natural drug products and with research on those products. Compounding those products into dosage forms that were safe, stable, effective, accessible, and palatable was the predominant role of pharmacists in the pre-industrial era.

These traditional roles changed with the establishment of the pharmaceutical industry. Pharmaceutical companies, which were often founded by pharmacists, took the key scientific knowledge of the pharmacy profession and developed large, efficient systems for producing a dizzying array of pharmaceutical dosage forms. Increasingly, pharmacists accepted the responsibility to assure that already-manufactured drug products were readily available to the public by maintaining systems of efficient, safe, and accurate drug distribution.

Change of major proportions is once again confronting the profession. The major expansion in the fundamental professional responsibilities of pharmacists— *that of caring for people and for the outcomes of their medication use*—represents a paradigm shift for practitioners, educators, and regulators. In short, all elements of the pharmacy profession are effected by this change.

The Concept of Role Expansion

While profound change has been and is occurring in the profession, pharmacy is not abandoning the responsibilities the public has historically conferred upon it. Indeed, pharmacy continues to promote the pharmaceutical sciences, which support research and development in the pharmaceutical industry. Increasingly, the clinical and biomedical sciences are directly applied to patient care. A growing area of scientific inquiry, that of outcomes assessment, will provide the foundation upon which much of contemporary clinical practice, including pharmaceutical care, will be built.

The profession has accepted new responsibilities in practice as well, without completely abandoning the old ones. Many pharmacists continue to compound finished dosage forms, although in some cases the types of products compounded are vastly different from those compounded in past practice. Radioactive pharmaceuticals for diagnostic and therapeutic use and intravenous admixtures and nutritional support products are examples of modern-day compounded products most often prepared by pharmacists. It is interesting to note that for both examples cited above, the Board of Pharmaceutical Specialties, the specialty-recognizing body in the profession, has recognized that practitioners involved in such practices possess specialized bodies of knowledge and skill that warrant certification.

Safe and effective systems of drug distribution are very much within the scope of responsibility of today's pharmacist. However, as will be noted in more detail later in this text, automation and technical personnel will play an increasing role in executing the drug distribution function, making it possible for pharmacists to apply their skills to the caregiving functions so essential to pharmaceutical care.

The continuing expansion of pharmacists' professional roles and responsibilities into clinical specialties, long-term care, home health care, and a myriad of other areas reflects the consistent response of the profession to the changing needs of society. It also underscores the unique knowledge and services that pharmacists can bring to the health care system.

Signposts on Pharmacy's Road of Change

In a century filled with change of the magnitude and pace of that which pharmacy has experienced, it is not surprising to note that the profession's leaders have dedicated considerable effort to studies and reports that chronicle the status of the profession and how practitioners have met the needs of society. In the first half of this century, such reports were primarily concerned with the nature of the services pharmacists were providing and how those services were perceived, received, and appreciated by the public. In the middle of this century, it was clear that changes in the practices of pharmacy and drug manufacturing had called into question what the societally sanctioned role of the pharmacist truly was. Toward the mid-eighties, pharmacy turned its attention to strategic planning by inquiring about the future and by asking what the public's existing needs were and how the unique knowledge and skills of pharmacists could be useful in addressing those needs.

A brief summary of these chronicles, which were originally published as survey findings, key speeches, or study commission reports, provides a roadmap of the philosophical journey of the pharmacy profession toward pharmaceutical care. The summary will show that the leaders of the profession have made a transition from documenting practice to strategically envisioning how practice must be transformed to secure a professionally viable role for pharmacists.

The earliest report in this chronology, *Basic Material for a Pharmaceutical Curriculum,* is a report of the Commonwealth Fund Study and Survey of Pharmacy (Christensen 1927). Dr. W. W. Charters and his team visited hundreds of pharmacies throughout the United States to investigate and tabulate the duties and functions of the pharmacist. Thousands of prescriptions were checked for ingredients and frequency of ingredients. Colleges of pharmacy and boards of pharmacy were encouraged to use the report as a foundation for both curricula and state board examinations to insure that individuals entering practice were equipped with relevant and adequate knowledge and skill to perform their socially sanctioned duties.

In reporting on the survey in his report to the American Pharmaceutical Association (APhA), National Association of Boards of Pharmacy Secretary H. C. Christensen noted that the profession should not depend on the results of this survey indefinitely and alluded to a concern that the profession was not evolving as rapidly or consistently as necessary. He called for continued surveying of the activities of pharmacists as a mechanism for continuously moving the boundaries of pharmacy practice forward and remaining in step with societal needs.

The Great Depression and World War II stalled subsequent analyses of the status or functions of pharmacists until 1948, when the American Council of Education published The Pharmaceutical Survey, also known as the Elliott Report. The purpose of the survey was to ensure that pharmacy continued to occupy its proper place among the health professions in a post-war era marked by expanding opportunities for greater service to the public.

The survey covered all phases of the practice of pharmacy, with particular emphasis on professional education. Unlike the Charters' study, which truly addressed the need to document the practice of pharmacy itself, the Elliott Report contained recommendations directed toward increasing the pharmacist's prestige and standing both in the community and among his fellow heath care professionals. This difference in study goals reflects a profound change in pharmacy practice. This change was brought on by the explosion of prefabricated medications and increased sophistication and profitability in the pharmaceutical industry. These developments altered the day-to-day functions of pharmacists markedly, and, called upon much less frequently to prepare or compound dosage forms, pharmacists began to struggle with a clear definition of their new role.

The Elliott Report devoted a considerable amount of attention to the supply and preparation of manpower for the pharmacy profession's emerging roles and to the quality of faculty and curricula at colleges and schools of pharmacy. The report recommended that the four-year program of education and training be fortified with a stronger base in both the pharmaceutical sciences and economics. Curricular emphases noted in the study spanned the entire spectrum from drug procurement and preparation to preparing students to provide "professional services to the public appropriate to the basic functions of pharmacy in its role as a health profession." The report also recommended that the American Association of Colleges of Pharmacy and the American Council on Pharmaceutical Education take steps to develop an educational program leading to the professional Doctor of Pharmacy degree (Elliott 1949). Significantly, the concept of "clinical pharmacy" was not recommended as the focus for the Doctor of Pharmacy degree program since the development of clinical pharmacy was still 15 years off.

Donald Brodie articulated a key concept which can be credited with shifting the inquiry of pharmacy's leaders from the question of "what do pharmacists do?" to "what is the mainstream of pharmaceutical service (Brodie 1967)?". Brodie's concept of "drug-use control" was the keystone to pharmaceutical service, the mainstream of pharmacy. Brodie noted that while many felt that dispensing pharmaceuticals was the main activity of pharmacy professionals, this was not necessarily true. Brody quoted from the *Mirror to Hospital Pharmacy* to point out the frailty of this belief: "the dispensing function of the pharmacist, while important and even vital for patient care, is essentially a superficial practice of the profession which, by itself, does not utilize knowledge or skills sufficiently basic to merit professional recognition to the depth that lies within the grasp of hospital pharmacists (Francke et al. 1964, 6)." This argument applies to all pharmacists, regardless of where they practice.

Brodie defined drug-use control as that system of knowledge, understanding, judgments, procedures, skills, controls, and ethics that assures optimal safety in the distribution and use of medication. It is patient-oriented and applies to the practices of all pharmacists, educators, journalists, and regulators. It extends from the point of drug discovery on scientist's bench, to the pharmacy, and ultimately to the point of drug administration. Certainly Brodie brought the vision of the profession markedly closer to and more in line with the modern vision of pharmaceutical care.

Did Brodie's vision reflect the perception of the American public regarding the role their pharmacists played? Another key study, this one of the perceptions of consumers, revealed, troublingly, that people did not view the average pharmacist of the 1970s as the same kind of professional as the physician or dentist. A businessman with primarily commercial motivations, more closely aligned with pharmaceutical manufacturers than patients and other professionals, was the common vision held by respondents to APhA's Dichter Institute Study (What Is the Dichter Institute Saying About You? 1973). These beliefs were fortified by the environment in which most community pharmacists practiced. The study did not examine the public's perception of hospital pharmacists.

A lack of public awareness of the services pharmacists could and often did offer was noted as a compelling reason for the pubic's lack of trust in their pharmacist. The public took for granted that pharmacists packaged and labeled medications properly and maintained the appropriate quality of products in inventory. Failure to provide personal attention and establish a personal relationship with patients decreased customer confidence that pharmacists could provide professional services warranting professional status in the community. The research did reveal, however, a strong public desire for such a relationship, while noting that the rebuilding effort would not be an easy one for the profession.

A 1975 report entitled Pharmacists for the Future (Millis 1975), commissioned by the American Association of Colleges of Pharmacy, signals more change both within and external to the profession of pharmacy. The report begins by noting the tremendous concern among all elements of society regarding drug purity, efficacy, and safety, as well as the misuse and the cost and benefits of drugs. Commission chairman John Millis notes further that while pharmacists are naturally concerned about these issues, they are also concerned about their role in society. Impressions of the role the pharmacist might fill in efforts to improve the drug-use process spanned from no role for an obsolete profession to a key role in filling the gaps in health services involving drugs.

The Millis Commission report noted a discontinuity regarding the generation of new knowledge about pharmaceuticals and the application of that knowledge in clinical use. Much drug research is done within the proprietary boundaries of the pharmaceutical industry, and findings are disseminated to busy therapy prescribers via vehicles of the industry's making. This process leaves a true gap in a system of optimal drug use. The commission proposed that "pharmacy should be conceived as a knowledge system which renders a health service by concerning itself with understanding drugs and their effects upon people and animals." As they make up an integral subsystem of the larger national health service delivery system, pharmacists, armed with essential information about drugs and their use by patients, should be fully engaged in applying their professional judgment to weighing the expected benefits against possible risks of drug therapy (Millis 1975). This commission's wide-ranging recommendations for pharmacy education and practice are still being studied and implemented today.

In keeping with the profession's desire to periodically examine what pharmacists do in the course of their practices, the American Pharmaceutical Association and the American Association of Colleges of Pharmacy conducted a pharmacists' task analysis in 1977 and 1978. The Standards of Practice for the Profession of Pharmacy (Kalman and Schlegel 1979) provided a comprehensive definition of pharmacy practice. The standards were used by the National Association of Boards of Pharmacy as the basis of its NABPLEX licensing examination and by schools and colleges of pharmacy as the basis for building a pharmacy curriculum.

Perhaps motivated by the stark realization, articulated by the study commission, that the future of the profession was insecure unless aggressive steps were taken to redefine the role of pharmacists, the profession turned its attention in the 1980s to first defining and then strategically charting the future course of pharmacy practice and education. Brodie again articulated the need to capture the essence of pharmacy in the form of "a theory of practice" in his Harvey A. K. Whitney Award Lecture in 1980 (Brodie 1980).

Brodie called for an articulation of the theoretical base of pharmacy and, in doing, so underscored the evolution that had been occurring in the profession for decades (Brodie, McGhan, and Lindon, 1991). The theories that make up this base reflect the evolution from drug product focus to patient focus and ultimately state that the pharmacist is *responsible for the outcomes of drug therapy* used by patients and other professionals in the health care system. The four theories noted by these authors include:

- Theory of pharmacy as a drug-use control system
- Theory of pharmacy as a knowledge system
- Theory of pharmacy as a clinical profession
- Theory of pharmacy as the interface between mankind and drugs

The profession embraced the concept of "clinical pharmacy" in the 1970s and 80s. While this term carries many definitions, it is often used to distinguish those functions that are primarily informative and advisory from the more standardized, distributive functions of drug-use control. Hepler challenged the participants at the 1985 ASHP conference Directions for Clinical Practice to understand that limiting the scope of clinical pharmacy to just informative and advisory functions does not allow for conveyance of the maximum value of pharmacy's professional services to the public. Defining pharmacy in terms of responsibilities to the public for the appropriate use of drugs in patients more clearly suggests the social value of pharmaceutical services (Hepler 1985).

The pharmacy profession was concerned that clinical pharmacy, often cited as the secure future for the profession, might fail to secure pharmacists' place beside physicians and other recognized professionals. A series of strategic planning efforts, actually beginning as early as 1984, unfolded over the next decade. While some were professionwide and others focused on a single area of practice, all shared the commitment to clearly articulate a vision for pharmacy and to set forth strategies to enable pharmacists to achieve that vision.

Schwartz (1990) reviewed the considerable effort invested in the late 1980s by the profession's leaders in shaping the future of the profession. While noting that developing a strategic plan is a difficult undertaking for a large and diverse profession, the author suggested several mechanisms for strategically moving the profession forward.

The first of a series of profession-wide strategic planning efforts began in 1984 with a conference entitled Pharmacy in the 21st Century, Planning for an Uncertain Future (Bezold et al. 1985). Five years later, a second Pharmacy in the 21st Century Conference was sponsored by 17 major national professional pharmaceutical organizations. The purpose of this conference was to identify and prioritize the major issues that would confront the profession during the next 15 to 20 years (Cocolas et al. 1989). At this conference, the keynote speaker, C. Douglas Hepler, challenged participants to identify pharmaceutical care as the profession's major societal purpose and to establish standards and models of such care.

Participants clearly embraced this challenge, as evidenced by the strength of the consensus on key statements generated by work groups. Key statements receiving a score of greater than 4.5 on a 1 to 5 scale included:

• The need to develop a mission statement for pharmacy
• The need to develop standards for pharmaceutical care
• The need for pharmacy to demonstrate and communicate its value in health care

The American Society of Consultant Pharmacists also convened a strategic planning conference in 1989. This conference resulted in the articulation of a mission statement for consultant pharmacy and five strategies to guide the society and provide leadership to consultant pharmacists. The outcome statements from this conference reflected a strong desire to assist consultant pharmacists in realizing their role in optimizing pharmaceutical and related care and to help develop broad recognition for the value of pharmaceutical care.

These national conferences spawned several state and regional strategic planning efforts, and pharmacy's leaders increased their efforts to help practitioners and educators understand the importance of enunciating a new mission for the profession. These subsequent planning efforts encouraged participants to identify obstacles to pharmacy's advancement and set forth strategies that would allow the practice of pharmacy to meet contemporary societal needs.

Recognizing the importance of keeping pharmacy education positioned to produce graduates whose knowledge and skills meet the needs of contemporary society now and in the future, the American Association of Colleges of Pharmacy (AACP) initiated its own planning process. The Commission to Implement Change in Pharmacy Education began its work in 1989 and a year later issued the first of four background papers reflecting its work. The first articulated a mission for pharmaceutical education which, in general, is consistent with the concept of pharmaceutical care. The three additional papers examine the core competencies needed to prepare pharmacists for contemporary practice, the structure of the degree program, and post-graduate training and education needs of the profession in light of the profession's chosen mission (American Association of Colleges of Pharmacy 1993).

The American Pharmaceutical Association also charged a task force with examining the needs of society, ways the profession should prepare to meet these needs, and obstacles that stand in the way. The report, entitled An APhA White Paper: The Role of the Pharmacist in Comprehensive Medication Use Management (American Pharmaceutical Association 1992), describes the drug use problems in today's society and defines pharmaceutical care as the services provided by pharmacists which can address those problems. Three broad areas preventing pharmacy from delivering these services were identified along with a series of 20 principles, or areas for action.

In 1993, the American Society of Hospital Pharmacists (ASHP) and the ASHP

Research and Education Foundation conducted a conference entitled Implementing Pharmaceutical Care in San Antonio, Texas. The objectives of the conference included identifying the implications of pharmacists' assumption of the responsibility for the outcome of drug therapy, the barriers to and opportunities for implementing this practice, and practice-level processes for pharmaceutical care implementation in organized health care settings. The national conference was to establish the basis for regional, state, and department-level planning efforts and catalyze the widespread adoption of the pharmaceutical care practice model.

Another professionwide conference carrying the "Pharmacy in the 21st Century" title was convened in October 1994 to continue the effort of identifying obstacles to the delivery of pharmaceutical care and designing strategies to overcome them. This conference addressed obstacles in all venues of practice and took advantage of the emergence of models of pharmaceutical care practice in ambulatory, managed care, acute, and long-term institutional settings.

Pharmacy has moved, in the span of approximately 65 years, from being a profession proud of and comfortable with a scope of practice limited to the preparation of pharmaceutical products, to being a profession whose scope of practice includes creating and implementing quality drug distribution systems, and whose leaders are undertaking an aggressive attempt to redefine what practitioners do in terms of delivering pharmaceutical care to patients. This effort stems from the realization that unless it defines a role that is societally necessary and valued, the profession of pharmacy, which has served society for centuries, will cease to exist.

Changes Affecting the Health Care System

Each of the recent strategic planning activities has been an exploration of the environments in which pharmacy is currently striving to define its role. Issues include trends in demography, epidemiology, technology, and economics and the status of drug use in the United States. Each of these major trends impacts on the practice of pharmacy. On balance, the current direction of change within each broad area lends credibility to the advancement of pharmacists' practice and support to the emergence of pharmaceutical care.

Demographic Trends

The American population is aging and becoming more diverse. Those aged 65 and older will soon constitute 15 percent or more of the U.S. population. While the majority will maintain their independence, the elderly as a group suffer more chronic ailments than the young. Moreover, the elderly frequently suffer from multiple chronic illnesses. The management of one or more chronic conditions typically involves the use of prescription and nonprescription medications.

A poor clinical research base supporting the appropriate use of medications in the elderly and a poorly developed model of chronic health care delivery often leave this population vulnerable to unintended, negative consequences of drug therapy.

Cultural changes are also occurring in our society in at least two dimensions. More Americans are prepared to take responsibility for their own health and wellness, leading to more self-care for routine and nonurgent health conditions. In addition, immigration has led to a more ethnically and economically diverse population. Within different ethnic and socioeconomic groups, health professionals find different medical care needs, and some of these medical care needs require nontraditional strategies for managing health and illness.

Epidemiologic Trends

Major diseases, which were once predominately acute, are now predominately chronic. This change is largely a result of immunization, improved public health practices, and demographic changes in the population, chiefly the aging of the American population.

Consequently, new and different diseases have taken the place of the acute illness prevalent earlier this century. Cardiovascular diseases, metabolic illnesses, immune disorders such as HIV/AIDS, and mental health disorders are the conditions that will impact markedly on the delivery of health care in the future. Genetic research, such as the isolation of the gene which marks a predisposition to certain forms of cancer in late 1993, may also significantly change the patterns of disease in the future.

These changes in the patterns of illness pose a problem for America's health care system, which is already under siege for its inadequacies and high cost. The model of care currently most prevalent in the U.S. remains an acute-disease-oriented model. Episodic care, which is not necessarily related to the patient's previous medical history, can be delivered without integrated and reliable medical records. The acute-care health-care delivery system also spawned a proliferation of medical specialties. In today's specialty-oriented system, chronic care is often inadequate due to the lack of integration of medical information and poor communication between multiple providers of care.

Health care providers, who have historically been trained in an acute care model, are poorly equipped for the philosophical and practice transition from curing illnesses to managing illness in a caring way with emphasis on the quality of a patient's life. Also, it is easy to monitor the outcomes of an acute illness, that typically has a short duration of therapy—the patient either responds or does not. When patients with one or more chronic ailments receive care from multiple providers, it is much more difficult to monitor the progression of the diseases and the outcomes of care over prolonged periods of time.

Economics

No matter what the final outcome of the debate over the need to reform the nation's health care system, one idea has been universally accepted by the American public. The country's economic profile and the ability to increase U.S. international competitiveness depend substantially on reigning in increases in the cost of medical care.

Paul Starr described the economic issues propelling changes in health care financing and delivery in his book *The Logic of Health Care Reform* (Starr 1993). He noted that according to numerous polls, over 90 percent of Americans believe that fundamental health care reform is essential. This view was also held by most American business executives in 1993.

Business spending on health benefits climbed from 2.2 percent to 8.3 percent of wages and salaries and from 8.4 to 56.4 percent of pretax corporate profits between 1965 and 1989, (Starr 1993, 22). These increases translated to lower real wages, as dollars which might have gone to increase salaries were diverted to health benefits.

Government faced the same dilemma. Resources were shifted to health care at the expense of education, roads, bridges, transportation, and defense. The end result of these shifts is a weaker infrastructure for America and a less prepared workforce, compounding the country's problems of competitiveness.

The investment made in health care does not translate into a healthier society. Comparing the health of America with that of other developed nations, which spend considerably less per capita for health care, proves that Americans are not healthier and, in fact, by some measures Americans are less healthy.

At one time, pharmaceuticals constituted a relatively modest percentage of overall health care costs. Yet pressure was brought to bear on this segment of health care costs for two significant reasons. During the 1980s, prices of existing drugs rose sharply and introductory prices for new, innovative products were higher than they had been in the past. Increases many times higher than consumer prices indices and higher than overall medical cost inflation drew attention to pharmaceutical manufacturers' and providers' pricing practices. Drug prices also attracted more attention from consumers and payers because medications were often an out-of-pocket expense. For many consumers, drug costs were the highest out-of-pocket medical expense. Consumers and payers became anxious for relief from increases of 10 to 20 percent annually for certain products.

Technology

Striking technological advances are markedly affecting the organization, delivery, and cost of health care. Some areas where advances have been significant are biotechnology, information processing technology, applications for patient records, automation of service delivery, and clinical decision-making.

Pharmacy is integrally involved with these technological advances. As Francke said as early as 1967, "[t]oday's drugs may be likened to ballistic missiles with atomic warheads, while we prescribe, dispense, and administer them as if they were bows and arrows (Francke 1967)." This was long before the discovery of the genetically engineered compounds such as monoclonal antibodies, human hormones and immunomodulators, and sophisticated yet potentially toxic pharmaceuticals for treating cancer, heart disease, and infectious diseases. The appropriate use and monitoring of such products are essential for clinical, economic, and ethical reasons.

Pharmacists are struggling to adopt professional responsiblity for the outcomes of drug therapy while maintaining a reliable distribution system. Technology is enabling this transition, although the expense of new technology certainly slows the pace of its integration. Dispensing technology, bar coding, and robotics free professionals' time from routine drug distribution responsibilities and allow pharmacists to embrace a more important role at the patient interface. Computers and other communication technologies allow for the capture and exchange of patient-specific information and provide clinical decision-making assistance for pharmacists, physicians, and other health professionals. Computer-driven direct patient education is also becoming increasingly available, in many cases tailored to the gender, educational level, ethnicity, and health profile of the patient.

Drugs as Tools in an Increasingly Sophisticated System

As pharmacists at state and national planning conferences listened to the experts' descriptions of the social, economic, technological, and other forces affecting drug use and heard their forecasts for the future, an easy consensus was reached that pharmaceuticals are and will increasingly be looked upon as important tools for the prevention, cure, and management of acute and chronic illness. The effectiveness of those tools depends on both the skill of the user and the quality of the system in which they are used.

The inability of the health care system in general and the pharmacy profession in particular to effectively systemize the drug-use process in a way that responds to the trends and changes noted above has created a major drug problem for the U.S. health care system. (See Chapter 4 for a more in depth analysis of drug-related problems in the current system.) Of all the health professions, pharmacy is best positioned to take the lead in resolving this problem. To support this contention, one needs simply to contrast the education and training of pharmacists with that of other professionals with regard to the science and application of pharmaceuticals. In addition, the distribution of pharmacists and pharmacies throughout the country, including inner city and rural America, is unparalleled by other professions. Therefore pharmacists have access to patients in ways most health care professionals do not.

It should be noted, however, that improving the drug-use process will require to a very great extent the cooperation of other professionals with a stake in the outcome of patients' care. Should pharmacy choose not to assume the responsibility for optimal drug use or decide that obstacles to this change of role are too difficult to overcome, the profession should recognize that other professions will take on this new responsibility. The cost of failing to manage medication use to produce better medical and economic outcomes is simply too great to be ignored by a society whose resources have become severely constrained.

A Paradigm Shift for Pharmacy

Role of Professions

As Buerki and Vottero discussed in substantial detail in Chapter 1, professions are sanctioned by a society to provide a service which members of the society, as a general rule, can not provide for themselves. Supporting the profession's status are a specialized body of knowledge, recognition by licensure, an ethical code, internal controls, a professional culture, and a system of organization.

The clear articulation of exactly what contemporary problems the profession of pharmacy is sanctioned to address is therefore critical to its transformation. Also, it is insufficient for the pharmacy profession alone to identify these problems. The lay public, other professionals, and society itself must agree on pharmacy's societal purpose.

One of the difficulties pharmacy has confronted in making the transformation to its new professional role is the lack of public appreciation for the need to apply pharmacists' skills to activities beyond the preparation of medications for patients' use. The historical role of the pharmacist-as-apothecary, charged with the almost mystical responsibility of preparing medications, changed markedly with the advent of prefabricated medications and increased commercialization of the environment in which pharmacy was practiced.

The public has also been led to believe that pharmaceuticals are highly safe and universally effective. Their allies have been their physicians and the government, and advertisers lent credence to both these allies. Physicians certainly did not want their patients to think that the prescriptions they so readily wrote to cure diseases and ameliorate symptoms could induce any harm, and, of course, physicians believed that their patients were equipped with the knowledge to ensure proper drug use. Federal regulators ensured, through a long and expensive approval process, that only safe and effective drugs reached the market. Advertising for the nonprescription drugs which were available in almost a half-million retail establishments lulled consumers into the belief that an armamentarium of highly safe and very effective products was available to treat every ailment. What need could society see for "the druggist"?

Manasse characterized that need in his examination of "drug misadventuring" (Manasse 1989), which is profiled in this book in Chapter 4. Adverse drug reactions, suboptimal response to therapy, and unnecessary institutionalization are all examples of societal problems which compound our nation's health care emergency. Pharmacy's redefined professional mission, which some call a mandate because of the increased complexity of drug use in America, seeks to address these problems.

One challenge facing the pharmacy profession is assisting the public in understanding the potential severity of the health care problem without weakening the confidence they have in their health professionals and further eroding their notion of the integrity of the health care system. Perhaps directing more attention to describing those services that pharmacists perform in an effort to achieve positive outcomes from drug therapy will serve to educate the public about the availability of the services and the implications the services have for individual and public health.

Pharmacists' Efforts to Intervene in the Drug Use Process

As noted by Strand, Cipolle, and Morley (1992), much of the drug use problem is not in the drugs themselves, but rather in the way the drugs are prescribed, dispensed, and used. Strand identified the major reasons why drug therapy goes awry. They are:

- An error is made in the drug therapy decision-making process. A drug is prescribed when none is indicated; no drug is prescribed when one is indicated; or the wrong drug is prescribed.

- The implementation of the therapeutic process is faulty. The patient is not administered the drug because the drug isn't delivered to the patient care area; the patient doesn't pick up the drug at the pharmacy because the patient cannot afford the medication; or the pharmacist makes an error in the dispensing process.

- Patient behavior is faulty. The patient does not comply with therapy.

- Monitoring fails. Monitoring for compliance, therapeutic effect, or for adverse effects does not occur or is lax.

Several studies specifically examine the application of pharmaceutical care practice models in ambulatory care (Mitchel 1993). An examination of these studies reveals a diversity in approach and expected outcome which is not surprising given the fact that pharmaceutical care as a concept is still relatively new to most practitioners and researchers. Outcomes research examining the scope of drug-related problems and the impact of interventions is needed in three key dimensions; clinical, economic, and humanistic outcomes.

Over the past several decades, pharmacists have undertaken significant efforts to expand the nature of the services they provide both to patients and to other health professionals. These were enumerated by Brodie in his 1980 Whitney Award Lecture. Described broadly, they encompass:

- Participating in therapeutic decision-making (rounds, formulary/P&T activities, therapeutic clinics, reviewing prescription orders, OTC drug selection)
- Selection of dose, dosage form, and dosage schedule using the scientific applications of biopharmaceutics and pharmacokinetics
- Preparing the dosage form (compounding)
- Providing the medication for the patient or caregiver
- Educating the patient or caregiver
- Monitoring the patient for compliance and clinical outcomes (including adverse effects)

When examined and studied, each of these pharmaceutical functions results in positive patient outcomes. Yet drug-related problems continue to plague patient care.

Why Do Drug-related Problems Persist?

Studies of individual pharmaceutical functions show the function's positive effect because all other functions are generally controlled in the study. In real patient-care situations, such controls don't exist. If a pharmacist ascertains that the drug prescribed is the best for the patient but the drug is not delivered in time to be administered, then further participation by the pharmacist in the drug therapy decision-making process would contribute little to the care of the patient. Moreover, if the drug is correct and the patient receives the drug at the proper time, but the dose or dosage schedule is wrong, harm would come to the patient. If all functions were performed perfectly, but no one monitored the patient to ensure that the patient was complying with therapy, harm could come to the patient.

Drugs must be used within a system that assures that consideration is given to providing *all* of the pharmaceutical functions needed for patient care. Assuming responsibility for the outcomes of drug therapy in patients and adopting a caring attitude toward patients ensures that pharmacists will consider performing all possible pharmaceutical functions to achieve the desired outcomes of therapy.

Pharmacists must *focus their attention on the PATIENT*. Pharmacists must CARE for and worry about the patient. Pharmacists must act on the knowledge that they share in the responsibility for the success or the failure of therapy. To quote Strand, Cipolle, and Morley (1992, 6), "*pharmaceutical care is that component of pharmacy practice which entails the direct interaction of the pharmacist with the patient for the purpose of caring for that patient's drug-related needs.*" Pharmacists must evaluate patients needs, determine whether there are actual or potential problems, and work with patients and other professionals to design, implement, and monitor pharmacotherapeutic plans.

It must be admitted that until very recently, pharmacy practice and education has not been focused on the patient but rather on drug products. Until recently, the bulk of the curricula in schools and colleges of pharmacy dealt with the nature of disease (biochemistry, anatomy, pathophysiology) and the physical properties of drugs (pharmaceutics, medicinal chemistry). Not until late in the course of study were students exposed to the application of pharmaceuticals to patients. Students did not enter the patient-care setting until their final semester or year of study. Many practitioners would be quick to admit that they have neither the skills nor the confidence to interact with patients beyond the superficial "How are you?" greeting that serves more as civility than caring.

The previously cited APhA white paper on the role of the pharmacist calls for the integration of pharmacists' practice with other components of the health care system (American Pharmaceutical Association 1992, 5). However, there first must be an integration of pharmaceutical care services within the pharmacy practice environments themselves. As Strand noted in the introductory work on pharmaceutical care, different care models will evolve to match the differing needs of patients in different settings (Strand, Cipolle, and Morley, 1992). However, the full range of services needed to provide pharmaceutical care must be integrated within a system to ensure that complete care is provided every patient. Many cite the division of drug distribution and clinical pharmacy services as they emerged in many hospitals as an errant model that should not be perpetuated as pharmacy moves toward a redefined practice. All pharmacists and support personnel in a pharmaceutical care system should be either working to deliver care or supporting its delivery by providing drug information, drug distribution, or other services. Mechanisms for the communication of patient information and referral between pharmacy providers in different settings and specialties is also an issue for the profession.

Just as important is the integration of pharmacy services into the mainstream of services provided by other health care providers. This integration begs for improvements in communication technology and the commitment on the part of all providers of patient care to fully utilize the unique knowledge and skill of other providers. The isolation of traditional community pharmacies, which are often located in shopping areas, discount stores, and supermarkets rather than in medical environments, is also an issue which must be considered as pharmaceutical care models emerge.

Needed: A Philosophy or Theory of Practice

As has been noted previously, Brodie first called upon the profession to articulate a theory of practice in the mid-60s and finally proposed a multiple-theory concept of pharmacy 25 years later. His theories recognize the need for a drug-use control system using the "knowledge, understanding, judgements, procedures, skills, controls, and ethics that assures optimal safety in the distribution and the use of medicines." They also encompass the interface between mankind and drugs and argue that pharmacy should be responsible for the outcomes of care, the promotion of health, and the prevention of disease (Brodie, McGhan, and Lindon, 1991, 539).

Chapters 8, 9, and 10 review in detail three keys to translating these theories into practices that impact significantly and positively on individuals. Caring (Chapter 8) must be the new practice paradigm. Caring pharmacists are not only concerned about their patients but also make an emotional commitment to and establish a covenant with each individual to whom they provide care.

Redirecting the pharmacist's focus from drugs to patients and drawing the pharmacist's attention to the outcomes that drug therapy achieves in individuals are fundamental to the new practice of pharmacy (Chapter 9). Failure to accept responsibility for helping patients to achieve optimal outcomes (Chapter 10) will limit the professional role of pharmacists in the future and perhaps even threaten the existence of this profession.

Pharmaceutical Care: A Philosophy or a Process?

Is this paradigm shift, now broadly referred to as pharmaceutical care, a philosophy of practice or is it a new process for practicing an age-old profession? Clearly, it is both. It represents a fundamental change in perspective for practitioners, educators, and regulators, who must stop defining what they do in terms of the drug products within the profession's control and begin identifying with the needs of the individual patient.

In order to make this change, however, a complete restructuring of the manner in which pharmacies practice is needed. Relinquishing direct control for drug distribution and entrusting this task to adequately trained technical personnel and automation (and perhaps another pharmacy), is an essential first part of the process of change. The caregiving portion of the pharmaceutical care process has been defined as "the pharmacist's workup of drug therapy (PWUDT) (Strand, Cipolle, and Morley, 1992)."

Redefining both the philosophy and practice models of a profession is a herculean task, and leaders in the profession of pharmacy do not underestimate that fact. Evidence of this understanding can be found in their commitment to pharmaceutical care. This commitment is reflected in mission statements, study commission reports, conferences, and research materials which have been released during the last five years or so and universally supported by pharmacy practice organizations. An examination of this evidence and a review of work yet to be completed forms the remainder of this chapter.

The Response of the Profession

Mission Statements of Professional Organizations

In strategic planning, the mission statement defines the core business of an organization. Considering the challenge by Hepler to adopt pharmaceutical care as the new mission of pharmacy, it is not surprising that an outcome statement of the Pharmacy in the 21st Century Conference in 1989 was the call for the profession to articulate a new mission. Before that conference had even adjourned, one of the work groups presented a draft mission statement to the conferees.

Subsequently, a subgroup of the Joint Commission of Pharmacy Practitioners (JCPP) began the process of drafting a mission statement for pharmacy. Finding common language acceptable to the leaders of such diverse groups of pharmacists as those represented at the JCPP table proved difficult, but ultimately consensus was reached on a relatively simple statement of pharmacy's mission which read, "the mission of pharmacy is to help patients make the best use of medications."

The boards and deliberative bodies of numerous national associations have adopted the JCPP mission statement and several have gone on to articulate, within their own organizations' strategic plans, missions which reflect their commitment to pharmaceutical care. Likewise, the results of state and regional strategic planning activities have universally demonstrated the broad commitment to this paradigm shift within the profession.

NABP Model State Pharmacy Practice Act

Licensure is one mechanism to distinguish a group of professionals from society at large. Pharmacy in this country has been licensed for more than a century through state boards of pharmacy. At the national level the boards are represented by the National Association of Boards of Pharmacy (NABP) which provides a uniform licensing exam used by almost all states, assists with reciprocity, and provides leadership on emerging issues confronted by the states as they strive to protect the public interest by regulating the practice of pharmacy.

A major effort was undertaken in the late 1980s and early 90s to prepare an updated model state pharmacy act. NABP, with significant input from state boards and state and national practitioner organizations, released the model act in 1992 with model rules for many specific aspects of practice (e.g., nuclear/radiologic pharmacy, sterile practice, and continuing education).

The NABP model act included model rules for pharmaceutical care which establish minimum requirements for facilities, personnel, and practice. The inclusion in state law of language which at least acknowledges the pharmacist's responsibility to provide pharmaceutical care is one step toward establishing a new standard of practice.

Pharmacy Education and AACP Policy on Entry Degree in Pharmacy

A lack of emphasis on the patient in pharmacy curricula was previously noted as one of the impediments to improving the drug use process and reducing patients' drug-related problems. Reference has also been made to the AACP Commission to Implement Change in Pharmaceutical Education which issued four background papers. Pharmacy education's commitment to making the changes in education needed to support pharmaceutical care is clear.

A significant step towards making changes in education came in 1992 when the AACP House of Delegates adopted the recommendation of the Commission and supported curricular changes that include the institution of the Doctor of Pharmacy degree as the single, entry-level degree for the practice of pharmacy. As outlined in other background papers from the Commission, this degree would provide the patient focus, communication skills, and problem-solving ability so critical to pharmacist's ability to deliver pharmaceutical care. United in philosophy over the appropriate entry-level training model, pharmacy education leaders defined specific competencies for graduates and current practitioners, made curricular changes in both undergraduate and post-graduate training and education programs, and identified the human, fiscal, and clinical resources that will be needed to change pharmacy education.

ACPE Revised Standards and Guidelines

The American Council on Pharmaceutical Education (ACPE) is charged with establishing standards and guidelines for pharmaceutical education and surveying schools and colleges of pharmacy to certify adherence to these standards. Periodically, ACPE undertakes a revision of its standards to ensure that they continue to produce graduates equipped to meet contemporary and future societal needs.

A revision of ACPE standards and guidelines began in 1989 with a declaration of intent to undertake such an action. Reflected in the declaration was the belief of the council that the new standards should recognize the Doctor of Pharmacy degree as the single entry-level degree for the practice of pharmacy. The initial draft of the standards and guidelines, which was subject to numerous open hearings at national meetings, also stated that schools and colleges of pharmacy should adopt the philosophy of pharmaceutical care as the framework for curricular design.

APhA White Paper on the Pharmacist's Role

The previously cited APhA white paper was commissioned by the APhA Board of Trustees and directed to all pharmacists in the United States in an attempt to define pharmacy's mission in the 21st century and determine what the profession must do to achieve its goals. It was intended to both stimulate pharmacists' thinking and challenge their professional beliefs and practice behavior. It is considered a blueprint for action aimed at moving the profession toward its new roles.

ASHP Statement on Pharmaceutical Care

The American Society of Hospital Pharmacists (ASHP) issued a statement on pharmaceutical care which was adopted by its House of Delegates in June 1993 (American Society of Hospital Pharmacists 1993). Its purpose was to assist pharmacists in understanding pharmaceutical care, as such understanding must precede efforts to implement the concept. The ASHP statement defines pharmaceutical care, articulates its principal elements, and examines its implications for pharmacists, patients, other providers, information systems, educators, and researchers.

Scope of Pharmacy Practice Project

Fundamental to defining the emerging roles for pharmacists as pharmaceutical care providers and to charting the course for achieving those roles is the question of what pharmacists and pharmacy technicians do today. A major study exploring the contemporary practice of pharmacy in all settings, the Scope of Pharmacy Practice Project, was completed in early 1994. The intent of the four national sponsoring organizations (AACP, APhA, ASHP and NABP) is to use the outcomes of the study for a variety of credentialing activities, to understand better how pharmacists apply their knowledge and skills in the care of patients, and to see how technical personnel support those efforts.

Reaction of Individual Practitioners to Pharmaceutical Care

How are concepts as new and different as those associated with pharmaceutical care accepted by pharmacists in practice? One need only look at the number of continuing pharmacy education programs at local, state, and national meetings and the attendance by pharmacists at those sessions to understand how the concept has captured the imagination of today's frontline practitioners.

More significant is the experimentation with new practice concepts that has begun within pharmacy practice settings in recent years. Michel profiled those associated with various research and demonstration projects in 1993 (Michel 1993). Some of the pharmaceutical care models are comprehensive in nature and others are focused on care of patients with specific diseases. All projects have incorporated the development of an expanded patient database which will be used by the pharmacist to assess patient's drug-related needs, establish a care plan, and document the services given. Each model finds the pharmacist involved in a significant amount of individualized patient care aimed at helping the patient achieve optimal outcomes from their drug therapy.

Conclusion

In spite of the positive evidence of pharmacy's commitment to redefining its role and applying the talents of pharmacists to pharmaceutical care, it is clear that the pharmaceutical care concept is not yet a fully embraced philosophy or standard of practice. The concept represents an ambitious and incomplete agenda for professionals and their organizations. The agenda has many components, including legislative issues, credentialing activities, public understanding, financial matters, and issues of liability. Many of these will be addressed in detail in subsequent chapters.

The agenda has become increasingly clear, however, and has been accelerated by the current debate over reforming the nation's health care system. It seems that pharmacy must simultaneously establish the new standard of pharmaceutical care practice and begin assessing the capability of practitioners to deliver this level of care. There are some who feel that the way to approach this is through the legislative process, inserting a mandate to provide pharmaceutical care to the public in a universal health care system.

What if only a fraction of those currently practicing pharmacy are prepared, or even willing to become prepared, to deliver pharmaceutical care? How can the profession, its organizations and educational institutions, undertake the enormous task of retooling 150,000 or more practitioners in a reasonable amount of time? Given the litigious nature of our society and the mindset that only limited resources are available to support and compensate providers as they adopt new roles, is it even practical to believe that pharmacy can successfully undertake the arduous journey ahead?

These are hard questions that the profession has been asking itself for several years. Perhaps it is time to begin a serious dialogue with other stakeholders in the drug use process, specifically with the patient. After all, it is society, made up of individuals, who deems that the activities and contributions of a group warrant recognition as a profession. Ultimately it will be the public that accepts or rejects pharmaceutical care on its merits.

References

American Pharmaceutical Association. 1992. *APhA White Paper: The Role of the Pharmacist in Comprehensive Medication Use Management*. Washington, DC: American Pharmaceutical Association.

American Society of Hospital Pharmacists. 1993. ASHP Statement on Pharmaceutical Care. *American Journal of Hospital Pharmacy* 50:1720–3.

Brodie, D. C. 1967. Drug-Use Control: Keystone to Pharmaceutical Service. *Drug Intelligence* 1(2):63–5.

Brodie, D. C. 1980. Need for a Theoretical Base for Pharmacy Practice. In *Harvey A. K. Whitney Award Lectures: 1950–1992*, 260–9. Bethesda: American Society of Hospital Pharmacists.

Brodie, D. C., W. F., McGhan, and J. Lindon. 1991. The Theoretical Base of Pharmacy. *American Journal of Hospital Pharmacy* 48(3):536–40.

Christensen, H. C. 1927. Dr. Charters' Commonwealth Survey Report. *Journal of the American Pharmaceutical Association* 16(4):351–3.

Cocolas, G. H. Winter 1989. Proceedings of the Pharmacy in the 21st Century Conference: Executive Summary. *American Journal of Pharmaceutical Education* 53(S):1S–5S.

Elliott, E. C. 1949. The Pharmaceutical Survey, A Resume. *American Journal of Pharmaceutical Education* 13(1):230–44.

Francke, D. E., et al. 1964. *Mirror to Hospital Pharmacy*. Washington, DC: American Society of Hospital Pharmacists.

Hepler, C. D. 1985. Pharmacy as a Clinical Profession. *American Journal of Hospital Pharmacy* 42(6):1298–306.

Kalman, S. H., and Schlegal, J. F. 1979. Standards of practice for the profession of pharmacy. *American Pharmacy* NS19(3):21–35.

Kremers, L., and Urdang, J. 1976. *History of Pharmacy,* 4th ed. Philadelphia, PA: Lippincott.

Manasse, Jr., H. R. 1989. Medication use in an imperfect world. Baltimore, MD: ASHP Research and Education Foundation.

Michel, N. E. 1993. Projects study pharmaceutical care outcomes in ambulatory patients. *American Journal of Hospital Pharmacy* 50(8):1524–7.

Millis, J. S., et al. 1975. *Pharmacists for the Future: The Report of the Study Commission on Pharmacy*. Ann Arbor: Health Administration Press.

Schwartz, M. A. 1990. Envisioning Pharmacy's Future: A Further Commentary on Strategic Planing. *American Journal of Pharmaceutical Education* 54(Summer):1–8.

Starr, P. 1993. *The Logic of Health Care Reform: Transforming American Medicine for the Better*. Knoxville, TN Grand Rounds Press.

Strand, L. M., R. J. Cipolle, and P. C. Morley. 1992. *Pharmaceutical Care: An Introduction. Current Concepts*. Kalamazoo: The Upjohn Company.

What Is the Dichter Institute Saying About You? 1973. *Journal of the American Pharmaceutical Association* NS13(11):638–41.

8

The Nature of Caring

Charles D. Hepler, Ph.D.
David M. Angaran, M.S.

The term pharmaceutical care was introduced in its modern sense by Brodie, Parish, and Poston in 1980.

> Pharmaceutical care includes the determination of the drug needs for a given individual and the provision not only of the drug required but also the necessary *services* (before, during, or after treatment) to assure optimally safe and effective therapy. (Emphasis added)

According to Hepler (1987) pharmaceutical care is a type of pharmaceutical practice that revolves around "a covenantal relationship between a patient and a pharmacist in which the pharmacist performs drug use control *functions* . . . governed by awareness of and commitment to the patient's interest." (Emphasis added.) The term was intended "to invoke analogies with the ideals of medical care and nursing care (Hepler, 1987)." Hepler and Strand further defined pharmaceutical care as, "responsible provision of drug therapy for the purpose of achieving definite outcomes intended to improve a patient's quality of life (Hepler and Strand, 1989)."

This chapter will explore the ideas of professional *services, functions* consistent with patient interests and the ideals of medical and nursing care, and the *provision of drug therapy*. The chapter will also examine how pharmaceutical *care* differs from pharmaceutical *services*. The first part of the chapter will describe the idea of caring from an outcome-oriented perspective. From this perspective caring contributes to the formation and maintenance of professional relationships that lead to outcomes desired by both the professionals and his or her clients. The second part of the chapter will describe and demonstrate behaviors consistent with care.

Care and Service

Professional care encourages the relationship that is needed by both the professional and the client for the professional to provide services that succeed in improving the client's situation. The idea of professional care goes beyond the idea of professional service. While both refer to actions, *care* adds a dimension of concern and commitment. *Service* is cooler, more detached, and perhaps less focused on outcomes.

Among the usual dictionary meanings of the noun *care* are: "a disquieted state of blended uncertainty, apprehension and responsibility," "watchful attention," "maintenance," and "supervision." Care can also mean "regard coming from . . . esteem," which is problematic, as will be described below. As a verb, *care* means (inter alia) to maintain or supervise (as in care of the sick), and "to be concerned about." Again, it can also mean, "to like."[1] According to Gilligan, "The activity of care is an activity of relationship, of seeing and responding to need, . . . sustaining the . . . connections so that no one is left alone."

Service, as a noun, means (inter alia) help, usefulness, benefit, and "useful labor that does not produce a tangible commodity." Among the meanings of the verb *service* are "to perform service for: as . . . to perform any of the business functions auxiliary to production or distribution."

These definitions raise a fundamental issue: whether pharmacy is an occupation that distributes drug products with "business functions auxiliary to . . . distribution" or an occupation that provides care, with drug products auxiliary to care. Understanding the nature of professional work is necessary to fully appreciate the significance of the distinction between *pharmaceutical care* and *pharmaceutical service*.

The Nature of Professional Work

Professional services have three major characteristics: valued object, complexity, and specificity (Hepler 1985). See also chapter 1. The professions serve human values that are beyond price, as illustrated by the three classical professions: medicine, law, and clergy. Medical professions are supposed to support our physiological and psychosocial functioning. The law should encourage relationships among people based on logic instead of force and touch our basic civil rights. The clergy (and professorate) should serve the spirit and the intellect.

Professionals provide services that are beyond the capacity of an ordinary person to perform or to evaluate in advance. Medicine and pharmacy are technically complex (think of surgery or pharmacokinetics), the law is factually and logically complex, and religion is philosophically and spiritually complex. All

---

[1]All definitions are from *Webster's Ninth New Collegiate Dictionary*

have arcane vocabularies, customs, and procedures. All require the application of judgment at the limits of knowledge. If the service is performed inadequately, full recovery of one's biological function, legal rights, or spiritual health may be impossible.

Professional services are also intimate and individualized. They stand in contrast to standardized, mass-produced products or services. Some aspects of modern pharmacy practice embody such specificity. For example, an assessment of a patient's progress toward therapeutic objectives is inherently specific to one patient at a particular moment in a changing treatment process. It is far from standardized.

A second aspect of the dimension of specificity is personal commitment and the use of personal skill by the professional. Two members of the same profession might have different styles and methods of work. Their exercise of judgment may lead to different courses of action, *both of which may be correct*. Professional work involves the individuality of both the client and the professional. Both processes and outcomes of professional work may differ according to who is involved. This is a defining characteristic. If the practice of a profession could be standardized, its work would no longer be professional.

Science and Professional Practice

For a number or reasons, some professions, including medicine and pharmacy, claim to be scientific. This claim is illustrated by common terminology like "scientific medicine." This claim can also cause some confusion, especially with regard to care. For example, one of the valued attitudes of science is scientific objectivity, which includes emotional detachment, "dealing with facts . . . as perceived without distortion by personal feelings, prejudices or interpretations." Although professional care and professional objectivity are not complete opposites, an attitude of scientific objectivity does appear incompatible with professional care.

The difficulty lies in the attempt to describe professional practice as scientific. Although professional work should be based on accurate (scientific) knowledge, professional practice and scientific research differ in a number of ways:

1. Science constructs generalizations from particular observations, while professional practice applies generalizations to particular circumstances.

2. Scientists serve an abstraction called Knowledge with objective impartiality for the benefit of many. For a scientist to make a scientific conclusion prematurly, even if someone needs an answer, is at least bad form and at worst could lead to charges of scientific misconduct. (For examples, see Pool 1988; 1989) In contrast, professionals serve specific people, not the idea of universal Knowledge. They often must act on the basis of limited data, within time constraints. They should

be advocates of their clients, not neutral observers. While professional objectivity should include open-minded respect for reality, it need not, and arguably should not, include emotional detachment.

3. Scientific knowledge is valuable in itself. The test of scientific data is verifiability or non-falsifiability. Professional knowledge and skill are valuable not in themselves but only to the extent that professionals can use them to improve clients' quality of life. The test of profession is successful intervention.

Professional Decision Making

A patient's life is the result of biological, psychosocial, and environmental interactions that are so complex that every patient—indeed every patient encounter—is virtually unique. Patient care therefore results from decisions that depend on the details of each relationship and each encounter (Nortvedt 1993). Professional judgment is necessary in part because of the uniqueness of the patient's circumstances and needs. Although professional decisions should be based in part on scientific knowledge, the uniqueness of each patient requires an "unscientific," professional decision-making process.

Consider the following medical example of professional decision making.

> A man brings a three-year-old child to a hospital emergency room. He describes the child's problem as a bad cold but says that the fever is worse and the child has started to vomit. He says that he can't stand the child's crankiness and crying. The physician records that he appears uncooperative and defensive.

> Physical examination of the child shows fever, general irritability, headache, nuchal rigidity, Brudzinski's sign, and equivocal Babinski sign, all symptoms consistent with meningeal irritation, which suggest bacterial meningitis. The physician learns that the child has been symptomatic for 24 hours and requests the father's permission to perform a lumbar puncture. The father refuses and asks to take the child home.

> Although the ER is full (Friday night in a big city), the physician sits with the father and discusses the child's symptoms and what they mean. The man is clearly frightened, not only of his child's illness but also that he may be accused of stupidity or child neglect. He is also "afraid of doctors" and wants to leave. Finally he consents to the lumbar puncture.

> Smear of the CSF is negative but the biochemistry is consistent with bacterial meningitis. The physician advises immediate hospitalization. After another discussion, the father consents. The physician orders fluid and electrolytes, intravenous chloramphenicol and ampicillin. Culture of the CSF later confirms meningococci sensitive to Penicillin G.

Should the physician have waited to perform the lumbar puncture until the symptoms of meningitis were clearer? Should she have withheld antibiotics until a culture of cerebrospinal fluid had confirmed the diagnosis and revealed the antibiotic sensitivity of the causative organism? That would show appropriate scientific objectivity and deferred judgment but would not be appropriate care. The child might have died or suffered irreversible damage while the culture was in process. In this and many other cases, care requires immediate action based on reason and professional authority.

Specifically, professionals should interpret incomplete data about a patient by applying *professional judgement* and assert a conclusion as the basis for action by applying a unique kind of authority called *cultural authority* (Starr 1982). Cultural authority is the legitimate power to define reality and to impose values. In the example, the physician exercised cultural authority when she asserted that the diagnosis was bacterial meningitis and imposed a value judgment that the risk of waiting would outweigh the risk of mistake. In the example, the hospital admitted the child not because he really had bacterial meningitis (that was not confirmed until later) but because the physician *decided* and *asserted* that the child had bacterial meningitis. Given enough time, second opinions are possible, but they always come from another professional's application of professional judgment and cultural authority. Professional decision making often crosses the border between knowledge and mystery in the interest of the patient.

Professional decision making should be based upon scientific theory and, whenever possible, scientific knowledge (theory verified by controlled observation). However, to be effective in reaching its goal of improving the quality of a person's life, professional decision making must also take into account (Wulff 1986; Thomasma 1986):

1. Knowledge of customary practice (e.g., professional guidelines)
2. How the client experiences his life
3. The client's preferences or basic values
4. Therapeutic feasibility including risks, benefits and efficiency
5. Care (i.e., commitment to the interests of the client)

The logic of clinical decision making is not the hypothetico-deductive logic of science but rather hermeneutics (Wulff 1986), an interpretive application of science through a "logic of dialogue" between general principles and the patient's specific circumstances (Gatens-Robinson 1986).

Caring in Professional Relationships

The preliminary to pharmaceutical care is establishing or renewing a professional relationship. A primary purpose of a professional relationship is the support of professional services intended to improve a client's quality of life. A pharmacist might have "service relationships" (see introduction) with his patients, which support dispensing medicines, offering essential product information, and answering questions. However, he might need to modify those relationships if the purpose and functions of the practice changed to improving a patient's quality of life through the appropriate use of medicines.

The buying and selling of professional services requires "trust between strangers (Larsen 1977)" to a degree that the usual business doctrine of *caveat emptor* (let the buyer beware) cannot support. The nature of the relationship between client and professional is important to both. It is important to the professional because trust and cooperation by the patient may be a prerequisite to desired outcomes. For example, for a trial lawyer to be effective, her client must help her learn the truth about his past actions and must participate in his own defense. For a pharmacist to be effective, the patient must give an honest medication history and often must participate in her own therapy. For example, successful management of a diabetic patient might require appropriate injection technique, injection site rotation, performance of urine tests, and keeping a diary.

Some patient information (e.g., laboratory data), can be obtained with mere permission from the patient, that is, passive cooperation. Other information, such as an accurate medical history, requires more active cooperation, and often risk, by an already stressed patient. In order to decide what to do, the physician in the earlier example needed to know how long the child had been symptomatic. That physician would be more likely to get an accurate answer if the parent trusted the physician not to interpret a delay in seeking assistance as child neglect or parental stupidity.

Caring behavior is a way for the professional to initiate and to sustain the development of an appropriate professional relationship. In the example, the physician's treatment plan required the consent of the patient (or parent in this instance). There are legal ways to proceed without consent in an emergency, but it is much easier for the professional if the patient trusts the professional's competence and cooperates in care.

Caring Transforms Relationships

Caring behavior is much more than an interpersonal technique, although it is valuable in that respect alone. Caring behavior may transform an otherwise "objective" professional encounter into a relationship in which each member is able to recognize the humanity of the other. Just as patients want to feel known and understood by the professional, a professional wants to be known and understood by her clients (Engel 1988). Just as the client wants to believe (one hopes realistically) in the professional's virtue, a professional wants to know and understand those things that are essential to helping her clients. Presumably, a professional also wants her clients not only to believe that she has knowledge and understanding but also to accept the limitations of what a professional can do for a client.

Caring relationships with clients may also increase professional competence (see below) and enrich the professional's understanding of the goals and functions of practice. In Dossey's (1984) poetic image, the wounded healer meets the healthy patient in a caring relationship, and the healer's respect for the realities of illness in the context of people's lives increases, while the patient comes to understand the pharmacists professional struggle. The pharmacist may develop a more complete understanding of the human meaning of health and disease. This would push her knowledge far beyond the abstractions of biological and behavioral science and challenge her to develop greater skills in applying the new knowledge.

Finally, caring behavior by a professional may lead to caring behavior by the client. That is, the client may behave as if he understands the difficulty and uncertainty of professional work and have realistic expectations. The client's behavior may, in turn, lead to therapeutic partnership and to genuine mutual regard and concern. That is, professionals and clients may become covenanted. This concept is discussed below and again in Chapter 16.

Professional Covenants

Social scientists use descriptions of "ideal types" in the study of professions to clarify ideas. Action oriented people can also use a description of an ideal as a goal to work toward. Many ideals are unattainable in reality, just as a building may not exactly match its blueprint. Even so, an ideal provides direction for effort and a benchmark for assessing progress.

One ideal for professional relationships is a covenant. As used here, a covenant is a solemn, secular, binding agreement between people (usually two) for the performance of unspecified actions or the exchange of unspecified gifts. There may be a contract contained in a covenant, but a contract is legally enforceable, while a covenant is not. Covenants transform relationships in ways that contracts cannot.

Marriage is a familiar example of a personal covenant. Marriage is a solemn, binding agreement between two people to love, honor, and cherish one another for life. It is solemnized by a civil or religious ceremony. Marriage may contain legal obligations, (i.e., spousal support), but loving, honoring and cherishing are not legally enforceable. This secular covenant lasts as long as the parties to it continue to exchange those gifts.

A covenant is a useful context within which to understand the nature of professional care (Cooper 1988). A professional covenant is a solemn and binding agreement between a professional and a client in which the professional promises the client *competent care,* which involves use of the professional's knowledge and skill, and commitment to the patient's major interests. In return, the client promises both to give the professional *cultural authority* to define the problem (e.g., to diagnose) and to cooperate during care (Veatch 1981; May 1975).

The covenantal ideal is less moralistic for both the professional and the client than, for example, the ideals of professional philanthropy and beneficence. The covenential ideal is an alternative to professional paternalism on the one hand or consumerism on the other. The covenantal ideal places the professional and the client on an equal footing and emphasizes the dynamic process of exchange. In contrast to the paternalistic view, the professional covenantal ideal does not attempt to substitute professional values for client values. Professional altruism, as self-abnegation or sacrificial concern for the welfare of others, is not a virtue in a professional covenant. A covenant does not oblige the patient to be grateful, nor to follow the professional with blind obedience. Rather, patients choose to accept professional authority because it is in their own self-interest. Patients are not expected to be compliant but rather to participate in their own care as much as they can. In a covenant, the professional sees cooperation by a client as "a gift not wholly deserved," which he can only accept gratefully (May 1983).

On the other hand, a covenant does not reduce the professional to a skilled technician who is obliged to cater to the desires of a sovereign customer, as the "consumerist" view does. Caring means that the professional attempts to look beyond a consumer's wants and into a client's need.

The professional who recognizes the full extent of his dependency on the client would choose if possible to offer care as opposed to services. The client who trusts a professional and sees him as a caring, competent human would choose if possible to cooperate. In a covenant, the professional continues to give competent care and the client continues to accept professional authority when, among other things, each sees more long run benefit from doing so than from not doing so. Specifically, the professional needs the client in order to practice his profession just as much as the client needs the professional to solve his problems (May 1975).

Issues Raised by the Idea of Caring

Brody (1988) has proposed that care is "the central virtue for nursing." When one tries to place caring at the center of the professional relationship, as we have done here for pharmacy practice, some philosophical problems arise. Some of these problems are fairness or distributive justice, from both an objective and subjective perspective in the allocation of care (Nortvedt 1993) and sufficiency of care for a professional relationship. In other words, is caring enough?

Justice and Fairness

Caring takes into account the particulars of a situation and fits well into the specific nature of professional relationships, as described in an earlier section. However, that specificity can also raise questions about the consistency and appropriateness of caring. For example, if there is no standard, how can a professional decide how much care and what kind of care are appropriate for a particular patient? Given limited resources (e.g., time), how can one decide how to distribute caring resources among patients?

A related problem involves the emotional component of caring. Dictionary definitions of caring include the senses of "regard coming from esteem" and "a fondness or liking for." Such emotions can motivate and organize care, but they also raise the concern that care may be withheld, perhaps in subtle ways, from those who the professional does not esteem or like. Both of these issues seem to be ameliorated by the idea of care occurring within the context of a covenant. Having promised care, the professional has accepted special obligations to the client to which he must be faithful (Cooper 1988). Clearly, then, the giving of promised care should not depend on the professional's fondness for, approval of, or emotional dependency on the client.

> Mr. Stone, a 55 year old white male, brings all his prescriptions to pharmacist Susan Brown. Today, he brought a new prescription for nitroglycerin patches. He explained that he received the prescription from his family doctor after he was taken to the ER of Community Hospital by paramedics who came after a passerby called 911.
>
> Chewing an unlit cigar, Mr. Stone said to Susan Brown, "I guess I was riding my bike too fast for such a hot day, so I got dizzy and lost my balance. Big deal. So they gave me some tests at the hospital on a treadmill but would not let me finish the test. Now they say I have angina and I'm supposed to stop smoking and go on a diet and take medicine. Once they get their hooks into you, they don't want to let go. Now I suppose you'll be putting your hand in my wallet, too."
>
> When Mr. Stone heard that his prescription cost $60, he said to Pharmacist Brown, "Look, sweetie. Why don't you just keep the medicine? It would be a lot cheaper for me just to walk to the store or ride my bike a little slower."
>
> Brown replied, "First of all, Mr. Stone, my name is not Sweetie, its Ms. Brown, just like on my nametag. I'm a licensed professional and I think that you should show me the same respect that you would show a man in my position. Second, your doctor thinks you should take this medicine. It's for your heart. I'm sure that we can work out something so you can. . . ." (The last sentence was said to Mr. Stone's departing back.)

Perhaps unlike personal covenants like marriage, a professional covenant should not depend on friendship, approval, or other emotional interdependency, although feelings of dependency can appear in professional covenants for brief periods. Medical relationships have included a certain amount of emotional discord since the time of Hippocrates (Freidson 1989). There are several reasons for this: the emotional effects of illness on patients, differences in professional and lay constructions of illness, and possible social status differences (Freidson 1989).

Furthermore, emotional attachment to the client is not even a professional "virtue" in this view. Curzer has described the problems associated with care motivated by fondness (Curzer 1993). Fondness, or any judgment of whether a client is worthy of care, would require the patient to somehow satisfy the professional's values, but in professional care the patient's values should be primary.

Although Mr. Stone seemed unpleasant to Ms. Brown, he needed advice and support about his angina a lot more than he needed a lecture on courtesy. This simple example represents a larger class of differences involving major values, goals of therapy, culture, or socioeconomic status. This class includes many contemporary, morally sensitive issues such as, whether a professional is obliged to continue to care for persons who have objectives to which the professional conscientiously objects. The special obligations of a professional covenant suggest that the responsible professional who does not share the values or objectives of a client must weigh his preferences against the duties of covenant.

Competence and Other Professional Virtues

The care of one person for another surely has intrinsic value, both to the carer and the person cared for. Brody (1988) has called care a virtue and proposed a virtue-based ethics for nursing practice. She offered three overlapping perspectives on virtue: as a personal attribute, as actions which reflect a person's moral nature, and as the ability of people to "meet the moral obligations of a collectively defined role they have assumed." The last of these, especially, suggests that caring is a necessary virtue for the maintenance of professional covenants. However, maintenance of a covenant would appear to require additional virtues.

The classic, Platonic virtues are wisdom, courage, temperance and justice. To these we may add the Christian virtues of faith, hope, and charity. We suggested above that professionals promise their clients *competent care,* which implies the ability to provide valued, complex, and specific services with an attitude of commitment to the client's interest. Now we can suggest that *competence* is a familiar and modern collective name for a number of professional virtues necessary to complement the attitude of care.

Competence is the ability to use personal and environmental resources to reach one's objectives. People need competence to satisfy their other needs. Moreover, the need to feel competent may be as strong as any other need. To temporarily maintain the illusion of mastery or competence in their daily lives, people may do things that may damage them in the long term, such as deny and escape, as Mr. Stone did in the example above. Fortunately, most people are competent to satisfy most of their needs (Waters and Lawrence 1993; Hepler 1990).

Just as personal competence is essential in daily life, professional competence is essential for a professional. Professional competence, the ability to use available resources to achieve the objectives of professional practice, requires knowledge of a subject, wisdom, basic communications and problem solving skills, judgement, and a practice model for applying that knowledge and skill. Temperance is required to maintain each of the other virtues.

Professional competence has precise meaning, but, only in a given context of professional purpose. Purpose in this sense includes both a specific intention, such as the provision of care, and a specific objective, such as a therapeutic objective for a patient. Therefore, professional competence is not a personal attribute but rather depends on the circumstances of professional purpose.

Courage and temperance are often required for a professional to see what is real and articulate it, grow professionally, choose an objective based on patient need instead of professional convenience or opportunity, and help a patient choose the course of his own care. Fidelity is required when the professional disagrees with a patient's choice of treatment, especially if the treatment happens to fail. People build competence by courageously extending their abilities outward from a secure center. Relationships, either with mentors or colleagues, encourage this growth (Waters and Lawrence 1993).

To clarify the concept of competence, it may be useful to discuss some related concepts. Most importantly, competence is not a matter of heredity or personality but rather must be learned, practiced, cultivated, and habituated (Fowler, quoted by Brody 1988). Competence is not mere knowledge or skill but the ability to apply them purposely. Competence is not academic degrees or self-esteem. Most importantly, competence is not the absence of incompetence. Competence is not like a classroom test score, the remainder left over after enumerating everything a person cannot do. Competence is measured by what one *can* do to reach one's objective. Many pharmacists are already competent to provide pharmaceutical care. They can talk to every patient to find out if he understands how to take his medications; call a patient at home a day or two after he starts a new medication, just to ask how he's doing; send an occult blood test kit home with a patient receiving long-term NSAI therapy; look for evidence of drug-induced dementia or depression in elderly patients; monitor blood pressure; and look for bruises and nail-bed bleeding in patients receiving anticoagulants.

Summary

Once a professional aims for an outcome, the necessity of client cooperation usually becomes apparent. Once the professional recognizes the need for cooperation, care becomes necessary. Furthermore, care can take both the professional and the client far beyond the level of professional services provided with scientific detachment.

However, care is not sufficient for a professional relationship. Some philosophical problems with care can be ameliorated by understanding it in the context of a professional covenant. We have proposed a formulation, *competent care,* to denote a series of decisions and actions that would be made by a responsible, knowledgeable, and skilled professional toward improving a client's quality of life. Quality of life should be defined as the client would define it if he possessed the knowledge and skill of the professional along with his own basic values. In this context, *responsible* means moral trustworthiness and refers to the behavior of a disciplined person who expected to be held accountable for his/her contribution to the outcome. Caring and competence are mutually supportive and may well be synergistic. Care may be rooted in the motivation to successfully provide professional service, but its leaf can be the transformation of practice.

Enacting Care

Pharmaceutical care is equally a philosophy manifested by action and a set of actions guided by a philosophy. That is, because pharmaceutical care is an idea about helping people make the best use of their medicines, its meaning depends upon its being enacted.

The nursing literature lists a number of caring behaviors that can guide nursing care: attentive listening; comforting; accepting responsibility; informing; touching; behaving sensitively, honestly, respectfully, and patiently; and calling a person by his name (Sprengel & Kelley 1992).

Another, more formal, way to describe the enactment of care is to propose that it would include the actions of continuous improvement. The theory of pharmaceutical care is similar in some ways to the theory of continuous improvement (CI). Likewise, the actions of pharmaceutical care are, in many ways, the actions of CI applied to individual patient outcomes. For example, the CI formulation called PDSA includes four steps: Plan, Do, Study, and Act (Batalden and Stoltz 1993; Gitlow and Melby 1991).

Consider the following example:

When Mr. Smith gave his prescription for cimetidine to Mr. Jones, the pharmacist did not just take the prescription "in the back" to fill it. Instead, Jones asked Smith some questions and wrote the answers down on a card. Smith did not feel too comfortable about the questions. No pharmacist had ever asked him questions before, other than his name, address and the name of his doctor. This pharmacist wanted to know whether Smith had taken this medicine before (He had not.), what medicines he had tried in the past (He had taken antacids.), and whether Smith's symptoms were more like a pain in his side or more like heartburn (They were more like heartburn.). He also seemed really curious about Smith's other medical problems and what medicines Smith used. Smith wondered why Jones wanted to know these things. He thought about asking, but instead he just answered the questions and added, "How long is this going to take? I'm really in a hurry."

After about 15 minutes, the pharmacist brought the filled prescription to Mr. Smith. Smith had not expected this visit to the pharmacy to take this long and was worried about missing his bus. Jones started to explain some things that

Smith did not really listen to, but one thing stood out very clearly. Jones had called Smith's doctor and the doctor had changed the prescription. This made Smith a little nervous because the doctor now knew that Smith had carried the prescription around for a week before bringing it in. Smith wondered why Jones would do that. Smith wanted to know if his doctor had made a mistake, but there was no time left to find out. He repeated that he was in a hurry, paid for the prescription, and left.

The next day, Jones telephoned Smith at home. After identifying himself, Jones said, "I had the feeling that you did not get your questions answered when you left yesterday, so I thought I'd give you a call to see how you are doing." Smith was a bit concerned and asked if anything was wrong. Jones replied that everything was OK from his perspective, but he wanted to know how Smith was doing. Smith said that the medicine was not helping, and he asked the questions that he had not asked before. Jones explained that there had been no mistake. Another medicine Smith was taking for his blood pressure would not go well with the cimetidine, so Jones had suggested to Smith's doctor that he switch to ranitidine, and the doctor agreed.

Finally, Jones said, "Well, it will take a while longer for you to really find out if the medicine is helping you. I recommend that you give it at least a week more. It would be best if you avoided using antacids within an hour of taking the medicine. Call me if you have any questions. Let me or Dr. Brown know right away if you notice any dizziness. Next time you are in the neighborhood, stop in and see me or, if it's OK, I'll call you in about a week to see how you are doing."

Each person should see a professional relationship as mutually beneficial. A patient may not be able to correctly interpret a pharmacist's actions or questions in the context of the past "dispensing and advising" relationship. Or, a patient may not want a pharmacist to provide pharmaceutical care and may therefore not want a new relationship with a pharmacist for that purpose. There are several possible reasons that a patient may not want to take part in pharmaceutical care. The patient may tacitly assume that the pharmacist would provide services limited to dispensing and advising, as in the past; the patient may simply not appreciate the dangers of drug therapy or recognize the pharmacist's possible contribution; or the patient may worry about the pharmacist getting in the way of the patient's relationship with his physician.

According to normal business-consumer views, the pharmacist should let the customer decide what their relationship will be and what services will be provided. On the other hand, philanthropic, paternalistic professionalism would suggest that the pharmacist tell the patient what services and what relationship the pharmacist thinks is appropriate. Care is a third option, in which the pharmacist makes a professional decision, as described in the previous section, and then asks a question or recommends an action, either to the patient or the physician. The objective is not to please the customer or to please the pharmacist. The initial purpose is to establish a relationship that facilitates effective services. In the example, Jones seems to have focused on information essential for the effective management of Smith's problem.

The desire to explain an exciting new idea like pharmaceutical care to patients can be quite strong. Wanting to be accepted as a caring professional and an apparent misinterpretation of the pharmacist's actions by the patient may push the pharmacist toward giving a mini-lecture on pharmaceutical care. Sometimes, this may be advisable. For example, the pharmacist may have professional credibility with a patient. If the pharmacist is proposing a major change, such as an asthma management program or a diabetes education program, a written description like a brochure followed up with oral discussion may be exactly what is needed. In other circumstances, however, the pharmacist may decide simply to enact, that is, to demonstrate, his or her side of the new relationship. For example, suppose Jones noticed Smith's confusion about the transaction. An explanation of pharmaceutical care might have been counterproductive under those circumstances, unless it included a ride home. However, a telephone call to ask how the medicine was working served two important purposes. It helped pharmacist Jones achieve his therapeutic objectives for Mr. Smith, and it helped Mr. Smith to understand what Jones was trying to accomplish. At least it offered an opportunity for questions and discussion.

The following discussion is an outline of the topics and basic questions involved in enacting a caring professional relationship. Although the activities frequently take place in the order they are listed, the order and timing of addressing these topics requires judgment about specific circumstances at hand. Some questions may be inappropriate in some circumstances. Furthermore, effective professional communications require knowledge, skill, and attitudes that are beyond the scope of this chapter. For example, a respectful manner, demonstrations of empathy, and active listening all are important. Basic questions should be framed and worded appropriately for the circumstances.

Establishing a Caring Relationship: Joining

Joining is the process of establishing relationships based on common interest. Pharmaceutical care to outpatients requires at least a brief medical and medication history. Joining should begin when the pharmacist takes the patient's history, as long or as brief as that needs to be. Questions like the following are essential in pharmaceutical care not only because they give the pharmacist vital information about the patient but also because they demonstrate and initiate the relationship that the pharmacist wants to have with the client. The pharmacist should ask these questions when taking a history, perhaps interspersed with more specific medical and pharmaceutical questions, and at other times during the care of the patient.

1. What do you hope to accomplish with this medicine? What do you really want this medicine to do for you? Examples of responses are cure, control of disease or symptoms, control of life, ability to function.

2. What are your symptoms like to you? The objective in asking this question is to learn about the patient's subjective illness experience.

3. What effect, if any, does this illness have on your life? For example, some asthmatic or heart patients give up second-floor sleeping quarters because they cannot comfortably climb the stairs.

4. What aspects of therapy with this medicine are you unsure about?

Relationships can be enhanced by actively taking in and acting on information. Active listening requires providing verbal evidence that the listener is processing information. Other behaviors consistent with acting on information are taking notes, referring to past events, and reaching conclusions. An example of acting on information is the response, "My notes reminded me that last year a medicine like this one made you really sleepy, and you just said that you wanted this medicine to help you enjoy your children when they visit next week."

Some clients may not understand why the pharmacist is asking questions about their treatment. Sensitivity to such concerns is very important. It can take time to develop the necessary relationship. However, caring, as respectful commitment to the patient's welfare, requires that the pharmacist obtain the necessary information. Collecting from a patient information that you confidently believe is necessary for the successful management of therapy is an eloquent indication of both your competence and your interest in the patient's best interests.

Obtaining a History

The quality of the care provided by the pharmacist depends in two major respects on the information that the pharmacist has about the patient. First, the specific care activities to be provided should depend upon the patient's needs, as assessed from patient information (Strand et al. 1991). Second, the appropriateness of care provided depends on the completeness and accuracy of patient information. What information the pharmacist should obtain directly from the patient depends on the practice environment. In a hospital practice, for example, a lot of the necessary information may already be in the medical record. In community pharmacy, the pharmacist may need to collect and document more necessary information. In some instances, a patient referral form, similar to those used to refer a patient for home care, will provide some information.

Both structure and professional judgement are necessary prerequisites to obtain an acceptable history. A history should include basic demographic, administrative, medical, pharmaceutical, and sociobehavioral questions. The structure can be provided by a standardized form. In community practice, many patients can complete such a form themselves, without taking up the pharmacist's time, although there should always be some face-to-face communication about the patient's history to verify and complete the information. Both subjective and objective information may be important. Subjective information includes the patient's symptoms, values, disease experience, and objectives, as described above. Objective information is all verifiable facts.

Despite some pharmacists' academic bias toward collecting all available information, collecting unnecessary information is inefficient; may delay collecting necessary information; and may obscure the significance of necessary information. The objective is to collect information that is reasonably likely to be relevant to care. Meeting this objective requires a process similar to the professional decision making process described above, where the pharmacist taking the history interprets information already received, such as information from a history form, to guide subsequent requests for information.

Recognizing Therapeutic Objectives and Alternatives

The next step in enacting care is the evaluation of the therapeutic plan in the context of therapeutic objectives. This is a process of reconciling, as much as is necessary and possible, clinical objectives; values, such as quality of life objectives; and therapeutic possibilities. This step is one of the pharmacist's major opportunities for professional decision making. It requires implementing the professional decision making process described above and the exercising professional judgement in a dialogue between general principles and the patient's specific circumstances. In the example above, the pharmacist asked about other medicines that Smith was using and got information that caused him to reconsider the therapeutic plan. In another example, the pharmacist may know something about a patient's therapeutic objectives or concerns or idiosyncrasies.

Strand, Cipolle, and Morley have proposed eight categories of pharmaceutical problems which provide a structure for evaluating a prescription or therapeutic regimen (Strand, Cipolle, and Morley 1988; Strand, Cipolle, and Morley, 1990). This evaluation process requires the pharmacist to collect and to evaluate possible outcomes of therapy.

Developing a Monitoring Plan

After the medication regimen or therapeutic plan is established, the next step is the construction of a written monitoring plan. The central issues are what information will be needed for monitoring, why it is necessary, how it will be used, and how it will be obtained.

The objective is to develop a simple written plan to obtain the information that is needed, but only the information that is needed, to monitor the patient's progress toward clinical and quality of life therapeutic objectives.

The monitoring plan should briefly state what information will be collected, how it will be collected, when it will be collected, and who will collect it. If the appropriate use of the information would not be obvious, the plan should also describe that use. For example, if the monitoring plan included collecting information on peak flow readings, the plan might state, "consult Dr. Brown if maximum daily PFM readings are below _____."

Discussing Objectives and Responsibilities

Changing a familiar professional relationship introduces ambiguity about the respective duties of the participants. For example, suppose a pharmacist begins to move the familiar dispensing and advising relationship toward a pharmaceutical care relationship as described above. The client and the physician (and others) may become unsure of what changes in the usual pattern of duties may be necessary. (Relationships with colleagues are discussed in Chapter 11.)

The pharmacist who is accepting new responsibilities should make these duties explicit to others and also be prepared to demonstrate the corresponding responsibilities that others, especially the patient are expected to take on. This step should follow the development of a monitoring plan so that the pharmacist knows exactly what actions and information will be needed and when. Armed with this information, the pharmacist can ask the patient or caregiver for the necessary assistance. In the example above, pharmacist Jones stated what he would do and what he expected Smith to do. Normally, this would happen as a part of the dispensing and advising process.

Advising a patient in pharmaceutical care might have quite different objectives than advising a patient in some traditional relationships. In pharmaceutical care, the patient or caregiver is a partner in care, to the extent possible given the patient's circumstances, and the nature of the drug therapy. Therefore, advising is an activity of patient empowerment rather than of information transfer. The pharmacist would be more interested in what the patient actually *did* or was *able to do* than in what the patient knew or was able to recite. Informing the patient to achieve outcomes, rather than as an outcome in itself, requires a focus on action. In the example, Jones asked Smith to let him know if Smith noticed any dizziness and to check with him in a week or so. A pharmacist who is monitoring a patient should routinely follow up with a note to the physician describing significant findings and actions. For example, pharmacist Jones might send a note saying, "I spoke to Mr. Smith today on the telephone. He reported that the ranitidine 'was not helping' his heartburn. I recommended that he continue the medicine for a week but to call you or me if he noticed any dizziness. I will check him in a week."

Implementing the Monitoring Plan

Pharmaceutical care requires a reliable means of carrying out the monitoring plan. For example, when the monitoring plan is written or updated, the patient's name could be placed in a log book under the date of the next follow up. Then, when that date arrived, each record could be consulted and the plan carried out.

Pharmaceutical care involves more than therapeutic drug monitoring, that is, monitoring clinical effect. Monitoring should always include questions about the patient's subjective response to therapy, including ability to carry out desired activities, ability to meet social role obligations, satisfaction with care, and future intentions. In some cases this should be done formally with specific questions designed for this purpose (e.g., the SF-36) (Bungay and Ware 1993).

The pharmacist should evaluate the patient's progress toward definite outcomes according to a systematic process. The pharmacist should follow up possibly significant evidence of treatment success or failure. There are three basic questions:

1. Is the patient actually receiving the medicine? For example, does the refill history appear consistent with intended use? Can the patient correctly use administration devices, such as metered-dose inhalers or syringes?

2. Is there evidence that the medicine is achieving the intended result in an appropriate time?

3. Is there evidence of a new medical problem, such as a side effect, toxicity, or an adverse drug reaction?

Resolving Pharmaceutical Problems

Information processed by the pharmacist is worthless to the patient unless it is followed by behavior. The final step in the process of enacting pharmaceutical care is to resolve any pharmaceutical problems that were detected in monitoring and to document all relevant information obtained, problems identified, actions taken, and recommendations made.

The pharmacist can choose the extent of his participation in pharmaceutical care. There are two basic stages. The pharmacist can detect evidence of possible pharmaceutical problems as described above and then notify the physician of the evidence, or, the pharmacist can proceed to define and resolve the detected problem and recommend action to the physician, patient, or caregiver. The first stage can be called *drug therapy monitoring* and the second *drug therapy management*. How far the pharmacist proceeds should depend on the problem, the pharmacist's competence and confidence, and the nature of the specific professional, collegial, and ministerial relationships involved. For example, suppose Mrs. Hubbard, an asthmatic patient, requests a refill of her albuterol metered-dose inhaler. Pharmacist Joan Grey notices that the last inhaler refill was two weeks ago. One inhaler has typically lasted four weeks for Mrs. Hubbard. Joan Grey knows that increased beta-agonist use been shown to predict increased risk of asthmatic crisis (Spitzer et al. 1992). In a caring relationship, Grey is obliged *at least* to notice this indicator of possible trouble and to take some action. To simply refill the prescription without considering the patient's welfare would violate the professional relationship between Hubbard and Grey. However, a variety of actions are possible. Four examples may illustrate the range of possibilities:

1. *Basic Monitoring*. Pharmacist Grey could advise Mrs. Hubbard that her increased MDI use could indicate a problem and recommend that she consult her physician, Dr. Brown.

2. *Thorough Monitoring*. Grey could assess Mrs. Hubbard's present condition. For example Grey could ask whether she is coughing more lately, having more frequent attacks, or waking up at night because of asthma, and whether asthma is interfering with normal activities. Grey could then refer Mrs. Hubbard to Dr. Brown or to an emergency room based on that assessment.

3. *Dosage Form Management*. Pharmacist Grey could ask Mrs. Hubbard to demonstrate how she uses the inhaler and assess her technique. It is possible that Mrs. Hubbard's asthma is not worsening but that her inhaler technique is. If that were the apparent problem, pharmacist Grey could train Mrs. Hubbard about proper MDI use.

4. *Therapeutic Management*. Grey could follow alternative two with a specific recommendation to the physician. For example:

   Doctor Brown, I have just seen Mrs. Hubbard and I'm concerned that she is having an asthma flareup. I advised her to see you in the next day or two—I hope you can work her in. After you have seen her, it is possible that you will want to consider a short course of steroids. I would recommend 40–60 mg of prednisone daily for seven days and then re-evaluation in your office. If it is OK with you, after this flareup is over I would like to train Mrs. Hubbard to use a peak flow meter so that we can see her exacerbations coming a bit sooner.

Conclusion

Many people feel a spontaneous impulse to help another person when they see a problem. The "man on the street" would pull a young child who had strayed into traffic back onto the sidewalk without thoughts of his own convenience or qualifications to act. The obligations of a professional are similar but go further. The point of a professional relationship is to actively seek solutions to problems and to take action within the limits of competence. Improving patients' quality of life by improving the outcomes of drug therapy requires that the pharmacist seek opportunities to improve outcomes among patients and then take those opportunities.

Relationships are an essential means to reaching this objective. Caring behavior goes on as long as the relationship lasts—regardless of whether the patient knows enough to ask for care or whether others agree. Pharmaceutical care is action oriented. It need not be technically complex. It does not necessarily require knowledge of clinical pharmacology beyond that of a typical, competent pharmacist. It does require action. The professional is in an unique position to see opportunities and to act. Even small steps, taken often enough, will lead to large advancement.

References

Batalden, P. B., and P. K. Stoltz. 1993. A Framework for the Continual Improvement of Health Care: Building and Applying Professional and Improvement Knowledge to Test Changes in Daily Work. *Journal of Quality Improvement* 19:424–52.

Brodie, D. C., P. A. Parish, and J. W. Poston. 1980. Societal Needs for Drugs and Drug Related Services. *Am J Pharmacy Education* 44:276–8.

Brody, B. A. 1988. *Life and Death Decision Making*. New York, NY: Oxford University Press.

Bungay, K. M., and J. E. Ware. 1993. *Measuring and Monitoring Health-Related Quality of Life* Kalamazoo: The Upjohn Company.

Cooper, M. C. 1988. Covenantal Relationships: Grounding for the Nursing Ethic. *Advances in Nursing Science* 10:48–59.

Curzer, H. J. 1993. Is Care a Virtue for Health Care Professionals? *J Medical Philosophy* 18:51–69.

Dossey, L. 1984. *Beyond Illness*. Boulder & London: New Science Library.

Freidson, E. 1989. *Medical work in America: Essays on Health Care*. New Haven: Yale University Press.

Gatens-Robinson, E. 1986. Clinical Judgement and the Rationality of the Human Sciences. *Journal of Medicine and Philosophy* 11:167–78.

Engel, G. L. 1988. How Much Longer Must Medicine's Science Be Bound by a Seventeenth-century World View? In *The Task of Medicine—Dialogue at Wickenburg*, ed. K. L. White. Palo Alto: Henry J. Kaiser Family Foundation.

Gilligan, C. 1982. *In a Different Voice*, 62 Cambridge: Harvard University Press.

Gitlow, H. S., and M. J. Melby. 1991. Framework for Continuous Quality Improvement in the Provision of Pharmaceutical Care. *American Journal of Hospital Pharmacy* 48:1417–25.

Hepler, C. D. 1987. The Third Wave in Pharmaceutical Education: The Clinical Movement. *American Journal of Pharmaceutical Education* 51:369–85.

Hepler, C. D. 1990. The Future of Pharmacy: Pharmaceutical Care. *American Pharmacy* NS30:583–9.

Hepler, C. D., and L. M. Strand. 1989. Opportunities and Responsibilities in Pharmaceutical Care. *American Journal of Pharmaceutical Education* 53 (SUPPL):7s–15s.

Larsen, M. S. 1977. *The Rise of Professionalism*. Berkeley: University of California Press.

May, W. F. 1975. Code and Covenant or Philanthropy and Contract? Hastings-on-the-Hudson, Hastings NY *Hastings Center Report* 5:29–38.

May, W. F. 1983. The physician's covenant: Images of the healer in medical ethics. Philadelphia, PA: Westminster Press.

Nortvedt, P. 1993. Emotions, Care and Particularity. *Vard. Nord. Utveckl. Forsk.* 13:18–24.

Pierce, C. S. 1956. The Fixation of Belief. In *The Enduring Questions: Main Problems of Philosophy*, ed. M. Rader, 88–99. New York: Henry Holt & Co.

Pool, R. 1988. More Squabbling Over Unbelievable Result (Research News) *Science* 241:658.

Pool, R. 1989. Fusion Followup: Confusion Abounds (Research News) *Science*. 244:27–9.

Reichenbach, H. 1958. *The Rise of Scientific Philosophy*. Berkeley: University of California Press.

Spitzer, W. O., et al. 1992. The Use of Beta-agonists and the Risk of Death and Near Death from Asthma. *New England J Med* 326:501–6.

Sprengel, A., and Kelley, J. 1992. The ethics of caring: A basis for holistic care. *Journal of Holistic Nursing* 10(3):231–9.

Starr, P. 1982. *The Social Transformation of American Medicine*. New York: Basic Books.

Strand, L. M., et al. 1991. Levels of Pharmaceutical Care: A Needs-based Approach. *American Journal of Hospital Pharmacy* 48:547–550.

Strand, L. M., R. J. Cipolle, and P. C. Morley. 1988. Documenting the Clinical Pharmacist's Activities: Back to Basics. *DICP Annals of Pharmacotherapy* 22:63–6.

Strand, L. M., R. J. Cipolle, and P. C. Morley. 1990. Drug Related Problems: Their Structure and Function. *DICP Annals of Pharmacotherapy* 24:1093–7.

Thomasma, D. C. 1986. Philosophical Reflections on a Rational Treatment Plan. *Journal of Medicine and Philosophy* 11:157–65.

Veatch, R. M. 1981. *A Theory of Medical Ethics*, 110–38. New York: Basic Books.

Waters, D. B., and E. C. Lawrence, 1993. *Competence, Courage and Change. An Approach to Family Therapy*. New York: W.W. Norton & Co.

Watson, M. J. 1988. New Dimensions in Human Caring Theory. *Nursing Science Quarterly*. 1:175–81.

Wulff, H. R. 1986. Rational Diagnosis and Treatment. *Journal of Medicine and Philosophy* 11:123–34.

9

Outcomes of Drug Therapy

David M. Angaran, Ph.D.
Charles D. Hepler, M.S.

Three interrelated health care issues both influence the attractiveness of professional services and justify professionals' claims to serve the public interest: accessibility, cost, and quality. The ability of pharmacists to influence the conditions and value of their practices may depend to a large extent on their ability to maintain a market for those services. In turn, maintaining a market for pharmaceutical services may depend greatly on pharmacists' ability to influence accessibility, cost, or quality of health care.

Outcomes directly affect cost and quality of care. In fact, people and their governments may define quality of care in terms of outcomes. For example, the U.S. Office of Technology Assessment (OTA) defines *quality of health care* as, "the degree to which the process of care increases the probability of outcomes desired by patients and reduces the probability of undesired outcomes given the current state of knowledge (OTA 1988)." Also, outcomes are of fundamental importance to the people we care for and the people who pay for care, more important than the organizations and processes of care.

Pharmaceutical care is outcome oriented. One definition of pharmaceutical care includes the phrase, "definite outcomes intended to improve a patient's quality of life (Hepler and Strand 1990)." Hepler and Strand then enumerate four outcomes:

1) Cure of a disease
2) Elimination or reduction of a patient's symptomatology
3) Arresting or slowing of a disease process
4) Preventing a disease or symptomatology

This chapter will explore patient outcomes: ways to think about outcomes, how patients may experience them, and how professionals may recognize them. Finally, it will describe programs for the continual improvement of the outcomes of drug therapy.

Outcomes, Outputs, Therapeutic Objectives and Patient Progress

If a cure, control of symptoms, or retardation or prevention of diseases are outcomes, and if a patient's quality of life is also an outcome, the definition of pharmaceutical care involves patient outcomes on at least two levels of complexity. This may appear to be mainly a problem of terminology. However, vague terminology often conceals real problems of conceptual clarity. In such cases, professional purpose may be blurred and performance reduced.

To begin from a broad perspective, a person's life can be understood as comprising many *processes* (e.g., working, playing, eating, resting), that occur in one or more *structures* (e.g., the society within which the person lives, its cultures, institutions, and organizations). In this framework, health care is one group of processes occurring in one group of structures within the larger socio-economic environments. In health care, as in life, every outcome (e.g., chronic hyperglycemia as an "outcome" of diabetes) seems to give way to another outcome (e.g., chronic renal failure). An *outcome* is defined in plain English as, "the final result of complex or conflicting causes or forces (Webster's New Collegiate Dictionary)."

Avedis Donabedian has defined an outcome of health care as a change in state or condition attributable to antecedent health care. He includes changes in health states, changes in knowledge or behavior pertinent to future health states, and satisfaction with health care (expressed as opinion or inferred from behavior) in his definition (Donabedian 1992). (See Table 9-1 for a classification of outcomes.) A. Donabedian The role of outcomes in quality assessment and assurance. *Quality Review Bulletin* 18(11):356–60 1992 Nov.

Either definition of outcome is too vague to be useful in helping the clinician decide what events in the course of pharmaceutical care should be called "outcomes." Outcome is somewhat easier to define in acute, episodic illness than in chronic illness, because therapy within the episode usually has a clear end. Consider, for example, a patient receiving five days of norfloxacin for the treatment of a urinary tract infection (UTI). Cure of the UTI would be an outcome according to both definitions, as the cure would be a *change in status* which is the *result* of antecedent health care. Remission of symptoms or disappearance of bactiuria satisfies Donabedian's definition, but not the common definition. Because symptoms and bactiuria can return if treatment is too short, such an outcome would not be final in any sense.

Outcomes are even harder to define for chronic diseases. Consider for example Mr. A and Mr. B, who have been receiving drug therapy for hypertension for six months. Both have mean diastolic blood pressures (dbp) of 95. Mr. A is on a diet and exercise program, and his dbp is slowly falling. B's dbp has been approximately constant for the last three months. Should either person's blood pressure on a certain date or after a certain period of therapy be called an outcome? Shall we say, according to the common definition, that Mr. B's blood pressure

Table 9.1. Outcome Definition, Classification, and Listing of Some Outcomes of Health Care

A. Clinical
  1. Reported systems that have clinical significance
  2. Diagnostic categorization as an indication of morbidity
  3. Disease staging relevant to functional encroachment and prognosis
  4. Diagnostic performance—the frequency of false positives and false negatives as indicators of diagnostic or case-finding performance
B. Physiologic-biochemical
  1. Abnormalities
  2. Functions
    a. Loss of function
    b. Functional reserve—includes performance in test situations under various degrees of stress
C. Physical
  1. Loss or impairment of structural form or integrity—includes abnormalities, defects, and disfigurement
  2. Functional performance of physical activities and tasks
    a. Under the circumstances of daily living
    b. Under test conditions that involve various degrees of stress.
D. Psychologic-mental
  1. Feelings—includes discomfort, pain, fear, anxiety, or their opposites, including satisfaction
  2. Beliefs that are relevant to health and health care
  3. Knowledge that is relevant to healthful living, health care, and coping with illness
  4. Impairments of discrete psychologic or mental functions
    a. Under the circumstances of daily living
    b. Under test conditions that involve various degrees of stress
E. Social and psychosocial
  1. Behaviors relevant to coping with current illness or affecting future health, including adherence to health care regimens and changes in health-related habits
  2. Role performance
    a. Marital
    b. Familial
    c. Occupational
    d. Other interpersonal
  3. Performance under test conditions involving varying degrees of stress
F. Integrative outcomes
  1. Mortality
  2. Longevity
  3. Longevity with adjustments made to take account of impairments of physical, psychologic, and psychosocial function—"full-function equivalents"
  4. Monetary value of the above
G. Evaluative outcomes
  1. Client opinions about, and satisfaction with, various aspects of care, including accessibility, continuity, thoroughness, humaneness, informativeness, effectiveness, and cost

Adapted from Donabedian A. The Role of Outcomes in Quality Assessment and Assurance. QRB 1992: 18:356–360.

is an outcome because it is a stable result, but A's outcome is still in the future because his dbp is still changing? Or, shall we say, according to Donabedian's definition, that Mr A's blood pressure is an outcome because it has changed since his last visit, but Mr. B.'s is not because it has not changed? Furthermore, although we may be justified in assuming that drug therapy has lowered both men's blood pressures, how shall we know whether A's still-falling diastolic pressure is a result of health care, as required by Donabedian's definition, or lifestyle?

The processes of life and health care are indeed complex and conflicting, and they have many outcomes. There are few or no "final results" of health care (or life) as long as a person remains alive. It is much easier to define the *output* of a specific process, especially for a specific patient. *Output* is an engineering term denoting the immediate result of a process acting on an input. For example, the output of a radio circuit might be a.c. voltage from 0–6 volts, which can be converted to sound by loudspeakers. Figure 9-1 shows a diagram of a generic process in which inputs go through a process and are converted to an output.

For example, consider the patient receiving treatment for a UTI. Three significant inputs to drug therapy are: the patient with the symptoms of a UTI, the therapeutic regimen, and a drug product (in this case, norfloxacin tablets). The output is a patient receiving therapy with norfloxacin. The output of continued therapy is symptom resolution and disappearance of bactiuria, and the outcome (cure) results from many such outputs, only some of which are humanly controllable, and uncontrollable environmental circumstances, such as, the patient's genetic disposition, immune status, and general health.

The process view is consistent with an older view which describes health care

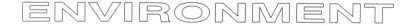

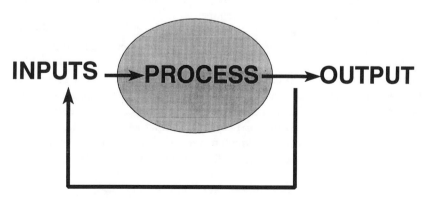

Figure 9.1.

as consisting of discrete episodes, such as office visits or hospitalizations. Figure 9-1 is a view which describes health care as a continuous process in which each output forms a part of the input to the next set of processes. For simplicity, the diagram shows only one generic process, which represents a large variety of specific processes that a patient might go through during care. To continue the UTI example, the output from one visit—a person beginning treatment with norfloxacin for a UTI—becomes part of the input to the next. The first process may be diagnostic services by a physician. The second process may be dispensing and advising by a pharmacist. The third process may be a followup visit or phone call, a prescription refill, or anyone of a number of possibilities.

The outcome of these continuous processes of care is the patient's health status either when care is terminated, for example when the UTI was cured or when the patient was discharged or transferred, or when health status stabilizes, that is becomes relatively constant over time. We could speak meaningfully of the outcome of continuing chronic disease management if the outputs of the episodes were relatively constant. Otherwise, we should think of them as outputs that can change in response to changes in the processes of care. (See Figure 9-3).

In health care, an intended patient-care output may be called a *therapeutic objective*. A pharmacist or physician may be unable or unwilling to definitely state what outcome of drug therapy should occur or when it should occur, but the pharmacist or physician should be able to specify a therapeutic objective, which is an intended, proximate result of therapy. For example, months of negative urine cultures may be necessary before one can announce the cure of a urinary tract infection. However, one *therapeutic objective* of antibiotic therapy is remission of symptoms and bacteriuria. This distinction between symptom remission and cure is important, and different terms would help keep the difference clear.

On one hand, reaching the therapeutic objective is not the same as reaching the outcome, merely a step toward it. On the other hand, not reaching the therapeutic objective in a few days may suggest that, even over time, no cure will occur in that patient with that regimen.

An outcome, such as a cure, is usually more valued than an output, but outcomes are harder for professionals to define and control and often require more time to be realized. Outputs, while less significant, are more achievable— that is, they are easier to define and to control and usually occur sooner. The term output is rarely used in health care to mean an achieved therapeutic objective, perhaps because it sounds too cold and objective. However, it is important for patients and professionals to avoid confusing output and outcome, just as it is important to avoid confusing symptom remission with cure. A term for an achieved therapeutic objective should distinguish it from both a desired objective and an achieved goal.

The closest term for an output in common use is *progress*, as in *progress notes* or, "the patient continues to make progress."[1] The terms *therapeutic result, intermediate outcome, process-outcome,* or *therapeutic outcome* may also be useful ways to express the precise outputs of a defined therapeutic process. These therapeutic results must be definite in order for drug therapy to satisfy the definition of pharmaceutical care given above.

Major elements in the management of drug therapy, therefore, are the identification, in advance of both desired and undesired possible or likely therapeutic results and the specification of approximately when the results should be expected to appear. For example, in a particular patient, first-dose dizziness from hypotension from ACE inhibitors, if it is going to occur, should be expected between one and four hours after administration. Symptom remission from antibiotic therapy of a UTI should appear within 24 to 48 hours. If symptoms persist beyond this time, a prompt change in therapy is indicated. Also, if the person who will notice these results, such as a patient or caregiver, may not be able to interpret the results correctly, then the significance of these results also should be specified in advance. This is common practice in inpatient care when a physician writes a chart note to the effect of, "Call me if. . . ."

In summary, pharmaceutical care includes the management of the processes of drug therapy. These processes can be managed by setting therapeutic objectives, which are intended to lead to therapeutic results, which in turn are the most likely to lead to desired patient outcomes.

Points of View: Perception of Therapeutic Results and Outcomes

Monitoring and managing drug therapy often require information available only from the patient or caregiver and actions that can be taken only by the patient or caregiver. Patients may have different therapeutic objectives than professionals and certainly may experience therapeutic results and outcomes differently. Furthermore, humane practice requires that caregivers respect patient values and preferences. For these reasons, professionals should recognize the different points of view involved in the management of therapy, in particular the patient's point of view, and negotiate, if possible, common goals.

Whose Therapeutic Objectives?

To have a patient as partner, the professional should accept that the patient's primary reality, his illness experience, may be different from the health professional's expectations. People with diseases do not always feel ill or act sick in

---

[1]Outside of psychiatry or rehabilitation, this is strange usage, as it seems to imply that progress is something the patient "makes." Patients who do not "make" progress are often described as having "failed therapy" when indeed it is the therapy which failed the patient.

the way we would expect. Sometimes, therefore, health professionals may expect the patient to follow instructions that have no basis in reality as the patient perceives it. This raises an important question that can be only be touched upon here: whose outcomes are important?[2]

Perhaps what the patient wants most from therapy is the ability to participate in certain activities, or perhaps he is willing to cooperate in care only as long as it does not interfere with such activities. This may not imply recklessness or foolishness. Difficult compromise is sometimes preferable to the theoretically ideal therapeutic plan. Suppose that a patient's blood pressure is not quite as good on thiazides as it had been on beta-blockers, but the patient has better quality of life. Whose outcomes is the team supposed to work for?

From a clinical perspective, the pharmacist should be actively monitoring medicine use and clinical results and keeping the team informed about these issues. However, she also has an opportunity to know how the therapy is affecting the patient's life and to keep the team informed about that.

Disease and Illness

A fundamental and essential distinction is made in the sociology of medicine between the personal experience of disease and its vicarious experience by a professional. This distinction is involved in the following example:

> Mr. Green, a regular patient in a pharmacy, asks to speak to the pharmacist. Mr. Green is holding a bottle of 250 ibuprofen tablets, 200 mg, which he intends to buy, but first he wants to know, "if ibuprofen can make you feel tired all the time and dizzy." Pharmacist Grey replies that although dizziness and drowsiness are reported side effects of ibuprofen, they may go away during treatment and usually do not require medical attention. She asks Mr. Green about other medicines that he might use (none) and then about his diet and sleep habits (normal). She politely terminates the discussion. Mr. Green buys the ibuprofen and leaves.

> A week after this conversation, Mr. Green's daughter calls 911 because his weakness and grey pallor frighten her. In the emergency room, his hematocrit and red blood cell count show that he is extremely anemic. He requires six units of whole blood. Fecal test for occult blood is positive. Endoscopy shows that Mr. Green has been bleeding from a gastric lesion.

Illness, Wellness, and Quality of Life

The terms *illness* and *wellness* refer to a person's subjective experience, such as, feelings and perceived ability to function. For example, a person may experi-

---

[2]This may be a difficult issue even with a highly symptomatic disease. It is even more difficult for asymptomatic diseases like hypertension. In addition to the "disease" and "illness" perceptions of reality, basic values and assumptions about responsibility for outcomes and autonomy are involved. These are important issues but happen to be outside the objective of this chapter.

ence chest pain and shortness of breath on exertion. Mr. Green knew that he felt tired and occasionally dizzy. Furthermore, the person may or may not act *sick*, that is change his activities, as a result of illness. Illness experience and sickness behavior are the primary realities of health care. That is, patients experience them directly. They often comprise the motivation for, and basis of, health care and they may powerfully influence a person's other life experiences.

Although there is no generally accepted definition for the phrase quality of life, the phrase refers to a person's satisfaction with life, their sense of well-being, and their subjectively experienced ability to perform certain activities (MacKeigan and Pathak 1992). These activities include pleasurable and recreational activities and those activities necessary to take care of oneself, activities of daily living and to meet social role expectations as a worker, spouse, parent, or friend.

> Quality of Life represents the functional effects of an illness and its consequent therapy upon a patient, as perceived by the patient. Four broad domains contribute to the overall effect: physical and occupational function; psychological state; social interaction and somatic sensation (Schipper, Clinch, and Powell 1990).

Diseases and Diagnoses

The term *disease* is reserved for the professional interpretation of the person's account of illness experience and any additional objective or subjective information the professional obtains, such as, from physical examination or laboratory tests results. A disease can be thought of as a professional's *secondary* perception of the primary illness experience. Disease is an interpretation of reality, the theoretical reality of diagnosis, pathophysiology, and therapeutics.

For example, a person experiencing chest pain and shortness of breath may visit a doctor for tests. After examination and testing, the physician may diagnose his condition as a recognized disease, perhaps angina pectoris or hiatal hernia complicated by obesity and poor physical conditioning, or as "essentially normal." If the doctor recognizes a disease or syndrome, she gains access to general knowledge that may be essential in managing the patient. In this example, although she may not know very much about this patient's angina, she may know a lot about angina from scientific studies and clinical experience. Nonetheless, this general knowledge, no matter how scientifically based, is abstract knowledge about people other than the patient. It is obviously not a valid substitute for the patient's primary experience.

Illness and Health-Related Quality of Life

Quality of life may be significantly influenced by non-health related issues like socioeconomic status. Furthermore, some peoples' health-related quality of life may be influenced more by their feelings of illness or wellness than by objective disease status. Therefore, it is possible for the treatment of disease to increase feelings of illness or reduce quality of life more than the disease itself. For example, Jachuk (1982) reported on the outcome of the treatment of hypertension from the perspectives of physicians, patients, and family members. Physicians reported that 90 percent of the patients were doing better. Only 50 percent of the patients reported that they were feeling better, while the family members felt that 95 percent of the patients were doing worse. This contrast among the "outcomes" the practitioner may focus on suggests that the distinction between health-related and non-health-related quality of life may be blurry.

Pharmacists should consider therapy's influence on the patient's illness/wellness experience and quality of life. Influence may involve simple or complex mechanisms, for example a patient may feel that drug therapy is reducing quality of life, perhaps by causing side effects, therapy may be affecting the lives of family and friends, and family and friends may affect a patient's quality of life.

Also, pharmacists and other health professionals should be careful not to ignore a patient's illness just because the patient does not appear to have a disease known to have a symptom or to be taking a drug known to have a particular side effect. While it is rare to openly deny a patient's illness experience, it may not be unusual to ignore symptoms like depression or to state that nothing can be done for symptoms such as chronic pain.

When the professional wants an outcome and the patient does not seem to cooperating in achieving that outcome, the patient, fairly or unfairly, is called "noncompliant." What should we call a professional who does not respond to a patient's illness in the apparent absence of disease? There is no equivalent term for a noncompliant professional, but "professional arrogance" might come to mind. That term may not be entirely accurate, however. Perhaps the cause of the professional's inattention is excessive preoccupation with scientific models of disease and inadequate attention to what the patient is experiencing and trying to describe. In the example above, if Mr. Green had asked pharmacist Grey about gastrointestinal bleeding from ibuprofen, she surely would have replied that it is quite common and recommended a course of action that might have avoided his collapse. The problem may have been that Grey was not concerned about weakness and dizziness unless they were *recognizable* symptoms of an adverse drug reaction. If she had been thinking about Mr. Green's health in general she might have referred him to his physician. As it was, she answered correctly in the narrow context of the direct side effects of ibuprofen, but incorrectly in the broad context of Mr. Green's health.

Systematic Improvement of Outcomes

The philosophy of systematic improvement of outcome originated in industrial production management. It has had various names, but we will refer to it as *continual improvement* (CI). CI is defined by the Joint Commission on Accreditation of Healthcare Organizations (JCAHO) as, "The combination of principles and methods that create both a quality and *customer* focused environment and the capability to identify, *assess* and constantly enhance the efficiency and effectiveness of those *processes* that determine important organizational results."

The origins of pharmaceutical care are in clinical practice, not industrial management. However, both CI and pharmaceutical care are continuous-systems approaches to achieving defined outcomes, and there are analogies between the philosophy of pharmaceutical care and CI, especially as CI is applied to health care. Pharmaceutical care is, in some respects, the application of CI principles to patient outcomes, one patient at a time.

Root Causes

Searching for "root causes" is an essential element of both patient care and CI. For example, a clinician may treat pain with analgesics. Chest pain due to angina can be relieved with analgesics, but pain caused by myocardial ischemia is inappropriate for treatment with analgesics. Instead, coronary vasodialators may be used. However, the ischemia is caused by underlying coronary artery disease, which is caused by elevated serum cholesterol, which is caused by improper diet and exercise habits, and so forth. Correcting causes is more permanent than treating symptoms but requires more understanding. Likewise, a rapid increase in medication errors in a hospital may not mean that the drug distribution system should be completely revamped. Analysis may show that the root cause lies in only part of the system. For example, the increase in errors may be attributed to a few people who did not follow safety guidelines because they were inadequately oriented.

Trigger for Action

A CI and a pharmaceutical care system may trigger corrective action according to different criteria. A pharmaceutical care system addresses one patient at a time. It may not advocate corrective action unless a problem, defined as an obstacle to a desired outcome, can be found.

The CI considers large aggregations or samples of outputs and assumes that the processes leading to those outcomes can be improved. The issue is not so much whether to take action but which action to take.

The components of a system applying the CI philosophy using a combination of performance indicators, guidelines, standards, and a data base is called a Performance Based Evaluation System (PBES). Pharmaceutical care systems at the patient level rarely use statistical standards. Figure 9-2 shows a generic systems diagram that shows some of the relationships between a patient-oriented pharmaceutical care system and a PBES which deals with aggregate data from many patient encounters or episodes.

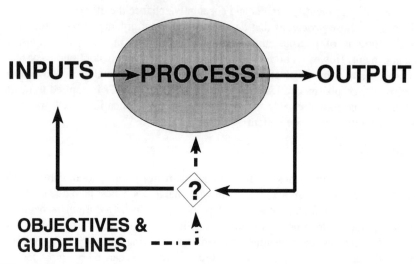

Figure 9.2.

A system consists of continuous processes as diagrammed in Figure 9-3. Each output forms part of the input to the next process. In a system, outputs are evaluated against some standard or expectation, as shown by the diamond-shaped box with a question mark in it. If an output appears satisfactory, no action is taken. If a problem is recognized, action is taken to correct it. For example, if, during a followup visit, the subjective and objective therapeutic results are consistent with desired progress, no action may be taken, and another followup visit may be scheduled for some weeks hence. If a problem is recognized, it is defined, root causes are sought, and a solution is implemented as soon as possible. Also, a followup might be scheduled in a shorter interval.

Guidelines

A guideline is a descriptive tool or standardized specification for care of the typical patient in the typical situation, developed through a formal process that incorporates the best scientific evidence of effectiveness with expert opinion. Related terms and synonyms include clinical criteria, practice parameter, protocol, algorithm, review criteria, and preferred practice pattern. Guidelines codify the care process to achieve uniformity and some degree of predictability in the patient care process. Deviation from guidelines may occur for individual patients (Joint Commission on Accreditation of Healthcare Organizations 1993).

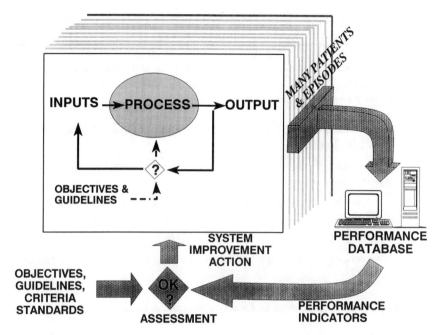

Figure 9.3.

Indicators

Both a pharmaceutical care system and a PBES may use indicators of performance or status. A performance indicator for use in a PBES is defined as "a statistical value that provides an indication of the condition or direction over time of an organization's performance of a specified process, or an organization's achievement of a specified outcome (Joint Commission on Accreditation of Healthcare Organizations 1993). According to an earlier definition,

> An indicator is a quantitative measure that can be used to monitor and evaluate the quality of important . . . clinical and support functions that affect patient outcomes. . . . An indicator is not a direct measure of quality. Rather it is a tool that can be used to assess performance and that can direct attention to . . . issues that may require more intense review within an organization (Joint Commission on Accreditation of Healthcare Organizations 1992)."

Similarly, a pharmaceutical care indicator may be defined as a therapeutic result that can be used to monitor and evaluate patient progress toward defined outcomes of drug therapy. A pharmaceutical care indicator is not a complete measure of therapeutic results (patient progress). Rather, it is a tool that can be used to assess progress and that can address attention to issues within the drug therapy of the patient that may require more intensive evaluation.

Two types of indicators for pharmaceutical care are therapeutic results and process indicators. Therapeutic results measure what happened or did not happen in care. They are, in principle, to be preferred to process indicators.

Process indicators measure definite activities that are a part of care, such as adjusting gentamicin dose based on serum levels. Process indicators of patient progress may be appropriate where:

1. No valid and reliable therapeutic result is available as when a therapeutic result is too complex to measure

2. Therapeutic result measurement is available but not economically or logistically feasible

3. The causes of the therapeutic result are not humanly controllable or are unknown

4. A process has a very strong, demonstrable link to outcome

5. The processes are of interest in themselves, as with, very expensive processes

Use of Progress Indicators in Pharmaceutical Care

Figure 9-3 and the associated discussion outline the general use of progress indicators to steer drug therapy toward desired outcomes. In order for this to work effectively in a pharmaceutical care system, however, monitoring must be planned, intelligent, coordinated, documented, active, communicated, and responsive. A monitoring plan should be written in a patient's care record after the pharmacist understands the therapeutic objectives and before the prescription is dispensed. This can be as simple as a note to telephone the patient in 48 hours to inquire about symptom resolution or early appearance of side effects. Intelligent monitoring is individualized. It emphasizes therapeutic results known to be significant in this patient's past therapy, like an idiosyncratic sensitivity to CNS side effects, or with this regimen, such as frequency of beta-agonist MDI inhaler use by an asthmatic patient. With active monitoring, the pharmacist would seek necessary data rather than wait for the patient to mention it. Active monitoring also includes active listening: asking the patient how he is getting along, expecting a real answer, and asking follow-up questions.

Coordinated monitoring would efficiently obtain information from the patient, caregivers, and professional colleagues. Each person involved in care may be better suited to get certain monitoring data than others. Regardless of who collects the monitoring data, it should be documented and communicated to others who may need it.

Finally, responsive monitoring would appropriately interpret and follow up the information obtained. If a pharmacist obtains information that an asthmatic patient is waking up more at night, coughing more, and having trouble getting up stairs that are usually not a problem, she might interpret this information to suggest that a serious exacerbation might be coming.

A pharmacist's response to learning about therapeutic results can end with notifying another responsible person, such as the patient, caregiver, or professional, of the possible significance of the results. This is the *monitoring* level, which entails collection of data and recognition of a potential or actual problem. In other cases, the pharmacist may chose to respond to such data by defining the problem, choosing a solution, and either implementing the solution or recommending the solution to another. This is participation in *managing* therapy. For example, suppose pharmacist Grey has learned that a patient is using his MDI more frequently than usual, coughing more, and waking up at night. Depending on how severe these results seem to be, she might recommend a visit to the physician without delay, telephone the physician's office herself to recommend an appointment for the patient on that day, telephone the physician with advice about starting a short-term course of corticosteroids, or arrange for transportation of the patient to an emergency room.

The Performance Based Quality of Pharmaceutical Care Evaluation System

If pharmaceutical care is the application of CI principles to individual patients, the Performance Based Quality of Pharmaceutical Care Evaluation System (PBES) is the application of pharmaceutical care to groups of patients. Both pharmaceutical care and the PBES are obligations of practitioners and not just a departmental or organizational function to be delegated to a select few. The purpose of the PBES is the creation of a measurement system to improve patient-care related processes that have a favorable impact on therapeutic results and on outcomes. Figure 9-3 illustrates the use of multiple patient experiences to create a database that provides information about the process and results of treatment. This approach may aggregate data from multiple practice settings, a single hospital, a patient care unit, or even an individual practitioner.

PBES Indicators

The perfect PBES indicator would be one which was technologically feasible; reliably collectable by various personnel; and validly related to quality of care issues important to patients, practitioners, third party payers, and other affected parties. An example of an indicator useful in a PBES is "Patients receiving appropriately timed intra-operative antibiotics for surgical prophylaxis."

Indicator Selection

According to *The Measurement Mandate,* a performance indicator should have the following nine properties:

1. Association with the quality of care. The JCAHO has proposed a Dimensions of Performance Model (See Table 9-2). Indicators should measure one or more of these dimensions. Pharmacy-related improvement efforts have focused primarily on the drug product appropriateness and efficacy. The challenge for a drug therapy PBES is to evaluate and improve all 8 performance dimensions.

2. A focus on processes and outcomes that are important and consistent with the organization's strategic plan. For example, if the hospital is a major cardiovascular center then CV-related drugs and diseases should be a high priority for treatment.

3. A relationship to results that are significantly and primarily influenced or explained by the actions of practitioners and organizations. For example, if the death rate from gram negative pneumonia in an organization is primarily attributable to patients' living conditions and nutritional status, it may not be a good indicator of practitioners' and hospitals' performance.

4. Quantitative measurability. For example, pain control is often measured subjectively and without a structured instrument, therefore the "Patients achieving adequate pain control" would be an uncountable indicator.

5. Clearly defined elements which allow for reliable data collection and comparison between sites. For example, a medication error due to mistiming must be precisely defined in minutes allowed before or after the scheduled time for administration.

6. Data collection that is both feasible and practical. Information management and cost of collection are factors that must be considered.

7. Acceptable specificity and sensitivity. False positive and false negative rates must be reasonable.

8. Uniform interpretation of a change in the rate of occurrence. For example, would an increase in the rate of reported preventable adverse drug reactions be interpreted as the result of poor performance, improved reporting, more patients at risk, or a combination of causes?

9. Improvement potential that is not obstructed by political or economic considerations of the organization.

Standards

A standard is a statement of an expectation that defines the organizations' governance, management, clinical, and support services' capacity to provide quality care. A standard specifies what is expected without exception, as with, "all requested pharmacokinetics will be completed within six hours of the availability of the necessary data" (Joint Commission on Accreditation of Healthcare Organizations 1992). Standards should ideally be based on empirical evidence from

Table 9.2. Definitions of Dimensions of Performance

I. Doing the Right Thing

The **efficacy** of the procedure or treatment in relation to the patient's condition

The degree to which the care/intervention for the patient has been shown to accomplish the desired/projected outcome(s)

The **appropriateness** of a specific test, procedure, or service to meet the patient's needs

The degree to which the care/intervention provided is relevant to the patient's clinical needs, given the current state of knowledge

II. Doing the Right Thing Well

The **availability** of a needed test, procedure, treatment, or service to the patient who needs it

The degree to which appropriate care/intervention is available to meet the patient's needs

The **timeliness** with which a needed test, procedure, treatment, or service is provided to the patient

The degree to which the care/intervention is provided to the patient at the most beneficial or necessary time

The **effectiveness** with which tests, procedures, treatments, and services are provided

The degree to which the care/intervention is provided in the correct manner, given the current state of knowledge, in order to achieve the desired/projected outcome for the patient

The **continuity** of the services provided to the patient with respect to other services, practitioners, and providers and over time

The degree to which the care/intervention for the patient is coordinated among practitioners, among organizations, and over time

The **safety** of the patient (and others) to whom the services are provided

The degree to which the risk of an intervention and the risk in the care environment are reduced for the patient and others, including the health care provider

The **efficiency** with which services are provided

The relationship between the outcomes (results of care) and the resources used to deliver patient care

The **respect and caring** with which services are provided

The degree to which the patient or a designee is involved in his/her own care decisions and to which those providing services do so with sensitivity and respect for the patient's needs, expectations, and individual differences

JCAHO AMH 1994, p 52.

comparable processes or published results. They should not be used to define minimum acceptable quality, and should not become an upper limit.

Performance Database

A performance database is a collection and counting of the indicator's, numerators, and denominators. In addition, a performance database should include data about major root causes of indicator variation. The relationship of indicators, the guidelines performance database, and standards is depicted in Figure 9-3. Compliance with a therapeutic guideline, like treatment of hypertension, can be measured through an indicator, such as patients achieving blood pressure control. The indicator results may document an opportunity for improvement through changes in the guidelines and raise the expected performance standards.

The identity of guidelines should influence the nature of indicators, and the nature of indicators (numerator/denominator) should determine the content of the performance database. The presence or absence of selected information in the database can itself be a performance indicator. For example, a lack of quality of life attributes associated with the drug treatment of hypertension may indicate inadequate attention to this area.

A PBES in operation is based on the following CI principles:

1. Understand the patient's and customer's needs
2. Focus on prevention of problems
3. Make decisions on data
4. Be managed in a cross-functional manner
5. Use statistical process control tools

The characteristics of the ideal pharmaceutical care PBES based on these principles are:

1. Measurement and monitoring of performance of organizations, teams, and individuals
2. Stimulating and facilitating continual improvement
3. Being cost-effective
4. Meeting accreditation and third-party performance requirements
5. Being an integral part of providing pharmaceutical care

Drug Use Evaluation Programs vs. PBES

Most hospital pharmacists are familiar with Drug Use Evaluation (DUE) or Drug Use Review (DUR) programs. DUE has been defined as, "a structured, ongoing, organizationally authorized quality assurance process designed to ensure that drugs are used appropriately, safely, and effectively (American Society of Hospital Pharmacists 1993)." The concepts of hospital conducted DUE apply to all practice settings.

DUE evolved from JCAHO accreditation requirements that focused on the usage patterns of high-cost antibiotics in the early 1980s. The emphasis was on appropriate use, which was narrowly defined as "the Correct Drug for the Right Bug." This concept of appropriate gradually evolved to include right dose, regimen, monitoring, and even cost effectiveness but still had a primary focus on the prescribing of drug products, especially high-cost products.

The underlying philosophy of DUE was called Quality Assurance (QA). DUE, as typically practiced, held individuals, usually physicians, responsible for appropriate prescribing and the pharmacy department responsible for data collection and, often, interventions. The QA philosophy served a useful purpose but had several shortcomings. It created an adversarial relationship between physicians and pharmacists, and it did not reflect the realities of patient care from multidisciplinary teams. It compartmentalized responsibility for improvement processes that included many departments. In contrast, where DUE emphasized prescribing, CI's emphasis was consistent with pharmaceutical care's philosophical emphasis on outcomes. Where DUE emphasized physicians, CI's emphasis was consistent with pharmaceutical care's philosophical emphasis on cooperation and shared responsibility. Where DUE emphasized individual action, CI emphasized system performance.

The transition from DUE to PBES can be accomplished by adopting CI principles. In conclusion, the application of a PBES to drug therapy leads to the development of a pharmaceutical care system. Who knows how far beyond pharmaceutical care CI can take drug therapy?

Summary

Pharmaceutical care is about achieving definite outcomes that improve a patients health-related quality of life. This discussion has emphasized outcomes that can be accepted as important and valuable to all parties in a health care system and serve as the focus of measurement and improvement efforts. Various definitions of outcome and quality of life may produce considerable confusion among health care providers and patients. This confusion can be resolved somewhat if the patient's primary "illness" perspective is harmonized with the practitioners "disease" orientation. For example, by considering professional and patient responses to, "What do you want to achieve from this therapy?" and "How can we improve it?"

Pharmaceutical care is about the measuring, monitoring and improving of an individual patient's quality of life. The PBES uses the pharmaceutical care data and associated processes from many patients to improve the care of future patients. Both pharmaceutical care and PBES are customer focused, require teamwork, use a feedback system, and are based on shared responsibility. They are indivisible and cannot be successfully practiced separately.

References

American Society of Hospital Pharmacists. 1993. The ASHP Guidelines on the Pharmacist Role in Drug Use Evaluation. *Practice Standards of ASHP 1992–93*. Bethesda MD: ASHP.

Angaran, D. M. 1991. Quality Assurance to Quality Improvement: Measuring and Monitoring Pharmaceutical Care. *Am J Hosp Pharm* 48:1901–07.

Donabedian, A. 1992. The role of outcomes in quality assessment and assurance. *Quality Review Bulletin* 18(11):356–60.

Creps L. B., et al. 1992. Integrating Total Quality Management and Quality Assurance at the University of Michigan Medical Center. *ORB* 18:357.

Hepler C. D., and L. M. Strand. 1990. Opportunities and Responsibilities in Pharmaceutical Care. *Am J Hosp Pharm.* 47:533–543.

Jachuck, S. J., Brrerly, H., Jachuck, S., and Wilcox, P. M. 1982. The effect of hypotensive dosage on the quality of life. *Journal of the Royal College of General Practitioners* 32(235):103–5.

Joint Commission on Accreditation of Healthcare Organizations. 1992. *Primer on Indicator Development and Application: Measuring Quality in Health Care.* Chicago: Joint Commission on Accreditation of Healthcare Organizations.

Joint Commission on Accreditation of Healthcare Organizations. 1993. *The Measurement Mandate: On the Road to Performance Improvement in Health Care.* Oakbrook IL.: Joint Commission on Accreditation of Healthcare Organizations.

Joint Commission on Accreditation of Healthcare Organizations. 1994. *Accreditation Manual for Hospitals,* 52. Oakbrook, IL: Joint Commission on Accreditation of Healthcare Organizations.

MacKeigan, L. D. and D. S. Pathak. 1992. Overview of Health-related Quality-of-life Measures. *Am. J. Hosp. Pharm.* 42:2236–245.

Schipper, H. J. Clinch, and V. Powell. 1990. Definitions and Conceptual Issues. In *Quality of Life Assessments in Clinical Trials,* ed. B. Spilker. Raven Press, NY.

US Congress, Office of Technology Assessment. 1988. *Quality of Medical Care: Information for Consumers.* Washington DC. Pub OTA–H–386.

10

Redefining Pharmacist Professional Responsibility

David B. Brushwood, J.D.
Charles D. Hepler, Ph.D.

Introduction

Within the pharmaceutical care model of practice, individual pharmacists provide drug therapy for patients and accept responsibility for the outcomes of the therapy they provide. The definition of pharmaceutical care begins with the phrase, "the *responsible* provision of drug therapy" (emphasis added) (Hepler and Strand 1989). Responsibility is an integral part of competent care, as that term is defined in Chapter 8. The competent provider of pharmaceutical care must be able to say, "I take responsibility for that," when a critical decision about a patient's drug therapy is to be made.

Responsibility is defined as an ability to answer for one's conduct and obligations, and as being morally trustworthy within a specific office, duty, or trust. *Trust* means assured reliance on the character, strength, ability, or truth of someone; *trustworthy* means worthy of confidence, dependable. In times past, *blind* trust has been the norm in health care, with obedient patients submitting to the orders of omniscient physicians, just as small children obey their parents. But in pharmaceutical care, *earned* trust is at the core of a provider-patient relationship. Earned trust is reciprocal. Providers trust patients, and patients trust providers, because each knows and respects the other. Earned trust is based not on traditions of power and obedience but on the richness of the relationship of caring (Katz 1984).

Responsibility arises in a relationship and depends on a relationship. Responsibility requires that a pharmacist intervene for a patient's benefit any time it is reasonable to do so. This requirement for intervention at any time is a key element of pharmaceutical care. Pharmaceutical care focuses on the needs of patients and requires action for the benefit of a patient even though a physician has not requested (and perhaps has even resisted) action by a pharmacist (Strand et al., 1991).

Responsible is related to *accountable, culpable, liable,* and *answerable,* but only *responsible* has a prospective sense of a duty yet to be fulfilled. Being responsible for patient care means that a care provider looks to the future and does what is necessary to improve the outlook for a patient. Responsibility is a characteristic of individualized patient care.

Responsibility is sometimes confused with *authority,* although the ideas are quite different. *Authority* is one basis that can be used to justify and legitimize the use of power to make something happen or to influence belief. Having responsibility may provide such justification. For example, a supervisor may request that an employee do something or believe something, using the justification that the supervisor is responsible for the employee's work. However, responsibility is only one basis of authority and often not the strongest.

Basic Concepts: Freedom and Obligation

A central feature of responsibility is that it is directed at a person, material, or idea, which called the object of responsibility. Responsibility entails a duty to respond when that object's interests are at risk of harm. To provide pharmaceutical care, as defined in this book, a pharmacist must respond whenever the circumstances of drug therapy present a significant risk of harm to a patient or present some other obstacle to reaching the patient's therapeutic objectives. Such circumstances may be termed "pharmaceutical problems" or "drug related problems (Strand, Cipolle, and Morley 1988, 1990)."

The pharmacist's duty to respond to potential or actual problems is limited by a number of factors. First, the duty to respond to a pharmaceutical problem arises only when harm to the patient is reasonably foreseeable. There is no duty to prevent adverse outcomes that are theoretically identifiable where a problem is undetectable or where harm is not realistically foreseeable for a given patient.

Second, responsibility implies capacity. In other words, "ought" implies "can." The pharmacist's duty to respond includes *all* of those actions that the pharmacist is legally obliged to perform and *some* actions that the pharmacist is legally permitted to perform and capable of performing, but the duty excludes *all* actions that the pharmacist is legally or otherwise incapable of performing and those actions that would be obviously futile given the circumstances. This chapter will be preoccupied with the second group of actions, permissible and feasible actions.

The pharmacists duty to respond may also be limited by competing interests, perhaps of different people. Being responsible requires the pharmacist to place a patient's interests above other interests, even at some cost to those other interests.

The Concept of Duty

Accepting responsibility connotes recognizing a duty to respond, react, or reply to certain problems. Duty means that there is a certain course of conduct that is due to others (Dukes and Swartz 1988). In pharmaceutical care, the duty of a pharmacist is to respond to pharmaceutical problems. This duty to respond is owed principally to the patient.

The concept of duty is not limited to one's professional role. In all walks of life we have duties such as meeting contractual commitments, supporting our dependents, and refraining from acts that would harm another person. However, a professional role carries with it a special duty to affirmatively act to promote the interests of those who establish a dependent relationship with us because of our professional status. The concept of duty has evolved primarily through litigation.

One view of duty is that in order for there to be an unmet responsibility, some specific requirement must have been violated. The duty to educate patients about medications and to monitor drug therapy are examples of specific requirements. However, duty is not limited to actions specifically required by law. It is generally considered preferable to view duty in terms of a general duty of reasonable care, with specific recognized exceptions being applicable when certain necessary conditions have been met (Dukes and Swartz 1988). Thus, if one is said to have a duty to prevent drug-drug interactions, it is preferable to interpret this as an example of the general duty of care. Duty should not be defined by listing an endless series of courses of conduct that must be followed for a responsibility to be met, but rather should be defined as a relationship between two parties.

A general duty of care arises out of a relationship and is circumscribed by the nature of the relationship. In determining the nature of a relationship-based duty, two issues are critical: the scope of the risk to the party who is owed a duty and the character of the interest that may be invaded if the duty goes unmet. The pharmacist's relationship with a patient has to do primarily with the prevention or minimization of the risks of drug therapy. Evaluating the risk that a drug will have an adverse effect on a patient is clearly within the scope of the pharmacist-patient relationship, and a pharmacist has a duty to prevent adverse outcomes for patients.

In addition, it is conceivable that the effects of a drug might cause a patient to become violent and attack someone. The question might then be asked, did the pharmacist who dispensed the drug to the patient owe a duty to the bystander to prevent violent drug-induced actions by the patient? While it would be possible to approach this question from a causality perspective, the duty issue addresses the question at a more basic level. The answer would likely be that the pharmacist had no duty to prevent harm to the bystander from an attack, because this type of harm is beyond the scope of the risks from which a pharmacist provides protection. If the same question were asked of a policeman who was assigned to protect the bystander, then the answer could be very different, because the risk of attack is well within the scope of the risks from which a policeman provides protection.

The character of the interest invaded is also relevant to the issue of duty. A provider of pharmaceutical care has a responsibility to uphold the interests of the patient, perhaps at the expense of the provider's personal, immediate interests. This may mean that a pharmacist would place himself or herself at some temporary inconvenience or risk (e.g., of economic or physical harm) in order to meet a responsibility to the patient. However, the interests of the patient are not all-encompassing. Within the pharmacist-patient relationship, patients have an interest in health and well being. They also have an interest in autonomy and bodily integrity.

Pharmaceutical care providers have a duty to act in a way that promotes these interests of the patient. Drugs, unfortunately, can be used in ways that perhaps may serve the patient's interests, yet are not justified. For example, anabolic steroids or growth hormones may assist a patient in gaining an advantage in athletics, and the patient may willingly accept the risks that these drugs present. Nevertheless, the pharmacist would have no duty to provide such drugs, because the interest in enhanced athletic performance is not an interest of a character that falls within the realm of health-related outcomes.

Controllable and Uncontrollable Harm

The second major distinction to be made in a discussion of responsibility in pharmaceutical care is the distinction between harm that is humanly controllable and harm that is not humanly controllable. Pharmaceutical care aims to soften the harsher realities of drug therapy but does not claim to abolish them. Responsibility is a human attribute. Humans can control the drug use process to promote some good outcomes and to prevent some bad outcomes from drug therapy. To accept responsibility does not mean that one has guaranteed a good outcome.

For example, prescribing errors, dispensing errors, and medication errors are usually humanly controllable, and there is a professional responsibility to prevent them. However, some adverse drug reactions may not be humanly controllable. Although the pharmacist has a professional responsibility to recognize problems and minimize adverse outcomes, there is no responsibility to absolutely prevent them.

Positive and Negative Freedom

In pharmaceutical care, the pharmacist has a responsibility to promote patient autonomy, that is self-directing freedom. Negative freedom is the absence of constraint, so that individuals are left alone to make their own personal choices. The argument for negative freedom is that it guarantees the maximization of utility, because individuals strive to improve their lot. An example of negative freedom in drug therapy is permitting or encouraging a patient's own goals for drug therapy, perhaps as manifested by obtaining the patient's informed consent to therapy. This assures that the patient is freely participating in decisions about care. One argument against negative freedom is that some people's freedom must be bridled so that all may advance. This requires the use of power by some in society to help improve or perfect other individuals.

Positive freedom, on the other hand, is the presence of real choices. It is meaningless to claim that a person is free in a certain thing if that person has no real choice. The rich and poor may both be "free" to sleep in doorways, but the rich are also free to sleep in beds. A pharmacist may increase a person's freedom by expanding the range of therapeutic objectives or treatment possibilities available.

Mandatory, Voluntary, and Prohibited Actions

A distinction must be drawn between behaviors that society requires, behaviors society allows at discretion, and behaviors society prohibits altogether. Behavioral restrictions can apply to certain people or perhaps all people in a society (Baier 1987). People who have not qualified for a profession are prohibited from performing the actions that make up the practice of that profession. For example, dispensing prescription medicines to the general public is an action that may only be properly performed by pharmacists. Even those who have qualified for a profession are prohibited from performing some actions associated with that profession. For example dispensing narcotic prescriptions without a valid prescription for a valid purpose is prohibited even for pharmacists. Some aspects of pharmacy practice, such as keeping certain records and offering to discuss medicines with patients, are required of all who would practice pharmacy. Other aspects, like, drug therapy monitoring, are permitted, but society requires that the activity be done well if it is done at all.

If a pharmacist did not perform a required act, or offered to take up a voluntary act and then failed to perform it properly, he or she would be responsible for an *omission*. If he or she did not refrain from performing prohibited acts he or she could be said to have failed a responsibility through a *commission*. For example, a provider of pharmaceutical care has a responsibility not to distribute controlled substances to a drug addict who has no therapeutic need for the drugs. A pharmacist who fails to meet this responsibility may be criminally prosecuted. However, a pharmacist who is inattentive in drug therapy monitoring, and who fails to meet recognized responsibilities in monitoring, probably would not be criminally prosecuted unless the omission were gross and outrageous. However, this omission might trigger a civil lawsuit—a social response to compensate a victimized patient.

Example

Perhaps the issues raised in the development of a theory of responsibility in pharmaceutical care can be better understood through reference to an everyday

200 / David B. Brushwood, J.D. and Charles D. Hepler, Ph.D.

hypothetical situation. Consider the decision faced by a person who, on a walk through the park, sees a stranger struggling to swim and apparently in danger of drowning in a pond. The basic question to ask in this situation is whether the passerby has a responsibility to jump into the pond and save the drowning swimmer. However, before that question can be answered, several other questions must be addressed. These questions include:

(1) How certain must the passerby be that the swimmer really is about to drown before there is a responsibility for the passerby to attempt a rescue? Maybe the swimmer is just pretending.

(2) If the passerby were to attempt to rescue the drowning swimmer, what cost might there be to the passerby. For example, the passerby might be in physical danger or miss a crucial business meeting. What mechanisms exist to reimburse the passerby for those costs?

(3) Is there another person present who is better able, and equally as willing, to save the drowning swimmer?

The prevailing view within American society probably is that the passerby has a responsibility to attempt to rescue the drowning swimmer, provided that the swimmer is obviously in grave danger, that the rescue is relatively cost-free to the rescuer, and that the passerby is able to swim at least as well as anyone else who is nearby. However, should any of these conditions not be met, there would be considerable controversy about the responsibility of the passerby.

In American culture, one's responsibility to strangers is conditional. We live in a society of individuals, who often gratuitously promote the interests of other individuals, but who are seldom recognized to have a responsibility to sacrifice their own interests to help others. If the passerby were to fail to rescue the drowning swimmer either because it appeared too risky to do so, or because the potential risk was difficult to determine, there would likely be little criticism of the passerby for having failed to meet a responsibility.

Yet changes can be made to the hypothetical situation to increase the likelihood that the person observing the drowning swimmer would have a recognized responsibility to come to the swimmer's rescue. For example, if the person seeing the drowning swimmer was a lifeguard, then there would clearly be a duty to rescue, because lifeguards are designated by society as having a responsibility to save drowning swimmers. If the swimmer had been pushed into the pond by the person who saw him struggling to swim, there also would be a clear duty to rescue, because one generally has a responsibility to alleviate circumstances that one has purposefully caused. It is generally recognized that a person accepts responsibility either by occupying a position of responsibility or by affirmatively acting to create a situation in which responsibility exists.

This chapter argues that, as a provider of pharmaceutical care, a pharmacist is not a mere passerby in drug therapy, and that, as a recipient of pharmaceutical care, a patient is not a stranger to a pharmacist. Just as a lifeguard has a socially imposed responsibility to rescue drowning swimmers, so too does a pharmacist have a responsibility to prevent harm to patients due to problems with drug use.

Furthermore, a pharmacist is an active participant in drug therapy. A pharmacist's purposeful action in providing pharmaceutical products creates a responsibility to prevent adverse outcomes that might be caused by either the provision of pharmaceutical products or the failure to provide them. Responsibility is not optional in pharmaceutical care; it is mandatory, both because responsibility is socially imposed, and because it arises out of the relationship between a pharmacist and a patient.

Dimensions of Professional Responsibility

Professional responsibility arises in professional relationships and depends much on the nature of the relationship. Responsibility and trustworthiness are familiar to practicing pharmacists, who know that they should behave in ways that merit patients' reliance on their knowledge, ability, and character. What is different in pharmaceutical care is that a pharmacist is offering to be responsible for *providing drug therapy*.

This suggests two important, interrelated differences between a practice of dispensing and advising and a practice of pharmaceutical care. First, the objectives of pharmaceutical care are the outcomes of drug therapy, in contrast to the more limited completion of the dispensing and advising process. Second, outcomes depend on both colleagues' actions and patient's actions, activities that are beyond a pharmacist's control. Therefore, a pharmacist can provide pharmaceutical care only in cooperation with others. This cooperation suggests in turn that pharmacists may often share responsibility for outcomes with other people.

The primary questions about professional responsibility are (Bosk 1979):

1. For what are you responsible?
2. To whom are you responsible?
3. What is a mistake, failure, error?

In a cooperative relationship like the relationship among patient, pharmacist, and physician, there is one more question:

4. How does a mistake by one member of the group affect the responsibilities of the others?

There are three major relationships in pharmaceutical care, professional, collegial, and ministerial. There are also three types of responsibility, technical, judgmental and normative. This yields nine possible interactions, as shown the following table outline.

Responsibilities to Patients, Colleagues, and Organizations

Responsibility to the patient occurs within the exchange of trust and competent caring described in Chapter 8 (Hepler 1985; Veatch 1981). These relationships can be called "covenental," or "fiducial," meaning they require trust. They are the foundation of professional service and normally take precedence over relationships with colleagues or organizations (Hepler 1985).

Collegial relationships occur between professional colleagues. They are valuable largely to the extent that they support short- and long-term cooperation for patients' benefit. Some collegial responsibilities are fundamental, such as truth telling or candor. Others are matters more of etiquette than ethics. However, since pharmaceutical care requires cooperation among all parties, collegial relationships are extremely important. The pharmacist can serve the patient's interests by actively supporting the patient's relationship with physician and pharmacist colleagues. Exceptions are those relatively rare instances in which the pharmacist suspects that a problem exists that has potential to harm or seriously inconvenience the patient and appropriate attempts to enlist the colleague's understanding and cooperation have failed.

Ministerial relationships are those between people and organizations. A pharmacist's employer or an affiliated organization, such as a hospital, nursing home, or insurance company, is responsible to its patients for some aspects of quality of care. If it is privately owned, it is also responsible to its owners or stockholders. Since an organization is incapable of providing professional services itself, it must rely on professionals to provide care and control the risks of care. The best examples of ministerial relationships, perhaps, are the policies of an organized medical staff in a hospital. Furthermore, an employee has ministerial responsibilities to the institution to protect its assets and to prevent injury to its patients.

Pharmacists' covenental, collegial, and ministerial responsibilities may overlap to a large degree, inasmuch as good patient outcomes are in the interests of all. For example, pharmacists can support the institution's desire to obtain good

Responsibility for Responsibility to	Technical (Details & Facts)	Judgmental (Decisions)	Normative ("Good Faith")
Patient	correct drug information	choice of information & presentation	review of therapy & warning
Colleagues	correct drug information	content & style of documentation	patient education & assessment of status
Organizations	accurate billing information	when to encourage non-formulary agent	encouragement of appropriate care

Examples of Pharmacists' Responsibilities: Responsibility Type by Object of Responsibility

patient outcomes, while the institution can support the pharmacist's desire for the same.

Pharmaceutical care, like all aspects of patient care, has as its primary goal the promotion of good outcomes related to a particular patient's health and quality of life. The responsible provider of pharmaceutical care does whatever reasonably can be done to promote the patient's best interests. Patient care activities are special because the caring provider enters into a relationship with a patient and serves as the patient's advocate. As an advocate for the patient, the pharmacist can only secondarily consider interests of colleagues, institutions, and others external to the pharmacist-patient relationship. This is not to say that a responsible pharmacist ignores those external interests. Rather, those interests are secondary to the interests of the patient.

Technical, Judgmental, and Normative Responsibilities

In pharmaceutical care, a pharmacist is not just responsible for drug products or drug advice, but also shares responsibility with the patient and physician, among others, for the outcomes of drug therapy. Each relationship enumerated in the preceding section involves the three types of responsibilities necessary for pharmaceutical care: technical, judgmental, and normative (Bosk 1979). Broadly, an *error* is a failure to achieve, through ignorance, deficiency or accident, that which should be achieved. That is, an error is a failure to meet a responsibility.

Technical responsibilities involve basic knowledge and skill, such as knowing the usual dose of a medicine and being able to recognize an unusual dosage. Most pharmacists are familiar with the major examples of technical responsibility: right drug, right dose, right time and route, and all in the right patient. An example of a "technical" responsibility owed to a patient or colleague would be providing accurate information about drug therapy.

Judgmental responsibilities involve decisions and other applications of knowledge and skill, such as, choosing an appropriate dosage for a specific patient. Judgmental responsibility also is being exercised when the pharmacist decides which information to provide to a patient, what aspects of the information to emphasize, how to present and reinforce the information, and also in the pharmacist's evaluation of the patient's comprehension of the information.

Normative responsibilities involve role obligations within relationships. For example, suppose physician Brown reasonably would expect pharmacist Jones to warn him if an ordered dosage were worrisome or if a patient's condition appears to be worsening (Bosk 1979). They might have discussed their relationship and informally agreed. For Jones not to warn Brown would be a *normative error,* that is, a breach of responsibility created within a relationship.

Normative responsibility to a patient would similarly consist of acting in good faith within the given relationship. For example, if a patient relied upon his pharmacist to review his drug history and to warn of possible drug interactions or side effects, and the pharmacist failed to do that, the pharmacist would have committed a normative error. If the pharmacist warned of a potential side effect with negligible probability or practical significance for a patient, that would be a judgmental error. If a pharmacist did not know that two medicines that the patient was taking could interact significantly, that would be a technical error. Technical and judgmental activities are part of professional decision making, as described in Chapter 8.

As clinical practice matures toward pharmaceutical care, one should expect the nature of a pharmacists' relationships with patients and with colleagues to change. Consequently, one should expect normative responsibilities to change. Also, the increasing importance of health care providers and third-party payers involves significant issues in the balancing of competing claims of normative responsibility. A basic issue for the future is whether pharmacists will develop further direct responsibility to patients or whether that responsibility will be subsumed under the responsibilities of the health care organization or the physician.

Interrelated Errors

The fourth primary question about professional responsibility, how a mistake by one team member affects the responsibilities of the others, depends on the relationship among team members and so is related to normative error. Each team member has a right to expect the others to meet their respective responsibilities to the patient. If a physician makes a wrong diagnosis, it is possible that nothing that the pharmacist or patient can do (other than discover the error!) can improve the patient's quality of life. Furthermore, such an error could lead to secondary errors by the patient or pharmacist. Imagine the pharmacist's confusion when attempting to monitor the therapeutic outcomes of a normotensive patient who had mistakenly been diagnosed with hypertension and treated with propranolol. Likewise, the others should expect the pharmacist at the very least to correctly dispense a prescribed drug product and to advise the patient appropriately. A dispensing error can confuse all concerned and cause secondary errors of its own.

Patients can commit each type of error described above. Examples of technical errors a patient would make include not reading or following label instructions or forgetting to take doses. Judgmental errors are perhaps the most difficult to discuss, since patients are not expected to exercise professional judgment. However, if a competent patient fails to exercise common sense and, for example, operates a motor vehicle after being warned that a new prescription might make him drowsy, or fails to notice an obvious new symptom, such as a skin rash, one might be justified in considering the patient to have made an error of judgment. Certainly, lying or withholding information from the pharmacist or physician would constitute a normative patient error.

It is clear that in a team, errors by one party can frustrate the work of others or even cause them to commit error of their own.

Shared Responsibility

Were they working alone, it might be feasable for a physician, pharmacist, patient, or caregiver to accept full responsibility for the use of medicines to improve the quality of a patient's life. However, since an error by one team member can frustrate the efforts of another, meeting responsibilities for outcomes often requires teamwork. Pharmaceutical care is both an idea about the practice of pharmacy and an idea about how medications should be used in a cooperative system (Hepler 1993).

Within a cooperative team, questions may arise about how responsibility should be shared. Sometimes such questions are really asking about apportionment of *liability*. That is, if someone is injured and found deserving of damages, how should the damages be apportioned among the members of the team? However, the questions can also be asked about responsibility.

Courts have held physicians liable for unacceptable outcomes of drug therapy, even in cases where another professional could have prevented the injury. This suggests a football metaphor for drug therapy. The physician is the quarterback, and he chooses and executes plays, takes credit for success and blame for failure, and accepts a few bone-crushing tackles along when another team member misses an assignment.

The courts have resolved questions of the professional liability of teams in hospitals and other formal organizations, and stable primary care teams could accept joint accountability in a similar model. These models, suggest that pooling of risk and written descriptions of team responsibilities are important steps in the implementation of shared responsibility.

We propose an approach to prospective responsibility which is easily articulated, even if its practical implementation can be difficult. Each pharmaceutical care team should have written practice guidelines that set forth the broad responsibilities of each team member, including patients and family caregivers. However, each team member should act as if he expected to be held accountable for recognizing the appropriate course of action and acting appropriately each time a significant opportunity to improve the outcomes of a patient's drug therapy presents itself.

If a particular opportunity is outside a team member's area of competence even to notice, then it has no effect. If the opportunity is noticeable but outside the team member's competence to resolve, then the team member is responsible for calling it to the attention of the team member who is responsible for solving that type of problem.

This arrangement might be easiest to illustrate with an example. Suppose a patient is competent to observe the subjective effect of a medicine. The pharmacist advises the patient to be aware of dizziness, especially during the second through fourth days of a new regimen. The patient should act as if he is responsible for mentioning his experience to a pharmacist or physician, even though the patient is not competent to adjust dosage.

The applicable metaphor for this arrangement is a soccer or basketball team. There is a captain who provides strategic and tactical leadership, but each member of the team may get the ball unexpectedly at any moment. At such moments, that member must decide how to advance the interests of the team based on skill and opportunity.

Retrospective Responsibility: Liability and Accountability

The idea that a health care provider has a responsibility for patient care carries with it the corollary ideas that a mechanism must exist for the health care provider to confirm that people have met their responsibilities, and that there must be appropriate corrective consequences when a health care provider fails to meet a responsibility. *Accountability* is a concept and it is related to responsibility. Also known as *answerability,* it primarily concerns activities undertaken to answer the question, "Why have things not gone well?" *Accountability* and *liability* imply the additional existence of an authority such as a court or review board. A responsible person would be culpable for harm that he could have avoided. *Liability* exists when the answers to the accountability-related questions are unacceptable, showing a failure to meet a duty of care that resulted in a bad outcome (Baier 1987).

While responsibility relates to individualized patient care, accountability is somewhat analogous to continuous quality improvement (CQI). The goal of CQI is to improve outcomes related to health and quality of life for all patients, not just one patient. The concept of accountability requires that an account or explanation be provided when less than optimal outcomes occur. People in responsible positions are called to account for what they did at a particular time if there is reason to believe that a responsibility was not met. Through examination of patient records, incident reports, a performance data base, or some other repository of information, it is possible to recognize sentinel indicators, or "red flags", of suboptimal performance or outcome. Accountability requires that those who were in a position of responsibility with regard to the patient for whom a sentinel indicator is identified account for their actions with regard to the patient.

Professionals cannot guarantee good outcomes, and the presence of an indicator does not in and of itself establish anything conclusive with regard to responsibility. An indicator presents a rebuttable presumption that a person or persons has not met his responsibility. To be accountable means simply that the accountable person(s) rebuts that presumption. Accountability, in retrospect, requires a show-ing that the standard of care was adhered to and that prospective responsibility was met at the time care was provided. If the account provided is unsatisfactory, then a pharmacist's care of a patient can be considered not to have been responsible.

The failure to provide responsible care, as shown by the inability to account for a suboptimal outcome, may lead to liability. The principal difference between accountability and liability is that legally enforceable sanctions accompany a finding of liability. The purpose of liability is not to improve the quality of patient care, or to promote a good outcome for a particular patient, as by the time liability is determined it is too late to pursue these goals. The purpose of liability is to compensate one party for harm caused by another party by requiring the party that caused harm to make a payment to the party that was harmed. Although a beneficial effect of liability is deterrence of further improper conduct, and in this regard overall quality of health care may improve as the result of the imposition of liability, the purpose of liability is simply compensation.

Thing Responsibility and Agent Responsibility

Culpability means *blameworthiness* and involves the ideas of cause and, perhaps, guilt. Identifying the "culprit" when things have not gone well with drug therapy is an engaging but perilous exercise. The concepts of duty and causation can be difficult to grasp, and the analysis can be further confounded when the facts of what happened are unclear. Pharmaceutical care usually includes the provision of both a product, although perhaps indirectly, and a service. When a bad outcome occurs during the provision of pharmaceutical care and there is a need to identify the culprit, it may be helpful to separately consider the responsibilities of the product and those of the care provider.

Max Baier has made a useful distinction between thing-responsibility and agent-responsibility (Baier 1987). The difference between the two concepts can be illustrated by citing a hypothetical statement. In explaining what happened following a bad outcome, any pharmacist might say, "I gave him Drug A, and, unfortunately, an adverse reaction occurred." Note the quick transition from the active voice, when describing what was done, to the passive voice, when describing the result. Is this pharmacist shirking responsibility? Is he unwilling to admit that he is at fault for what happened? Not necessarily. The statement more likely illustrates the distinction between thing-responsibility and agent-responsibility.

The traditional approach to ascribing responsibility for drug-induced injury has been backward-looking. The assumption has often been made that drugs cause adverse effects, not people or systems of drug use. When an adverse effect occurs, the approach has been to attempt to identify which (if any) of the drugs that the patient received caused the adverse effect. Yet the overall purpose of allocating responsibility must be to improve the quality of patient care. This is a forward-looking exercise. It would ordinarily be said that a drug *was* responsible for an adverse effect (thing-responsibility), but that a pharmacist *is* responsible for a patient's care (agent-responsibility). The backward-looking approach of agent-responsibility is necessary to the analysis of responsibility in pharmaceutical care, but it is not sufficient. Within pharmaceutical care it is people who are responsible, not things. Individuals and the drug use systems they devise are more likely than the drugs themselves to be the culprits when bad outcomes occur. Since the way people behave and the way systems operate can be changed more readily than the effects of drugs can, then when responsibility lies with an agent rather than a thing, useful modifications are more likely to occur.

Baier has described the difference between agent-responsibility and thing-responsibility thus:

> Ascribing agent-responsibility differs in several important ways. Although it is also backward-looking, it is not merely so; the consequences of the identification of the culprit are much more complex. The main reason for these differences is that agents, especially human agents, are extremely complex entities, particularly as far as their response mechanisms are concerned. Unlike things, human beings cannot only be blamed, they can be found blameworthy; not only have faults but be at fault; and not only be due for repair, but be culpable and deserving of condemnation or punishment or liable to pay damages (Baier 1987).

Baier explains that humans are *agents* rather than *things* because humans are moral beings. As moral agents, humans have a faculty of choice and they have the ability to understand what they ought to do. It is this basic ability to understand guidelines for action and to act on them that creates agent-responsibility. Whereas the analysis of thing-responsibility is an analysis of causation (it caused the harm, therefore it was responsible for the harm), the analysis of agent responsibility is an analysis of duty (I am responsible for the patient, therefore I caused the harm). Drug A may be considered thing-responsible for an adverse effect simply by virtue of being the significant causal factor. A pharmacist becomes agent-responsible only if the pharmacist has failed in, or was in breach of, a duty that arises out of agent-responsibility. The fact that a drug ordered, recommended, or dispensed by a pharmacist causes harm is not sufficient to establish such a duty. Pharmacists are agent-responsible in a forward-looking sense for a process of drug therapy that is free from drug-related diseases. They are agent-responsible in a backward-looking sense for the problems that drugs cause. As moral agents, pharmacists have a duty to patients, and this duty formalizes the pharmacist's responsibility.

Formalizing Responsibility Through Regulation

The notion of a professional responsibility to protect people from harming themselves through risky choices may conjure up images of paternalistic health care providers racing to the aid of patients just in time to provide protection from the patients' own foolishness. A government that would endorse or even permit such over-protectiveness would seem to threaten individual freedoms. Over-protective health care providers remove people's incentive to take responsibility for themselves. Why, then, would a government, through regulation, impose on care providers the responsibility to make appropriate decisions for patients and not imposing those same responsibilities on the patients themselves? After all, if one assumes that people tend to act in their own self-interest by making decisions that will increase their happiness rather than decrease it, then why does the government need to recognize professional responsibilities that take authority away from patients and give authority to care providers?

Regulatory recognition of responsibility for care providers can be justified because the free market does not always act efficiently to promote happiness-maximizing behavior by people (Weimer and Vining 1989). When market inefficiency like this occurs, it is often called a "market failure," and that serves as justification for regulatory recognition of professional responsibilities. The most significant type of market failure in a discussion of professional responsibility is known as information asymmetry. This type of market failure occurs when the consumer of a good or service is uninformed as to the true value of that good or service.

Some goods and services have characteristics that are obvious to a consumer prior to purchase. These are sometimes referred to as "pre-experience" goods and services. A chair or a tablet of paper, for example, can be examined and evaluated by most consumers. Other goods and services, however, can be evaluated only after they have been acquired and used. These are sometimes referred to as "experience" goods and services. A meal at a restaurant or a haircut are examples of these kinds of goods and services. Yet another type of good or service is sometimes referred to as a "post-experience" good or service, because consumers are unable to evaluate these even after they have been used. The value of a medication, for example, is very difficult to evaluate immediately and perhaps cannot be evaluated even after the passage of a considerable period of time (Weimer and Vining 1989).

Through experience and training, professional people can develop expertise with post-experience goods and services. Professionals are therefore able to help the users of these goods and services make decisions about them as if they were pre-experience goods and services. The responsibility of the health care provider is not to take away from a patient decision-making authority that the patient would otherwise have, but to give to the patient decision-making authority that the patient cannot otherwise have. Government regulation of professional responsibility does not intrinsically threaten individual freedom or discourage individual responsibility. It can, instead, enhance the independence of patients by imposing upon health professionals, among other things, a responsibility to involve patients in a way that they otherwise could not be.

Sources of Regulatory Responsibility

Society expects pharmacists to be responsible providers of pharmaceutical care, and this expectation is reflected in the regulations and judicial opinions that comprise the law of pharmacist responsibility. As with any area of evolving responsibility, the problem of setting limits has confronted regulators and jurists. The legal community is torn between the possibility that expectations might be set too low and not provide adequate protection for patients and the possibility that they might be set too high and unfairly require more of pharmacists than pharmacists are able to provide. The legal community has therefore struggled with the question of how to decide how much responsibility is enough responsibility for pharmacists (Dukes and Swartz 1988).

Several theories of pharmacist responsibility have been used by the legal and regulatory community, with varying degrees of success. These theories form the basis of four models of pharmacist duty (Brushwood 1993). The objective of theory development is to establish a means to consistently determine what conduct is responsible conduct. Theorists usually provide a framework for analysis by an unbiased evaluator whose only interest is in the fair and uniform application of the force of law. While it may not be possible to achieve universal recognition of a single theory over all others, the exercise of theory development and selection can help clarify issues and can lead to an understanding of why some legal and regulatory actions regarding pharmacist responsibility are more well conceived than others in terms of scope and rationale justification.

Policy Analysis, Consumer Expectation, and Professional Standards Models

The focus in the policy analysis model is social utility. Within this model, an expanded responsibility would be recognized for a pharmacist if the benefits of such a responsibility, for example, improved quality of drug therapy, would exceed the detriments of the responsibility, for example, damage to the physician-patient relationship caused by pharmacist intervention. Because it is so difficult to identify the benefits and detriments of establishing expanded responsibilities for pharmacists and to assign values to those benefits and detriments, this model has not worked well.

The consumer expectation model focuses on the patient's right of self determination. It reasons that if consumers want pharmacists to have a particular responsibility, then pharmacists should have that responsibility. Unfortunately, consumers do not know enough about what pharmacists can do to know what pharmacists ought to do, therefore a model based on consumer expectations is fraught with problems.

The focus of the professional standards model is on organized pharmacy. This model attempts to use professionally developed guidelines as the basis for determining legal and regulatory responsibility. But the pharmacy profession has not done a good enough job of developing meaningful practice standards, so the attempts to use pharmacy-produced standards and guidelines have been for naught.

Power Model

The most successful approach thus far to legal and regulatory recognition of expanded responsibilities for pharmacists is the power model of pharmacist responsibility. This model focuses on the capabilities of the individual pharmacist within the context of a specific patient care situation (Brushwood 1993).

The power model of pharmacist responsibility asserts that without knowledge there is uncertainty. Uncertainty leads to dependence, and dependence gives rise to a responsibility. A similar approach, that is more theological than sociological, is based on the principle of stewardship. Since one's personal knowledge and abilities are not inherent to one's self but instead are God-given, no person has the right to determine how their own skills are used. Skills must be used altruistically for the benefit of others.

Under the power model of pharmacist responsibility, knowledge is the key factor. A pharmacist has a responsibility to act for the benefit of a patient when the pharmacist knows or should know of a potential problem with drug therapy that places the patient at risk of harm. The knowledge that is necessary for expanded responsibility for pharmacists under the power model relates to pharmacological knowledge of drugs, medical knowledge of patients, and personal knowledge of patients.

Knowledge of a problem is the first factor that must be established for a pharmacist to have responsibility under the power model. Pharmacists know about drugs, and drug specific knowledge may be all that is necessary to identify a potential problem with drug therapy. A pharmacist's knowledge of drugs may cause the pharmacist to know that a prescribed drug regimen would pose a problem for any patient, no matter what their history or physical condition may be. For example, a prescription for digoxin 0.25 mg with directions to take one tablet four times daily poses a pharmaceutical problem that is obvious on the face of the prescription, irrespective of the patient's condition. Likewise, a prescription for ergotamine suppositories with directions to use one suppository every four hours and no caution about limitations on use over specified periods of time is a problem that can be recognized without knowing anything about the patient.

On the other hand, there may be problems that can only be recognized as significant by one who has patient-specific knowledge. For example, a drug may pose a problem only for patients who have frequent nose bleeds or high blood pressure. A pharmacist may not have that patient-specific information and would not be able to identify the problem. Although pharmacists sometimes do not have knowledge of a particular patient's unique characteristics, under many circumstances it will be possible for pharmacists to have patient-specific knowledge. For example, a pharmacist may know that a patient who has been prescribed an NSAID has reported an allergic reaction to aspirin or that a patient who has been prescribed a beta blocker suffers from COPD and is using beta agonists.

When they are knowledgeable of a specific patient's physiologic idiosyncrasies, pharmacists must use that knowledge. However, when it is not possible for a pharmacist to have such patient specific knowledge, it will be impossible to know of a problem.

A pharmacist is responsible only when the pharmacist has knowledge of a potential problem. The knowledge factor incorporates both actual knowledge and constructive knowledge. This means that a pharmacist is held legally accountable under the power model for what the pharmacist really did know (actual knowledge), or could have known using reasonable care (constructive knowledge). If a pharmacist knows less than what a reasonable and prudent pharmacist would know, then the pharmacist is held to the higher objective standard. If an exceptional pharmacist knows more than a reasonable and prudent pharmacist would know, then the pharmacist is held to the higher subjective standard. This approach prevents a pharmacist from deliberately remaining unknowledgeable of drug therapy and then escaping responsibility by claiming not to have known things that he or she should have known.

The foreseeability factor places a limit on the bad outcomes for which a pharmacist can be held legally accountable, even if the pharmacist had knowledge of a problem with drug therapy. Of course, if the facts of a case were to show that a pharmacist did not know of a problem, and could not have known of it, then there would be no reason to even consider the foreseeability factor because there would be no potential liability to limit. The foreseeability factor introduces the concept of reasonableness. When knowledge is defined to include both actual and constructive knowledge, there is a danger that the fictional concept of what a pharmacist should have known will be viewed too expansively. By requiring that knowledge be used only when potential harm is recognizable, pharmacists are protected from expectations that are unreasonable within the context of their actual knowledge. Action can be taken to prevent avoidable harm only if the actor recognizes a problem in time for a suitable response. The foreseeability factor, as a determinant of legal accountability, requires not simply that the actor did or should have knowledge of existing facts, but also that the actor believed or should have believed that a bad outcome would occur in the absence of a response to prevent it.

As with knowledge, foreseeability may be drug-specific as well as patient-specific. Some problems with drug therapy are so highly likely to occur that they warrant a response from a pharmacist no matter who the patient may be. Knowledge of drug's characteristics alone makes the problem foreseeable. Other problems may be equally well known but occur infrequently and only with patients who have unusual and difficult to detect characteristics. A pharmacist may have no way to know of a patient's peculiar susceptibility to the problem. Such a problem is ordinarily unforeseeable to a pharmacist, and a pharmacist would have no responsibility to prevent it, even though the pharmacist has knowledge of it.

Capacity is a final factor in the power model. A pharmacist should not be held legally accountable for failure to respond to a problem of which the pharmacist did or should have known, and which the pharmacist foresaw or should have foreseen, if the pharmacist lacked the capacity to prevent the problem. The law does not require that futile gestures be made. Pharmacists have a significant but correlative role in health care. Patients, physicians, nurses, pharmaceutical manufacturers, hospitals, and others share responsibility with the pharmacist for the outcomes of drug therapy. The pharmacist's power is based largely on the ability to persuade others that a problem exists and that action to prevent the problem should be undertaken. A pharmacist may fail in the effort to persuade. Should that occur, a pharmacist is under no legal responsibility to independently take full control of a situation and insist that his or her recommendation be followed. A pharmacist would not be held legally accountable for a bad outcome under such circumstances.

The power model of expanded pharmacist responsibility, which incorporates the knowledge, foreseeability, and capacity factors, has a solid foundation in the litigation of the 1980s and early 1990s. It establishes expectations of pharmacists that will protect patients from harm, and it sets limits that are fair to pharmacists. By focusing on the power model, a court can retrospectively apply theory to facts and distinguish those circumstances in which a pharmacist had no expanded duty from those circumstances in which a pharmacist did have an expanded duty. Pharmacists can prospectively apply theory to fact and recognize those circumstances in which they have a responsibility.

Summary and Conclusion

President Harry S. Truman is frequently praised for the sign he placed on his desk saying, "The buck stops here." That the public would revere a person for accepting responsibility so openly is no great surprise. The public places trust in certain people, recognizing that those trusted people have a responsibility to the public that transcends their responsibility to themselves. The acceptance of responsibility earns these trusted people respect and admiration. It may also earn them the privilege of practicing a profession if they have unique knowledge and skills. Society conveys upon these professional people the authority to do for other people things that most people are not trusted to do.

The responsible provider of pharmaceutical care earns the trust of patients by entering into a caring relationship with them. A hallmark of this relationship is the duty of the provider to respond to potential pharmaceutical problems that pose a risk of harm to the patient. The failure of a provider to act responsibly is a betrayal of trust. It leads to review activities in which the provider must account for his or her actions. Providers who cannot adequately explain their failure to respond to a potential pharmaceutical problem will be held accountable, and perhaps legally liable, for the harm they have caused.

Pharmaceutical care adds a quality-related responsibility to the pharmacist's traditional accuracy-related responsibility. The pharmacist must still perform correctly those functions that have been appropriately ordered by others for example, drug distribution and pharmacokinetic monitoring. However, the pharmacist must also take the initiative to do those things that are necessary for the patient, even though they have not been ordered by someone else. The pharmacist's quality-related responsibility is derivative of the pharmacist's relationship of trust with the patient, and it is not dependent on a relationship with any other person. In pharmaceutical care, the pharmacist has a primary responsibility, with the physician, for the outcomes of drug therapy. That responsibility is met by responding to potential pharmaceutical problems.

References

Baier, K. 1987. *Moral and Legal Responsibility*. In *Medical Innovation and Bad Outcomes: Legal, Social, and Ethical Responses*, ed. M. Stiegler. Ann Arbor: Health Administration Press.

Bosk, C. L. 1979. *Forgive and Remember—Managing Medical Failure*. Chicago: University of Chicago Press.

Brushwood, D. B. 1993. The Pharmacist's Drug Information Responsibility After McKee V. American Home Products. *Food and Drug Law Journal* 48:377–410.

Dukes, M. N. G., and B. Swartz. 1988. *Responsibility For Drug-Induced Injury*. Amsterdam: Elsevier.

Hepler, C. D. 1985. Pharmacy as a Clinical Profession. *American Journal of Hospital Pharmacy* 42:1298–306.

Hepler, C. D. 1993. Issues in Implementing Pharmaceutical Care. *American Journal of Hospital Pharmacy* 50:1635–41.

Hepler, C. D., and L. M. Strand. 1989. Opportunities and Responsibilities in Pharmaceutical Care. *American Journal of Pharmaceutical Education* 53(SUPPL):7s–15s.

Katz, J. 1984. *The Silent World of Doctor and Patient*. New York: The Free Press.

Strand, L. M., et al. 1991. Levels of Pharmaceutical Care: A Needs-based Approach. *American Journal of Hospital Pharmacy* 48:547–50.

Strand, L. M., R. J. Cipolle, and P. C. Morley. 1988. Documenting the Clinical Pharmacist's Activities: Back to Basics. *DICP Annals of Pharmacotherapy* 22:63–6.

Strand, L. M., R. J. Cipolle, and P. C. Morley. 1990. Drug Related Problems: Their Structure and Function. *DICP Annals of Pharmacotherapy* 24:1093–7.

Veatch, R. M. 1981. *A Theory of Medical Ethics*, 110–38. New York: Basic Books.

Weimer, D. L., and A. R. Vining. 1989. *Policy Analysis: Concepts and Practice*. Englewood Cliffs, NJ: Prentice Hall.

11

The Need for Pharmaceutical Care

Donna E. Dolinsky, Ph.D.
C. Edwin Webb, Pharm.D., M.P.H.

Health Care Reform and Pharmaceutical Care

The emergence of pharmaceutical care as the pharmacy profession's mission within the health care system coincides with fundamental changes currently underway in the organization, financing, and delivery of health care services in the United States.

In a speech before a joint session of Congress on 22 September 1993, President Clinton launched the first major health care reform policy debate since the introduction of the Medicare and Medicaid programs in 1964. In his speech, Mr. Clinton described the American health care system as "badly broken, and it is time to fix it (Bureau of National Affairs 1993, S-46)." Among the flaws most often mentioned by health policy experts were the following:

- Failure to guarantee and/or provide access to care for all Americans
- Emphasis on illness, treatment, and cure rather than wellness, prevention, and ongoing care
- Spending increases for health care far exceeding that of other nations as well as exceeding other important areas of the American economy
- Inability of patients and payers to evaluate and compare the quality and cost-benefit of services and providers
- Lack of correlation between increased health care expenditures and Americans' health status

While difficult to characterize as a flaw, the American health care system's unique emphasis on, and immense success with, the development of cutting-edge technology and highly sub-specialized care was also cited as one of the major contributors to the "crisis," particularly the cost component (Fuchs 1992).

The essential components necessary for effective health care reform were described by Simmons, Rhoades, and Goldberg and by Lundberg in 1992. These included:

- Universal coverage for a comprehensive package of health benefits
- Effective control of costs
- Initiatives to improve the quality of care
- Organized delivery systems
- Health insurance reform
- Malpractice reform
- Simplified administration
- System management and oversight

In addition to these systemic and structural issues, **concern** has been expressed regarding the de-emphasis of primary and generalist care, preventive care, and public health within the medical profession specifically (Politzer et al. 1991) and other professions generally. Many of the reform initiatives in the early 1990s sought to address this issue by re-orienting financial aid programs in health professions education, redirecting support for graduate medical education toward primary care disciplines, and enhancing support for communities to attract and retain primary care providers in rural and urban areas underserved by the existing health care system.

It is within this background of substantial change and significant uncertainty that the further development and effective delivery of pharmaceutical care is occurring. In her testimony before the Senate Finance Committee in October 1993, Hillary Rodham Clinton referred specifically to pharmaceuticals, *if properly used,* as an example of the potential for certain components of the health care system to provide solutions to the problems of cost, access, and quality in health care.

Is There a Need for Pharmaceutical Care?

The concepts and activities that define pharmaceutical care have been reviewed elsewhere in this text. (See Chapters 7 and 8.) Presumably, pharmaceutical care developed in response to either real or perceived needs of patients, pharmacists, the health care system, or some combination of all of these. What is the evidence that this so? And what is the quality and quantity of that evidence?

What Are Patients Health/Drug Related Needs?—A Needs Assessment

What is the *need* for pharmaceutical care in maintaining and promoting health? A need can be defined as "whatever is required to maintain something at a satisfactory or acceptable (not ideal) level (Scriven 1982, 57)."

When assessing needs, it is necessary to discriminate between performance needs and treatment needs. Performance needs, such as drug-related health needs, are desirable outcomes—a situation in which health is maintained at a satisfactory or acceptable level. Treatment needs reflect "a need for something that is supposed to bring the performance up to the necessary level (Scriven 1982, 58)." The performance need helps define the intervention or treatment need, as illustrated by the following situation.

A patient has taken a sub-therapeutic dose of a medication. That is a problem. The solution, or performance need, would be for the patient to take a therapeutic dose. The patient needs to take a therapeutic dose but is not doing so. The patient needs some treatment or intervention to help them achieve the desired outcome of taking the therapeutic dose. The treatment need is whatever motivates or otherwise helps the patient to meet the performance need of taking the therapeutic dose.

How are interventions or treatment needs identified, and how are preferred treatments selected? Performance needs can be met through alternative treatments, or interventions. There is more than one way to meet a need. To identify the appropriate treatment, it is necessary to be specific about what constitutes satisfactory or acceptable performance and to evaluate the cost, efficacy, and side effects of each treatment in meeting that need. By identifying specifically what health outcomes patients need or desire, we can begin to identify appropriate treatments.

To meet the need of the patient who took a sub-therapeutic dose, a number of interventions could conceivably be introduced by a pharmacist. Giving information about the mechanism of the drug is one intervention that may be effective with a patient who chooses to take a sub-optimal dose. Working with the patient to modify her health beliefs about her condition may be another. Helping her find ways to remember to take all doses may be another. These are treatment needs. The patient needs information on the mechanism of action of the drug or needs to modify her health beliefs about her condition, or needs to find ways to remember to take her medication. The choice of treatment should depend upon the reason for her problem.

We can identify performance needs (patients' drug-related health outcomes), problems (reasons patients are not achieving those outcomes), and treatment needs (things that need to be done to help patients achieve those outcomes). Treatment needs should target the problems that stand in the way of meeting performance needs, although this is not always the case. For example, information-giving has been a treatment for drug-related health problems in situations where lack of information was not the reason for the problem.

Health performance needs are often defined through consensus. Treatment needs, while often identified through consensus or a political process, are probably better defined through an analysis of problem-solution links based upon research.

How do we assess patients' treatment needs? What do patients need from pharmacists to help them make the transition from focusing on drug-related problems to achieving desirable drug-related health outcomes? What "treatments" should pharmacists engage in to help patients achieve those ends? What do patients need from pharmacists in order to be healthy? To answer these questions, we need to identify:

- Performance needs—desired patient drug-related health outcomes

- Problems—barriers between where the patient is and where the patient needs to be

- Reasons for the problems—why patients are not meeting performance needs

- Treatment needs—what patients need to help them reach desired drug-related health outcomes. Selection of these treatment needs should be based on the reason for the problem

- Cost, efficacy, and side effects of treatments—measurable criteria of success in meeting needs

What are drug-related performance needs? What are the problems that prevent those needs from being met?

Performance Needs: Drug-Related Health Outcomes

Hepler and Strand (1990) have offered clear definitions of satisfactory or acceptable drug related health outcomes, or performance needs. Drugs are given to:

- Cure a disease

- Eliminate or reduce symptoms

- Arrest or slow a disease process

- Prevent a disease or symptom

Performance Needs: Overall Health Outcomes

Health is broader than drug-related health and is defined in various ways. The World Health Organization has historically defined health as "a state of complete physical, mental, and social well-being, and not merely the absence of disease or infirmity (World Health Organization 1944, 29)." As a definition of a need, this may be idealistic and more than the "acceptable or satisfactory level" which we are using to define a performance need. "The well-working of the organism as a whole (Kass 1981, 4)" is considered a "more functional" definition of health (Banta 1990, 8).

Drug-Related Problems: Barriers To Performance Needs

The nature and extent of problems associated with medication use have been the subject of substantial literature coverage in recent years (Manasse 1989; 1988). A comprehensive review of the literature in this area is beyond the scope of this chapter. However, in his extensive review of the subject which he describes as "drug misadventuring," Manasse noted that despite the variety of care settings, age groups, severities of illness, and methodologies employed in studies on the subject, "several common themes emerge:

- Drug misadventuring was causally implicated in hospital admissions
- Drug misadventuring was causally linked to increased length of stay
- Drug misadventuring was causally linked to increased morbidity and, in some cases, to mortality
- Most cases of drug misadventuring could have been avoided (Manasse 1989)

Manasse noted that this substantial evidence had failed, at least at that point in time, to stimulate substantial national debate or calls for reform of the system within which medications are prescribed, dispensed, consumed, and monitored for positive or adverse outcomes.

Drug misadventuring, specific drug-related problems, and their causes, that may lead to drug related morbidity and mortality, are described below. Drug misadventuring, a term for drug related problems which can lead to drug related morbidity and mortality, is defined as "an iatrogenic hazard or incident

- That is an inherent risk when drug therapy is indicated
- That is created through either omission or commission by the administration of a drug or drugs during which a patient is harmed, with effects ranging from mild discomfort to fatality
- Whose outcome may or may not be independent of the preexisting pathology or disease process
- That may be attributable to error (human or system, or both), immunological response, or idiosyncratic response
- That is always unexpected and thus unacceptable to patient and prescriber (Manasse 1989)

Manasse also identified the actors in drug misadventuring. They included medication users, makers, distributors, prescribers, payers, regulators, and policy makers. The users' community, family, and cultural environment can also help prevent or contribute to drug misadventuring.

Strand et al. (1990) categorized eight drug-related problems that interfere with achieving acceptable or satisfactory drug-related health outcomes. Those problems are:

- Requires therapy but not receiving drug
- Wrong drug
- Too little of the drug
- A medical problem that is the result of not receiving a drug
- Too much drug
- Adverse drug reaction
- Interactions of drug with drug, food, or laboratory information
- Taking a drug for medically non-valid indication

Additional drug-related problems can occur when a patient is taking a drug when a non-drug treatment could be equally or more effective.

Causes for drug-related morbidity and mortality include:

- Inappropriate prescribing
- Inappropriate delivery
- Inappropriate patient behavior
- Patient idiosyncracy
- Inappropriate monitoring (Hepler and Strand 1990)

Performance needs—desired patient drug-related health outcomes and problems in meeting those performance needs—have been described. Treatment needs can be identified in two ways: through an analysis of reasons for problems, and through the research literature which describes what people think they need to solve their drug-related problems.

Assessing Patients' Medication-Related Treatment Needs—
A Problem-Solving Approach

We can begin to systematically identify causes of problems by looking at the intersection of drug-related health outcomes, drug-related problems, and people involved in the system of medication use in a matrix. (See Figure 11-1). A common drug-related problem is the failure of a patient to obtain medication when it is needed (upper left hand corner of the matrix). By examining the matrix, we can identify several actors who may be contributing to the problem and suggest some possible reasons for the problems.

Suppose it is the patient who is responsible for the inappropriate behavior. That is, the patient was non-compliant or did not adhere to the medical recommendations. This is a common medication problem. Patients are non-adherent about

Figure 11-1. *Drug Related Health Outcomes and Problems in Drug Use—A Matrix to Identify Patient Treatment Needs*

Actors	Drug-Related Problems								
	No	Wrong	Too Little	Med Problem from No	Too Much	ADR	Interactions	No Med. Valid Indication	Drug Instead of Non-Drug Treatment
User	Inappropriate patient behavior	Inappropriate patient behavior	Inappropriate patient behavior	Inappropriate patient behavior	Inappropriate patient behavior	Inappropriate patient behavior	Inappropriate patient behavior	Inappropriate patient behavior	Inappropriate patient behavior
Community									
Maker	Too expensive				Poor labeling	Poor labeling		Aggressive marketing	
Distributor	Inappropriate delivery, monitoring	Inappropriate delivery, monitoring	Inappropriate delivery, monitoring	Inappropriate delivery, monitoring	Inappropriate delivery, monitoring	Inappropriate delivery, monitoring	Inappropriate delivery, monitoring		
Prescriber	Inappropriate prescribing, monitoring	Inappropriate prescribing, monitoring	Inappropriate prescribing, monitoring	Inappropriate prescribing, monitoring	Inappropriate prescribing, monitoring	Inappropriate prescribing, monitoring	Inappropriate prescribing, monitoring	Inappropriate prescribing, monitoring	Inappropriate prescribing, monitoring
Payer	Not covered								
Regulator Policy maker									

20 percent of the time with short term therapy, 50 percent of the time for longer-term symptomatic chronic conditions and 70 percent of the time with long-term asymptomatic conditions requiring a life-style change (Sherbourne et al. 1992) These problems occur to an even greater extent in the elderly (Tett, Higgins, and Armour 1993). To identify that patient's treatment needs, we need to identify why the patient demonstrated inappropriate health-related behaviors. Otherwise we may intervene with a treatment that is inappropriate for that patient's problem, such as suggesting that the patient buy an electronic medication reminder.

An appropriate treatment should be selected and its cost, benefit, and side-effects should be analyzed. What, then, are appropriate drug-related treatments?

Assessing Patients' Medication-Related Treatment Needs—Research and Position Papers

Several drug-related treatment needs have been identified. Methods used to identify these needs include surveying patients about what they perceive their treatment needs to be; inferring needs from research on reasons for patients' non-adherence to medication regimens; research on physicians' prescribing practices (Rucker 1987); and position papers on pharmaceutical education. The results of these studies and papers are summarized below.

Patient-Identified Treatment Needs

What do patients' perceive their drug-related treatment needs to be? Patients or consumers may not always be conscious of what they need to do to maintain their medication-related and overall health at a satisfactory or acceptable level. What do they know about their medications and treatment? What medication-related therapy do they receive? What do they ask from pharmacists to meet their needs?

What do patients say they need?

In 1986, 92 percent of a sample of upper income households responded that a "pharmacist . . . readily available for personal consultation" is important or very important to them (Joyce and Hubbard 1988). Sixty percent of adults of all ages stated that they wanted pharmacists to counsel them on their medications (Molzon 1992). Over 50 percent of a sample of consumers surveyed in 1987 said they would pay five to ten dollars for a pharmacist's consultation (Spaulding et al. 1989).

Information on how to take and store medications, possible side effects and possible interactions was desired by 64 to 89 percent of consumers in the late 1980s (National Pharmacy Services Study 1988). Information on side effects was identified by patients to be most important (Columbia Broadcasting System 1984). Patients in a health maintenance organization rated precautions, drug interactions, and adverse effects as the most important information they wanted from their physician (Gardner et al. 1988). Patients would like both verbal and written counseling (Harvey and Plumridge 1991; Kimberlin and Berardo 1987). Thus in most studies reviewed, the majority of patients say they need medication information.

What do patients know about their medications?

Patients' knowledge of their medications is generally poor. Ley reviewed research on patient's understanding of what they had been told by their health professionals and concluded that patients often do not understand what they have been told, are reluctant to ask for further information, and forget information they have been given (Ley 1988). Crichton, Smith, and Demanuele (1978) found patients recalled only 27 percent of medication information presented to them by their physician. Questions about adverse reactions, nonprescription medications to avoid, and activities to avoid or perform with caution were answered correctly less than 30 percent of the time by ambulatory clinic patients who were 65 or older (Rosenberg et al. 1984). Thus, patients "know" about a third of what they have been told about their medications.

What drug related treatments do patients receive?

Community Pharmacies

Over 1,000 patients who had obtained new prescriptions during the previous month were surveyed as to what information they received from their pharmacist. One-third said they received information on how to use their medications, 16 percent received information on precautions, and 11 percent received information on side effects (Morris et al. 1984). In a national survey, 23 percent of people interviewed said they received medication use information from their pharmacist. About 15 percent received information on potential risks (Morris et al. 1986). Similar percentages were found in the Schering Report. Twenty-five percent of the patients were told how often to take their medication, down from 40 percent 5 years earlier. Of 2,000 patients who were interviewed, 52 percent received their prescription from the clerk (Schering 1982). In another study, Sixty-five percent of patients over sixty years of age were not given information or warnings about their medication from either their physician or pharmacist (Morris et al. 1987).

A survey of California pharmacists indicated that they spent from 6 to 12 percent of their time consulting patients, with community pharmacists spending more time than hospital pharmacists (Tootelian 1989). A literature review of 10 studies on verbal consultation by pharmacists yielded percentages of pharmacists' failure to provide verbal consultation ranging from 30 to 87 percent (Wiederholt, Clarridge, and Svarstad 1992). In a 1992 survey of 722 patients with a new prescription, 31 percent received information on the purpose of the medication, 32 percent received directions for taking the medication, 11 percent received information on side effects, 7 percent received information on drug interactions or precautions, and 3 percent received general information.

Hospital Pharmacies

Sixty-nine percent of 509 hospital pharmacies surveyed responded that they had patient education or counseling services. Twenty-nine percent had counseling services for inpatients only and 9 percent had only ambulatory care counseling. Thirty percent had both inpatient and outpatient counseling or patient education (Crawford and Meyers 1993).

Pharmacists can and do effectively counsel patients. Based upon studies of pharmacist interventions on medication management by the elderly, it was concluded that clinical pharmacist interviews and counseling of hospitalized patients returning to the community were effective in helping patients better manage their medications. It was further concluded that this counseling should be followed up by community pharmacists with individualized patient education (Tett, Higgins, and Armour 1993).

About one third of patients receive medication information from pharmacists. There is little research on additional drug-related treatments dispensed by pharmacists directly to patients.

What do patients ask from their pharmacist?

One-third of 779 college students reported that they asked their pharmacist for information about their prescription (Trinkaus 1991). An earlier study found that 85 percent of patients did not ask their physician or pharmacist questions about directions, precautions, or adverse reactions (Morris, Barkdoll and Gordin 1986). Ley (1988) reviewed 13 studies and found that 11 to 75 percent of patients did not ask their physicians for medication information, even though they wanted the information.

Patients' knowledge about their medication is quite incomplete. Most patients want medication information, though they are reluctant to ask either their pharmacist or physician for it. About 25 to 30 percent of them receive it from their pharmacist.

Research on Adherence to Medication Regimens and Identified Treatment

Medication-taking behaviors are related to knowledge of medications. As stated earlier in this chapter, patients do not take their medications 20 to 70 percent of the time. This non-adherence to medication regimens has been found to be related to the following factors:

- Perception of being over medicated (Cooper, Love, and Raffoul 1982)
- Health Belief Model variables of perceived susceptibility, severity, benefits over costs (side effects are costs) and efficacy, patient dissatisfaction with personal and financial arrangements, misunderstanding, forgetting, not meeting patients' expectations, duration and complexity of the regimen, level of supervision provided, and influence of family and friends (Ley 1988)
- Earlier non-adherence, avoidant coping strategies, and being distressed about health, (Sherbourne et al. 1991)
- Patients' representations or perceptions of their illness including identity of the disease, time line, consequences, causes, and potential for cure or control (Leventhal, Diefenback, and Leventhal 1992).

Treatment needs to modify non-adherence to medication regimens include:

- Verbal and written information which is necessary but not sufficient for compliance
- Enhancing the patient-practitioner relationship
- Patient education
- Behavior modification and teaching of self-regulatory skills (Meichenbaum and Turk 1987)
- "clear instructions for short term treatments and combinations of the following for long term treatments: clear instructions, simplified regimens, recalling non-attenders, patient self-monitoring of compliance and/ or treatment outcomes, enhancement of social support, 'contingency contracting' rewards or reinforcement for high compliance, group discussion, and supervised self-management (Haynes, Wang, and Da Mota Gomes 1987, p155)"
- Better patient-practitioner communication
- Modification of health beliefs and behaviors
- Understanding and modifying patients' representations of illness and medication use (Leventhal and Cameron 1987)
- Understanding decision processes
- Teaching better ways of making medication-related decisions (Morris 1990)

Increased knowledge, by itself, does not automatically lead to compliance (Fallsberg 1991; Rimer and Glassman 1984). Not all of the correlates of non-adherence have matching treatments, as we do not know how to treat all non-adherence behaviors, and not all of the treatments were based on understanding the underlying mechanism of non-adherence. For example alarm clock reminders may have been used for any adherence problem. Selection of the appropriate treatment should be based on the reason for the non-adherent behavior and the degree of commitment of the patient.

Patients' drug-related needs can be better met by introducing treatments to help the patient adhere to their medication regimen in a manner compatible with their own needs and schedule.

Research on Physician Prescribing Practices and Identified Needs

The way in which physicians choose drugs has been described as a rational process in which physicians systematically use criteria to make a decision about appropriate drug therapy (Denig, Haaijer-Ruskamp, and Zusling 1988). Another explanation is that physicians attempt to use logic, or the expected utility theory, to maximize benefits and minimize problems for the patient. But in reality, biases in thinking, such as difficulty in dealing with ambiguity, interfere in the decision (Hershey and Baron 1987).

External variables have also been implicated in influencing physicians' choice of drug. Rucker suggested that physicians may be influenced through promotional activities of pharmaceutical manufacturers (Rucker 1987). The gender and age of patients also correlates with prescribing practices. For example, women and older people receive more prescriptions for benzodiazepines (Isaacson et al. 1993). Physicians' interpersonal behaviors have also been found to be related to patient characteristics, with Anglo-American physicians responding more empathetically to Anglo-American patients than to Spanish-American patients (Hooper et al. 1982).

Patients' medication-related treatment needs may also include pharmacists' influences on physicians' prescribing practices. The combination of personal educational visits with physicians by clinical pharmacists and mailed drug information was found to reduce inappropriate physician prescribing of propoxyphene, cephalexin, and cerebral and peripheral vasodilators (Avorn and Soumerai 1983). The mailed information alone did not influence prescribing behavior.

Raisch (1990) reviewed methods of influencing prescribing and developed a model based on educational methods, persuasion, administrative influences, and human inference. The model can be used to decide on means of influencing rational drug therapy and also to direct research into physician prescribing.

Position Papers on Treatment Needs

Patients' medication-related needs have been addressed by pharmaceutical educators. In response to the need to deliver pharmaceutical care, the American Association of Colleges of Pharmacy Commission to Implement Change in Pharmaceutical Education advocated the following practice functions for pharmacists in every practice environment to meet patients drug related needs:

- Participate in the drug use decision making process
- Select the appropriate dosage form
- Select the drug product source of supply
- Determine the dose and dosage schedule
- Prepare medication for patient use
- Provide drug products to patients
- Counsel patients
- Monitor patients to maximize compliance
- Monitor patients progress with regard to therapeutic objectives
- Monitor patients to prevent adverse drug reaction and drug interactions

These functions represent things that pharmacists do *to* or *for* patients. This concept was supported by Manasse who proposed that one solution for dealing with drug misadventuring lies in pharmacists "becoming their brothers' keepers (Manasse 1989)."

Berger suggests that rather than doing *to* or *for* the patient, pharmacists should form a therapeutic alliance *with* the patient and work through that alliance to identify and solve patients' drug-related problems (Berger 1993). The therapeutic alliance requires mutual commitment from pharmacist and patient and gives definition to the covenant implied in the definition of pharmaceutical care. It requires "shared responsibility for drug therapy outcomes between the pharmacist and patient (Berger 1993)." The relationship is a non-reciprocal one—it exists solely to meet the needs of the patient. "Pharmacists must do the necessary work to create relationships in which their patients feel safe; safe to discuss concerns, problems with taking their medications, etc. (Berger 1993)." This relationship would permit exploration of the patient's emotional agenda (Campion, Butler, and Cox 1992). Berger emphasized that the pharmacist must be competent, trustworthy, and caring.

If caring implies "having a liking for," it may not be a virtue for health professionals. It could lead to withholding information for fear of (not wishing to hurt hurt someone one cares for, paternalism (deceiving someone for their own good), reciprocal relationship (fostering dependency in a patient to meet one's own needs), favoritism (not caring for patients one cannot like), burnout, and loss of objectivity. Curzer suggests that benevolence, which leads to caring behavior (different from caring), leads to fewer problems for health care practitioner and patient. A benevolent person can respect the autonomy of others and act in their best interest but does not have to form an attachment to the patient (Curzer 1993).

In summary, the research on patients' medication-related treatment needs indicates fairly strongly that patients need:

- Medication information
- Interventions to help them identify and solve their problems with medication use and to plan, carry out, manage, and evaluate their medication-taking behaviors
- Interventions to facilitate rational prescribing practices
- Monitoring of their response to therapy
- A therapeutic alliance with the pharmacist

An analysis of the matrix in Figure 11-1 suggests that pharmacists need to address not only drug misadventuring involving patients and prescribers, as outlined in the research above, but also drug misadventuring involving the patients' community, the pharmaceutical industry, payers, regulators, and policy makers. It would also require that pharmacists be cognizant of non-drug therapies and the results of their appropriate and inappropriate application.

Treatment Needs—A Summary

Strand, Cipole, and Morley have developed a plan for a pharmacist's evaluation of a patient's drug therapy which includes the steps indicated below (Strand, Cipolle, and Morley 1992). Drug-related treatment needs identified through research earlier in this paper are subsumed under Strand's headings.

Step 1 Establish relationship with patient
- therapeutic alliance with the pharmacist

Step 2 Collect, synthesize, and interpret information

Step 3 Identify drug-related problem(s)

Step 4 Establish desired pharmacotherapeutic outcomes

Step 5 Determine feasible pharmacotherapeutic alternatives

Step 6 Select and individualize best prescribing practices
- interventions to improve prescribing
  - modification of structural variables
  - education
  - persuasion
  - identification of biases in decision making
  - confrontation of clinical judgment with science
- interventions to improve compliance
  - medication information
  - patient education
  - behavior modification
  - teaching of self-regulatory skills
  - simplification of regimen

- clear instructions for short term treatments
- enhancement of social support
- contingency contracting
- rewards or reinforcement for compliance
- group discussion
- supervised self-management
- better patient-practitioner communication
- modification of health beliefs and behaviors
- understanding and modifying patient's approach to illness and medications
- understanding patient decision-making processes

Step 7 Design a monitoring plan

Step 8 Implement the selection and monitoring plan

Step 9 Manage and follow up

In summary, existing evidence strongly suggests a broad societal need for the provision of pharmaceutical care. While the need for pharmaceutical care will necessarily vary from one patient to another and from one clinical situation to another, the provision of pharmaceutical care can effectively address a set of significant problems within the nation's health care system.

Integrating Pharmaceutical Care into the Health Care System

Despite an expanding acceptance and understanding of the philosophy and importance of pharmaceutical care, both within and outside the profession of pharmacy, both its structural details and a clear picture of its "fit" within the health care system remain to be fully developed. This is made more complicated by the ongoing national debate on both the relative values and roles of specialized medical care and primary health care and their impact as either causes or solutions to the problems that exist in the nation's health care system.

Starfield (1992) has written extensively on the nature and essential elements of primary care. The elements of primary care include "first contact, longitudinality, comprehensiveness, and coordination (or integration)." The philosophy and focus of primary care services (as contrasted with "medical" services) are described in Table 11-1.

Starfield further suggests that there is a natural tendency for medical professionals to specialize as knowledge in a particular field accumulates. It is this specialization, however, that often leads to fragmentation of care and a focus on a disease process rather than overall health care. One of the major characteristics of the ongoing health reform debate is a significant shift in public policy away from unqualified support for medical specialization and toward enhanced emphasis on primary health care services, disease prevention, and health promotion.

Table 11-1. Comparison of Elements of Primary Health Care and Primary Medical Care

Medical Care	Health Care
• Illness	• Health
• Cure	• Prevention and Care
• Treatment	• Health Promotion
• Episodic Care	• Continuous Care
• Specific Problems	• Comprehensive Care
• Specialists	• Generalists
• Physicians	• Multiple Disciplines
• Isolated Practice	• Team
• Professional Dominance	• Community Participation
• Passive Patients	• Self-responsibility

Adapted from Starfield (1992)

Is pharmaceutical care a primary care function or a specialty function? And how and where will it fit into the evolving health care system? Clearly, many of the skills and abilities of pharmacists that facilitate the provision of effective pharmaceutical care derive from specialized knowledge in such disciplines as pharmacokinetics, pharmacology, pathophysiology, and the social and administrative sciences. Indeed, the early development of the role of the "clinical pharmacist" was firmly grounded in a "specialist" mentality within the profession. Many within the pharmacy profession continue to equate "clinical" practice with specialty training and "advanced" degrees.

Conversely, it has been suggested (American Pharmaceutical Association 1993) that many of the characteristics of contemporary pharmacy practice imply a "primary care" orientation. The widespread availability of pharmacists, in communities of all sizes and locations, together with essentially unrestricted access to and communication with pharmacists, are suggestive of the potential for pharmacy to assume a much stronger primary care role. Among the primary care activities recently described by the American Pharmaceutical Association (APhA) for consideration by pharmacists were the following:

- Provision of pharmaceutical care and essential drug therapy

- Health education programs

- Environmental sanitation

- Maternal and child health, including immunization programs and family planning

- Prevention and treatment of local endemic diseases

- Appropriate treatment of common diseases and injuries

- Promotion of sound nutrition

The likelihood of "turf battles" with other primary care professionals if pharmacists choose to expand their roles into these areas is acknowledged by APhA. Indeed, the background paper suggests that expansion into these areas, though feasible and perhaps logical in many settings of care, should be approached with caution. "Expansion of the role of the pharmacist into the arena of primary care is certainly possible, but the process begins with every pharmacist providing pharmaceutical care. Every pharmacist must accept responsbility for the provision of optimal therapeutic outcomes, and continually establish the profession as an authority on medication use in each patient. This establishes a place for pharmacy on the primary health care team, and once that place is created, the opportunity for expansion exists. Pharmacists may choose to expand their roles and their practice sites further . . ., but to be truly effective, pharmacists must first establish their role in providing pharmaceutical care" (American Pharmaceutical Association, 1992).

Collaborative Pharmaceutical Care In A Reformed Health Care System

It has been suggested (Trinca 1993) that the essential nature of pharmaceutical care allows it to fit very neatly into a collaborative primary health care model. Pharmaceutical care has as its essential elements continuity of care, prevention of medication-related problems, and active communication and collaboration between the pharmacist, the patient, and other providers and prescribers to achieve optimal outcomes from medication use. These core values and philosophy of practice help to define the "primary" versus "specialized" nature of pharmaceutical care.

The simultaneous emergence of health care reform efforts and pharmaceutical care provides a unique opportunity to explore and develop interdisciplinary, collaborative models of care delivery which increase the quality and cost effectiveness of pharmacotherapy. It provides an opportunity to break down traditional "prescribing and dispensing" paradigms and focus instead on effectively using the professional knowledge of several types of health professionals who can contribute to the design, implementation, monitoring, and assessment of a medication use plan for a patient which assures an optimal outcome. The pharmacist is a logical participant, perhaps even the appropriate leader, of such a collaborative team. Importantly, the patient is an integral part of the team as well.

Given the development of centralized standards of care, nationally developed clinical practice guidelines, and uniform measures of quality assurance, it is likely that the structure of health care delivery systems will be reconfigured to promote and utilize interdisciplinary, collaborative models of both primary care and pharmaceutical care. While leadership for this change should ideally come from the collective efforts of the education and practice communities of the various disciplines, change will no doubt take place, even in the absence of such professional leadership, because society, and particularly those who pay for health care services, expect it.

One can envision several models of care which would facilitate the delivery of more effective pharmaceutical care. Among these are:

- An evolving delivery system similar to the current "managed care" or "health maintenance organization" environment. In this setting, the organization employs a broad variety of health professionals to render comprehensive preventative, diagnostic, and therapeutic services. Pharmacotherapy, as well as other aspects of the treatment/care plan (e.g., physical therapy, outpatient surgery, etc.), would be decided upon and implemented collaboratively to achieve the therapeutic goals established by the patient care team. Computer-based records documenting both the diagnostic and treatment decisions would be available to all providers in the system. These records and care plans would replace the traditional paper "prescription" generated by a single individual. Such a model is adaptable to home care, long-term care, and similar forms of health care delivery that are currently emerging.

- Protocol-based pharmacotherapy managed by pharmacists in both outpatient and inpatient settings, based on clinical guidelines developed and/or adopted collaboratively among the disciplines. Such systems would enhance the efficiency of care for patients who are in physician-directed care by shifting appropriate pharmacotherapy management functions to the pharmacist.

- Specialized pharmacotherapy clinics staffed by pharmacists, pharmacy technicians, laboratory personnel, and other appropriate staff to which patients are referred by other health professionals for the management of complex pharmacotherapeutic plans, pharmacokinetic consultations, nutrition support, and similar specialized services

Regardless of the model or models that eventually emerge, the success of such approaches will ultimately depend on the development of a more collaborative philosophy of patient care than has existed traditionally in the U.S. health care system. True collaboration requires effective communication, mutual trust and respect, and common purpose. These characteristics are neither easily nor quickly developed. It is for this reason that the system for educating and training health professionals must establish the philosophical foundation and provide the practice experiences which allow such professional collaboration to develop and flourish. With the emergence of pharmaceutical care, the common purpose, at least, has been identified. It is patient care.

How then can pharmaceutical care be effectively integrated into the American health care system? A recent white paper examination of the subject of the implementation of pharmaceutical care (American Pharmaceutical Association 1992) addressed two key aspects of pharmaceutical care's integration: intraprofessional integration and integration into the larger health care system. The paper notes that, "Among the several differences that can be noted between pharmacy and other health professions, none is more notable or problematic than the lack of regular professional interaction and dialogue among pharmacists [in different practice settings] regarding the [coordination of] care of a particular patient." It is further noted in the paper that sharing of patient medication information and records between pharmacists in different practice settings (e.g., community and hospital pharmacists) as patients move from one care setting to another is "virtually non-existent." The paper suggests that the development of models of patient referral and consultation, *within the profession of pharmacy,* is necessary to improve the quality of medication use.

Similarly, the services and expertise of pharmacists providing pharmaceutical care must be melded with the other primary care services being sought by or provided to patients within the larger care system. A key to this integration is the "building [of] relationships and communication with other members of the [primary] care team." The paper suggests the need for the reorganization of pharmacy practice settings to receive, process, and utilize information from other providers. More critically, however, it urges the development of comprehensive pharmaceutical care record systems which can be shared with patients and other providers to document the provision of pharmaceutical care. In summarizing its recommendations on the integration of pharmaceutical care, APhA recommended the following:

- Pharmacists and organizations that provide pharmaceutical care must integrate their practices fully into the larger health care system.
- Pharmacists must restructure their activities to utilize the full range of technology, information systems, and supportive personnel essential to the delivery of pharmaceutical care.
- Pharmacists must document all aspects of the delivery of pharmaceutical care, utilizing comprehensive, patient-specific record systems. Further, the profession should develop guidelines and model programs which foster the inclusion of nonprescription medication use information into patient records
- The profession must develop, and pharmacists must utilize, a system of intraprofessional consultation and referral among pharmacists that assures continuity of pharmaceutical care for patients.
- Pharmacists must take primary responsibility for communicating with other health professionals involved in the patient's care in assuring the appropriate use of medications.

Patient Participation, Expectations, and Values

What Should Patients Be Doing To Meet Their Needs?

What should be the role of the patient as responsible partner, decision-maker, and actor within the care team? The covenant developed in the process of rendering pharmaceutical care implies "shared responsibility for drug therapy outcomes between the pharmacist and patient. . . . the pharmacist cannot take action to prevent or solve drug related problems without permission and involvement of the patient . . . requires asking patients what is in their best interest (Berger 1993)." This requires that the patient take an active role. Do patients want to take an active role in managing their medications? Are they capable of doing so? Does it make a difference in health outcomes when they do?

Research on the active patient concept in medicine provides some clues. Studies on teaching patients to ask questions, measuring the degree of negotiation in a medical encounter, promoting an active patient orientation, use of behavioral technologies, and surveys of patient preferences for an active role suggest the following:

1. Patients in general want to be informed about their illnesses and the treatment options available to them.

2. Information that permits patients to anticipate and prepare for an experience can be a potent resource for coping with the distress and discomfort of illness and treatment.

3. Information interacts with patient preferences and personality traits in producing outcomes. More information is not always better than less.

4. While there is evidence that some patients desire an active role in decision making and many benefit from such a role, there is little evidence that this is sought by most patients in most situations.

5. The links between patient autonomy and clinical outcomes tend to be weak, ambiguous, or mediated by unexamined variables.

6. Clinicians are often poor judges of patients' information needs and participation preferences.

Recommendations included identifying individual patient needs and designing the interaction to meet those needs and also engaging in better-controlled research. This concept has value for pharmacy and needs to be investigated within the framework of pharmaceutical care. One means of educating patients about their role in pharmaceutical care is through the use of "Package Stuffers." A monthly patient education column encouraging patents to establish a relationship with their pharmacist and suggesting questions to be asked could be handed to patients with their prescription and discussed (Flynn 1993).

Attention to cultural and gender differences in communication patterns should be addressed. For example, "teaching patients to be assertive with their practitioners may be quite a different matter for lower socioeconomic Hispanic women than for an upper middle class, professional group of white men and women (Scharf 1988)." A patient questioning the pharmacist may be perceived of as an interruption, as controlling (Tannen 1990).

Manasse's solution is to encourage patients to "make clearer and more emphatic demands on the health-care system for better management and supervision of their drug therapy. Patients should not allow their health-care professionals, whether physicians, pharmacists, or nurses, to walk away from their socially derived responsibilities and authorities. A higher order of caring than is customarily the standard in pharmacies is certainly called for, especially in those pharmacy settings where the primary emphasis is piecework applied to the prescription dispensing process (Manasse 1989)."

In short, patients need to become actively involved in their pharmaceutical care. They need to be data gatherers, problem identifiers, problem solvers, designers of solutions, self-managers, and self evaluators.

What are Patients' Views of their Pharmacists?

Studies on consumer satisfaction with their pharmacists indicate high satisfaction, even though patients do not receive the information they need and want. Seventy-four percent of 2,000 people interviewed said they were completely satisfied with the verbal and written instructions provided by their pharmacist (Schering 1992). More than 80 percent of consumers were satisfied with 8 of 14 pharmacy characteristics (Joyce and Hubbard 1988). The Gallup Survey found 83 percent of those seeking advice from a pharmacist were very satisfied (Gallup 1990). In a telephone survey, consumers rated their satisfaction with their pharmacist 2.6 on a 4 point scale, with a 4 anchored at very satisfied (Smith and Coons 1993). Twenty-five percent of older patients stated that they chose their pharmacists because they provided information without being asked (American Journal of Hospital Pharmacy 1990).

The Gallup Survey found pharmacists rated highest in terms of honesty and ethical standards (Gallup 1990). In a comparison of pharmacists and other professionals, pharmacists' social standing was lower than doctors', dentists', lawyers' and clergy's, but was higher than bankers' and professors'. Only clergy were considered more honest and ethical. Pharmacists were considered more important to society than professors, lawyers, or bankers but less important than doctors, clergy, and dentists. Only banking was considered less interesting and challenging than pharmacy (Lawrence, Stevens, and Das 1992).

Patient satisfaction with pharmacists may be high because expectations are low. Patients' beliefs, values, expectations, and previous experience are predictors of patient satisfaction with health care (Strasser, Aharony, and Greenberger, 1993).

If patients have not had previous experience with pharmacist counseling, they may not believe that pharmacists will counsel and thus not expect it.

What are Patients' View of Health Care Services?

Patient satisfaction with the quality and amount of information they received from hospitals and medical practitioners was studied through meta-analysis of 33 studies. Thirty-eight percent of the hospitalized patients, 26 percent of the ambulatory patients, and 39 percent of the psychiatric patients were dissatisfied (Ley 1988).

Summary

At best, this chapter only partly answers the question, "Is there a need for pharmaceutical care?" There is substantial evidence that medications are not always properly used. There is substantial evidence that the outcomes desired from medication use are not always achieved. There is substantial evidence that patients do not fully understand the proper use of their medications, and yet they often do not seek the information necessary to do so. There is significant concern among policy makers about the costs of medication but a much less clear appreciation for the costs and impact of medication misuse on other elements of the health care system.

Hopefully, this chapter will stimulate additional study and questions in this important area. Many questions indeed remain, such as:

- Has the profession done an adequate needs assessment concerning pharmaceutical care and its value in the health care system? Have we asked the right questions? Have we identified the most appropriate performance needs? Are we perhaps missing patients' other health needs by limiting pharmaceutical care's emphasis to medication-related health outcomes.

- Should we be limited by present practice models in redesigning what a pharmacist should do? Should we delay judging ideas until we design a few models and test them?

- Should we examine models from other professions and occupations to determine what others are doing that we might use or adapt? While the health professions may be one place to look, we certainly should not be limited to them. Engineering schools could offer ideas in troubleshooting (Woods 1990). Architecture could offer ideas related to the design process, which is essentially problem solving, which would counterpoint the traditions of science, which looks for explanations. Marketing could teach us about persuasion. Education could offer teaching models, while counseling and clinical psychology professionals could teach us about therapeutic communications.

- Should we be designing a new health professional who would be a drug expert, a patient care expert, and a designer of patient medication management systems (Dolinsky 1993)?

Readers, whether pharmacy students, practicing pharmacy professionals, or others, are challenged to participate in the search for answers to these important questions for the profession and the health care system. Much work remains to be done.

References

American Pharmaceutical Association. 1992. The Role of the Pharmacist in Comprehensive Medication Use Management. White Paper Issued by the Board of Directors, March 1992.

American Pharmaceutical Association. 1993. The Role of the Pharmacist as a Primary Care Provider. Staff Discussion Paper. October 1993.

Avorn, J., and S. B. Soumerai. 1983. Improving Drug Therapy Decisions Through Educational Outreach: Randomized Controlled Trial of Academically Based Detailing. *New England Journal of Medicine* 308:1457–63.

Banta, H. D. 1990. What is Health Care? In *Health Care Delivery in the United States,* ed. A. R. Kovner, 9. New York: Springer.

Berger, B. 1993. Building an Effective Therapeutic Alliance: Competence, Trustworthiness and Caring. *American Journal of Hospital Pharmacy* 50(11):2399–403.

Bureau of National Affairs. 1993. Summary of President Clinton's Health Care Reform Proposal. *Health Care Policy Report.* 1(29):S–46.

Campion, P. D., N. M. Butler, and A. D. Cox. 1992. Principle Agendas of Doctors and Patients in General Practice. *Family Practice* 9(2):181–90.

Columbia Broadcasting System. 1984. *Prescription Drug Advertising: Issues and Perspectives.* New York: CBS.

Cooper, J. K., D. W. Love, and P. R. Raffoul. 1982. Intentional Prescription Nonadherence (Noncompliance) by the Elderly. *Journal of the American Geriatric Society* 30:329–33.

Crawford, S. Y., and C. E. Meyers. 1993. ASHP National Survey of Hospital Based Pharmaceutical Services-1992. *American Journal of Hospital Pharmacy* 50(July): 1371–404.

Crichton, E. F., D. L. Smith, and F. Demanuele. 1978. Patient Recall of Medication Information. *Drug Intelligence Clinical Pharmacy* 12:591–9.

Curzer, H. J. 1993. Is Care a Virtue? *The Journal of Medicine and Philosophy* 18:51–69.

Denig, P., Haaijer-Ruskamp, and D. H. Zusling. 1988. How Physicians Choose Drugs. *Social Science and Medicine* 27(12):1381–6.

Dolinsky, D. 1993. The Patient Consultation Mandate: Is It Time for Collaborative Externship Programs? *American Journal of Pharmaceutical Education.* In press.

Fallsberg, M. 1991. *Reflections on Medicines and Medication—A Qualitative Analysis Among People on Long-Term Drug Regimens.* Linkoping Studies in Education. Dissertation No. 31. Department of Education and Psychology. Linkoping University, S–581–583. Linkoping, Sweden.

Flynn, A. 1993. For Your Good Health: Talk to Your Pharmacist. *Illinois Pharmacist* 19.

Fuchs, V. R. 1992. The Best Health Care System in the World? *Journal of the American Medical Association* 268 (7):916–7.

Gallup Organization. 1990. *Public Perceptions of Pharmacists and Pharmacies: NACDS/Gallup Survey.* Princeton: The Gallup Organization.

Gardner, M. E., et al. 1988. Study of Patients' Perceived Importance of Medication Information Provided by Physicians in a Health Maintenance Organization. *Drug Intelligence and Clinical Pharmacy* 22:596–8.

Harvey, J. L. and R. J. Plumridge. 1991. Comparative Attitudes to Verbal and Written Medication Information Among Hospital Outpatients. *Drug Intelligence and Clinical Pharmacy-Annals of Pharmacotherapy* 25:925–8.

Haynes, R. B., E. Wang, and Da Mota Gomes. 1987. A Critical Review of Interventions to Improve Compliance with Prescribed Medications. *Patient Education and Counseling* 10:155–86.

Health and Public Policy Committee, American College of Physicians. 1988. Improving Medical Education in Therapeutics. *Annals of Internal Medicine* 108:145–7.

Hepler, D. C., and L. Strand. 1990. Opportunities and Responsibilities in Pharmaceutical Care. *American Journal of Hospital Pharmacy* 47(3):533–43.

Hershey, J. C., and J. Baron. 1987. Clinical Reasoning and Cognitive Processes. *Medical Decision Making* 7(4):203–11.

Hooper, E. M., et al. 1982. Patient Characteristics that Influence Physician Behavior. *Medical Care* 20(6):630–8.

Isacson, D., et al. 1993. Factors Associated with High-quantity Prescriptions of Benzodiazepines in Sweden. *Social Science and Medicine* 36(3):343–51.

Joyce G. and Hubbard. 1988. Consumer Patronage for Pharmaceutical Services: A Comparative Analysis of Upper Income Households in urban areas. *Journal of Pharmaceutical Marketing and Management* 3(1):11.

Kass, L. 1981. Regarding the End of Medicine and the Pursuit of Health. In *Concepts of Health and Disease, Interdisciplinary Perspectives,* ed. A. Caplan, H. T. Englehardt, and J. McCartney, 3–30. Reading, MA: Addison Wesley.

Kimberlin, C. L. and D. H. Berardo. 1987. Comparison of Patient Education Methods Used in Community Pharmacies. *Journal Pharmaceutical Marketing and Management* 1(4):75–94.

Lawrence, L. W., R. E. Stevens, and S. Das. 1992. The Public's Image of Pharmacists Compared to Other Professionals. *Journal of Pharmaceutical Marketing & Management* 6(3):51–8.

Lawson, B. H. 1980. *How Designers Think*. London: The Architectural Press.

Leventhal H., and L. Cameron. 1987. Behavioral Theories and the Problem of Compliance. *Patient Education and Counseling* 10:117–38.

Leventhal, H., M. Diefenback, and E. A. Leventhal. 1992. Illness Cognition: Using Common Sense to Understand Treatment Adherence and Affect Cognition Interaction. *Cognitive Therapy Research* 16(2):143–63.

Ley, P. 1988. *Communicating with Patients*. London: Croom Helm.

Manasse, Jr., H. R. 1989. *Medication Use in an Imperfect World*. Baltimore: ASHP Research and Education Foundation.

Meichenbaum, D., and D. C. Turk. 1987. *Facilitating Treatment Adherence: A Practitioner's Guidebook*. New York: Plenum Press.

Molzon, J. A. 1992. What Kinds of Patient Counseling Are Required? *American Pharmacist* NS32(3):50–62.

Morris, L. 1990. *Communicating Therapeutic Risk*. New York: Springer-Verlag.

Morris, L., et al. 1984. A Survey of Patient Sources of Prescription Drug Information. *American Journal of Public Health* 74:1161–2.

Morris, L., et al. 1986. *A National Survey of Prescription Drug Information Provided to Patients*. OPE study 73, May 1986 Rockville, MD: Food and Drug Administration.

Morris, L., et al. 1987. Information Search Activities Among Elderly Prescription Drug Users. *Journal of Health Care Marketing* 7(4):5–15.

National Pharmacy Services Study. 1988. Chicago: Market Facts.

Politzer, R. L., et al. 1991. Primary Care Physician Supply and the Medically Underserved—A Status Report and Recommendations. *Journal of the American Medical Association* 266(1):104–9.

Raisch, D. 1990. A Model of Methods for Influencing Prescribing: Part II. A Review of Educational Methods, Theories of Human Inference, and Delineation of the Model. *DICP-The Annals of Pharmacotherapy* 24:537–42.

Rimer, B. and B. Glassman. 1984. How do Persuasive Health Messages Work? A Health Education Field Study. *Health Education Quarterly* 11(3):313–21.

Rosenberg, J. M., et al. 1984. Elderly Ambulatory Care Patients' Knowledge About Drugs. *Hospital Pharmacy* 19:289–301.

Rucker, T. D. 1987. Pursuing Rational Drug Therapy: A Macro View, a la the USA. *Journal of Social and Administrative Pharmacy* 5(3–4):78–86.

Scharf, B. F. 1988. Teaching Patients to Speak Up: Past and Future Trends. *Patient Education and Counseling* 11:95–108.

Schering Report XIV. 1982. *Improving Patient Compliance: Is there a PHARMACIST in the House?* Kenilworth, NJ: Schering Laboratories.

Scriven, M. 1982. Needs Assessment. *Drug Intelligence and Clinical Pharmacy* 16(1):57.

Sherbourne, C. D., et al. 1992. Antecedents of Adherence to Medical Recommendations: Results from the Medical Outcomes Study. *Journal of Behavioral Medicine* 15(5):447–68.

Simmons, H. E., M. M. Rhoades, and M. A. Goldberg. 1992. Comprehensive health Care Reform and Managed Competition. *New England Journal of Medicine* 327(21):1525–8.

Smith, H. A., and S. J. Coons. 1993. Patron Experience and Satisfaction With Pharmaceutical Services. *Journal of Pharmaceutical Marketing and Management* 7(3):81–93.

Spaulding, C. D., et al. 1989. Fee-for-service Consulting: A Consumer Marketing Survey. *Journal of Pharmacy Marketing and Management* 3(4):73–85.

Starfield, B. 1992. *Primary Care—Concept, Evaluation, and Policy.* New York: Oxford University Press.

Strand, L. M., R. J. Cipolle, and P. C. Morley. 1992. Pharmaceutical Care: An Introduction. *Current Concepts.* Kalamazoo: Upjohn Company.

Strand, L. M., et al. 1990. Drug Related Problems: Their Structure and Function. *Drug Intelligence and Clinical Pharmacy—Annals of Pharmacotherapy* 24:1093–7.

Strasser, S., L., Aharony, and D. Greenberger. 1993. The Patient Satisfaction Process: Moving Toward a Comprehensive Model. *Medical Care Review* 50(2):219–48.

Survey Examines Pharmacists' Role in Meeting Needs of Older Patients. 1990. *American Journal of Hospital Pharmacy.* 47:2158.

Tannen, D. 1990. *You Just Don't Understand: Women and Men in Conversation.* New York: Ballantine Books.

Tett, S. E., G. M. Higgins, and C. L. Armour. 1993. Impact of Pharmacist Interventions on Medication Management by the Elderly: A Review of the Literature. *Drug Intelligence and Clinical Pharmacy—The Annals of Pharmacotherapy* 27(1):80–6.

Tootelian, D. H. 1989. 1989 Economic Survey Reveals Statistical Trends in the Profession. *California Pharmacist* 37:25–36.

Trinca, C. E. 1993. Future Scenarios in Primary Care: How Will Pharmacists Join the Team? *American Journal of Pharmaceutical Education* 57 (Summer):193–4.

Trinkaus, J. 1991. Medications and Information for Patients: A Quick Look. *Psychological Reports* 68(3, Pt 1):911–4.

Wiederholt, J. B., B. R. Clarridge, and B. L. Svarstad. 1992. Verbal Consultation Regarding Prescription Drugs: Findings from a Statewide Study. *Medical Care* 30(2):159–72.

Woods, D. R. 1990. *The MPS Program.* Montreal: McMaster University.

World Health Organization. 1944. The Constitution of the World Health Organization. *WHO Chronicle* 1(20):29.

Implementation of Pharmaceutical Care

12

The Pharmacist and Pharmaceutical Care

Calvin H. Knowlton, Ph.D.
Richard P. Penna, Pharm.D.

Introduction

For the past few decades, at least, when patients walk into pharmacies in the United States they are greeted by an employee who accepts the prescription, validates the patient's name, takes the order back to the "pharmacy lab" and places it into some queuing order to be processed (i.e., filled) by the pharmacist. This system has been established over time and occurs religiously in independent and chain community pharmacies and in outpatient hospital and clinic pharmacies (e.g., the Veterans Administration), with few exceptions. In more recent years this process has been duplicated in mail order pharmacy operations, with the post office acting vicariously for "walk-in" patients. The purpose of this chapter is to portray how the advent of pharmaceutical care is fostering role changes for pharmacists, in how prescriptions are processed, what pharmacists do, and why they do it. This chapter, thus, will challenge the ongoing validity of the established practice model described above and, perhaps, determine it to be an anachronism.

What Pharmacists Do and Why: "How Are You?"

In the established model of pharmacy procedures, conversations between pharmacists and patients are perfunctory and frequently oriented around casual social discourse. Often, the motivation for the standard inquiry, "How are you?," that projects from pharmacists to patients, and is often hurled over the width of one or two countertops that separate the parties, is more sociological and cordial than professional. Frequently, the topics discussed by pharmacists and patients are sports, weather, community, and family rather than personal health issues. The lack of health care probing and feedback is ostensibly intended by pharmacists and expected by the patients. Conventional wisdom even notes that the most frequent reason people changed pharmacies was a breakdown of these social interactions (e.g., no one cared if I came to the pharmacy or not); rather than from any desire for enhanced competence, skills, or services associated with the health care treatment provided by the pharmacist (Huffman 1993). Pharmacy education, regulation, and custom have focused pharmacists' actions and tasks on the process of product movement.

The Focus on Process: Education

Pharmacy students were taught and inculcated that their tasks were done when they had assured that prescriptions were "filled" correctly—right quantity, right strength, right dosage form, at the right time for the intended patient. Little emphasis was placed on whether or not the medication was appropriate for the patient or even what was meant by appropriateness?

Appropriateness, under pharmaceutical care, takes on a meaning beyond right quantity, right strength, right dosage form, etc. Appropriateness has more to do with ensuring positive outcomes from the therapy than merely ensuring the exactness of the prescription filling process. It has to do with pharmacists using judgement and extending their roles in patient care. It even has to do with caring (see Chapter 8). Ensuring appropriateness, under pharmaceutical care, means pharmacists assure that the medication therapy is needed to resolve a problem; the medication therapy will not interact with other medications or diseases; the dose and duration of therapy make scientific sense (e.g., age-related changes, allergies); the dosage form and directions will fit the patients' lifestyle; and the patient has awareness of endpoints or outcomes expected of the medication plan or intervention.

This re-focusing on the medication *use* process and intended outcomes, instead of the medication *distribution* process, is a significant challenge for pharmacists and pharmacy education. It is not only changing the nature of pharmacy school curriculums, but also compelling practicing pharmacists to acquire new competencies. Pharmaceutical care is having a major impact on pharmacy's traditional aim of continuing education. Pharmacists have been accumulating numerous continuing education certificates since the 1970s in order to maintain licensure. Obtaining these certificates merely required physical attendance at a seminar. Pharmaceutical care practitioners yearn for those educational experiences that enhance their abilities and self-confidence to meet the pharmaceutical care needs of their patients. One marker to illustrate this trend is the exponential increase in the number of pharmacists sitting for the Certified Diabetes Educator exam (Miller 1994).

Pharmaceutical care education blends traditional product science with new patient centeredness (see Chapter 17). The effect on the practitioner is remarkable. A new energy is aroused in practitioners who genuinely sense a renewed need, utility, and significance in direct patient care. The pharmaceutical care movement has inspired an educational thrust, including curricular revisions, that extends pharmacists' scope of interest beyond provision of an accurately dispensed prescription order, to a concern for what happens to patients once they leave the pharmacy.

Educating for pharmaceutical care is conceptually similar to educating for total quality management. Instead of delimiting them to processing and distributing the prescription, pharmaceutical care education is reorienting pharmacists for involvement in the entire medication use process.

The Focus on Process: Regulation

From a regulatory perspective, the pharmacy profession has a rich history laced with structural and procedural overtones. Of paramount interest to state boards of pharmacy has been the enforcement and assurance of protection of the public's health by proxy. That is, each pharmacy has had to maintain an adequate inventory of dispensing tools, reference books and linear feet of unencumbered counter space. Prescriptions had to be filled and filed in a particular, methodical manner specified by Board regulations.

Pharmaceutical care, along with new technology, is exerting an impact on pharmacy regulators and by extension on pharmacists. The revised pharmacy practice acts permit and even encourage pharmacists to broaden their roles beyond prescription processing tasks. Pharmacists are impelled to advance beyond their mooring to the product and to interact with patients and even to assume co-responsibility for positive health outcomes. Empowering regulations are evolving to give legal blessing to the expanded patient care roles associated with pharmaceutical care. To wit:

> The "Practice of Pharmacy" means the interpretation, evaluation, and dispensing of prescription drug orders in the patient's best interest; participation in drug and device selection, drug administration, drug regimen reviews and drug or drug-related research; provision of patient counseling and the provision of those acts or services necessary to provide pharmaceutical care . . . (National Association of Boards of Pharmacy 1992).

The Focus on Process: Custom

Until recently, custom dictated that pharmacists were not to discuss therapeutic regimens or medication treatment with patients. Until the late 1960s, patients' questions relating to their prescriptions were to be redirected by pharmacists back to the prescribers. Pharmacy's Code of Ethics, through the late 1960s, advised pharmacists "not to discuss the therapeutic effects or composition of a prescription with a patient" (See Table 12-1). Yet even before the code was revised in 1969, farsighted pharmacists began to develop and maintain patient medication profiles to forewarn prescribers when prescription orders were incom-

Table 12-1. *Code of Ethics for Pharmacists, Excerpts*

1952–1969

The primary obligation of pharmacy is the service it can render to the public in safeguarding the preparation, compounding the dispensing of drugs and the storage and handling of drugs and medical devices.

The pharmacist does not discuss the therapeutic effects or composition of a prescription with a patient. When such questions are asked, he suggests that the qualified practitioner is the proper person with whom such matters should be discussed.

1969–1993

A pharmacist should hold the health and safety of patients to be of first consideration and should render to each patient the full measure of professional ability as an essential health practitioner.

1993–

A pharmacist respects the covenantal relationship between the patient and pharmacist. A pharmacist promotes the good of every patient in a caring, compassionate and confidential manner. A pharmacist respects the autonomy and dignity of each patient.

---

patible or redundant and to advise patients. By the 1980s the patient medication profile was routine in the profession.

By the early 1990s, practicing pharmacists were ordered by federal legislation (Omnibus Budget Reconciliation Act of 1990 [OBRA 1990]) to obtain, record, and maintain various pieces of patient-specific medication information and to talk with the patients when they dispensed prescriptions to them. In 1993, the code of ethics was revised once again to highlight the obligations the pharmacist has to the patient. The Commissioner of the Food and Drug Administration challenged pharmacists to shift their attention from the product to the patient.

> If you are a community or hospital pharmacist who views your relationship with your patient as a commercial transaction drawing on a specialized expertise—no different from a purveyor of computers or washing machines—then you are not a healer. If . . . you can respond only to the immediate transaction . . . well, a dispensing machine could take your place. It is the healers who fix their gaze upon the patient (Kessler 1993).

The harbinger of a profession entering a transition, from process and product fixation to caring appeared in the early 1960s with the "clinical" movement in hospital pharmacy. Some thirty years later the patient-focused care role was written into the preface of the 1990 OBRA legislation. The Federal directive discussing the rules and regulations of Section 4401 of the OBRA started: "The purpose of the DUR [Drug Use Review] program is to improve the quality of pharmaceutical care by ensuring that prescriptions are appropriate, medically necessary, and that they are not likely to result in adverse medical results."

This destabilization of custom has profoundly affected the role of pharmacists.

The shock waves caused by national and state health care reform debates also contribute to this opportunity for enhancement of professional responsibility. Society demanded positive health outcomes (See Chapter 9) from a cost-effective perspective. Value was calculated from inputs (numerator) and costs (denominator). Pharmacists were creating value in the managed care arena. Their inputs were remarkable and often under-utilized. Their costs were below those of many other health care providers. Pharmacists were well positioned for additional responsibility and authority.

Adding Value or Creating Value: Soccer and Pharmaceutical Care

Business shifted from a sequential "value chain" management motif to a "value constellation" motif where functional roles were reconfigured and traditional lines of managerial demarcation were blurred (Normann and Ramirez 1993). In health care this change was manifested in new, cooperative alliances between and among providers and payers. These alliances sought improved patient care at the lowest possible cost. Cross-functional roles evolved for pharmacists, nurses, and others in the institutional and ambulatory settings. Interdisciplinary value creation surpassed intradisciplinary value adding. Pharmacy had set off on its quest to become a fully integrated player in the health care system.

A sports analogy may help make this point. The first half of the 1990s underscored the profundity of power transformation in health care. In the health care system of an earlier era, the physician was presumed to be the pitcher for the health care baseball team. All of the other team members waited for the physician to throw the pitch before reacting. In the early 90s, the system entered the era of the health care soccer team. Many professionals held active positions, were fluid, interactive, and co-responsible, and moved in the same direction for the benefit of the patient.

Timing is everything. Due to solid planning on the part of the profession, pharmacists were able to make the transition to pharmaceutical care. Mission statements and guiding principles were in place. Reconfigured education, regulation, and custom enabled change. Yet the catalyst that sparked implementation, by one pharmacist after another, were the turmoil within the payer-driven health care system and difficulties meeting expenses in pharmacies relying solely on dispensing income. It was fortuitous serendipity that all these elements came together.

Pharmacists Implementing Pharmaceutical Care

For pharmacists to fulfill this new proactive mission, changes were made, and continue to taking place, in attitudes, organization, relationships, functions, and communications. This section describes how the transition appears.

Attitudes

The first step pharmacists had to take was a mental one. The old adage, "what we do is a function of our decisions more than our conditions," has some eternal verity. Each pharmacist has had to recognize that individual attitudes control behavior (Knowlton 1993). Pharmacists have wrestled with the contention that, on one hand, they are licensed practitioners who can choose to adopt the new pharmaceutical care mission of the profession; yet on the other hand, such a revolutionary transition causes personal anxiety and, perhaps, tensions in their relationships with their employers.

However, part of the impetus for an attitudinal shift comes from a review of the data associated with the negative outcomes of medication use. From this data one can discern the need for pharmaceutical care (See Chapter 11). Suboptimal use of medication therapy results in the inefficient use of resources, preventable adverse drug reactions, and therapeutic noncompliance. If pharmacy does not take steps to attack this problem, others in society will come forth as saviors.

> Pharmacy is well positioned to assume many new service and care roles as
> the health care system continues to change and expand. Such opportunities
> may be open only for short periods of time before other professional groups
> "lay claim" to them (American Association of Colleges of Pharmacy 1992).

Technology and economics have driven the quest to correlate misuse of medication with various negative outcomes. The analysis of large prescription and disease computer data banks has piqued the interest of many health care stakeholders, including pharmacists and various payers, such as managed health care administrators and public policy makers. The data reveal unnecessary and preventable morbidity and mortality along with cost-imprudent medication therapy. The Commissioner of the Food and Drug Administration noted that patients' misunderstanding of the proper use of medications continues to be an underlying cause of "many" adverse drug reactions (Bloom 1991) which lead to unnecessary illnesses, hospitalizations, and expenditures (Kusserow 1990; Kessler 1991; Grymonpre et al. 1988; Col, Fanale, and Kronholm 1990; Davidsen et al. 1988; Sullivan, Kreling, and Hazlet 1990).

The attitude change in pharmacists starts when they realize that they can be part of the solution. A 1990 report from the Office of the Inspector General concluded that, "there is strong evidence that clinical pharmacy services add value to patient care and reduce health care utilization costs . . . but clinical services are not widely provided in community pharmacy settings (Kusserow 1990, 1). As mentioned before, OBRA 1990 requires that pharmacists obtain, record, and maintain vast amounts of patient data for assessment of appropriateness of medication therapy and then consult with patients after a prescription is prepared. Documentation exists to indicate that such counselling can increase patient medication compliance and patient satisfaction (Berger et al. 1990).

Other studies indicate that pharmacists can detect prescribing errors thus avoiding drug-related problem sequelae (Rupp 1990) and that pharmacists in hospital settings have a favorable record of cost avoidance related to drug therapy (Forstrom et al. 1990; McGhan, Einarson, and Savers 1987; McKenney and Wasserman, 1979). There is also empirical evidence regarding the impact community pharmacists might have on prescription drug expenditures or on the larger picture of preventable adverse drug reactions in the non-hospital settings (Morrisey, Plein, and Plein 1991; Andrews, 1992; Knowlton and Knapp 1994). Continued documentation of the cost benefit of pharmaceutical care is expected to enhance that picture.

Even when the reasons to change are compelling and obvious, changing attitudes, values and behaviors—from focusing on dispensing to becoming a pharmaceutical care giver—is not an easy task. Going from point A (dispenser) to point B (pharmaceutical care giver) is often a scary, protracted process and certainly not an overnight event. The starting point for B is also the ending point for A. Between A and B is transition space. In the transition space associated with such a dramatic change lurk high anxiety, low motivation, confusion, frustration, and even signs of grieving. Anger, denial, and bargaining are frequently observed (Bridges 1991).

Successfully emerging from the transition wilderness as a new type of pharmacist occurs only after a thoughtful, deliberate, and often painful process. Yet the time of transition is also a time ripe for creativity. The pharmaceutical care initiative has fostered numerous remarkably innovative practices. However, a change in the individual pharmacist's attitude was the first step. Once the attitude shifted, the first tenet of pharmaceutical care emerged: the nature of the relationship between the pharmacist and the patient has to change.

Relationships

Pharmaceutical care's pivotal precept is the establishment of a new kind of relationship with patients—a covenant. Pharmacists' duty under this covenant is to hold patients' best interests paramount. In entering the covenant, pharmacists commit to a process that focuses on empowering patients to participate actively in and to receive appropriate information about the selection and monitoring of medication-related therapeutic regimens (See Chapters 7, 8, and 10).

This covenential relationship results in a pledge. In return for the trust society has given to the pharmacy profession, pharmacists undertake an obligation to provide patients with pharmaceutical care. Pharmacists promise to be dedicated to helping patients receive optimum benefit from medications, to be committed to the patient's welfare, and to maintain the patient's trust. Pharmacists pledge to maintain communication with patients as proactive health care providers, rather than as episodic health care responders.

Pharmaceutical care positions pharmacists as complements to other health care professionals, not as a substitutes for them. It is the job of pharmacists to let other providers know (in word and deed) that pharmacists are with them, on the side of patients. In adopting pharmaceutical care pharmacists do not intend to become turf-takers, autonomous advisors, or second-guessers of other health care providers.

This relationship of shared responsibility for positive health outcomes can be fostered in various organizational settings. Perhaps it is more accurate to say no particular organizational setting or edifice is best for fostering this relationship, since practicing pharmaceutical care relies more on where the patient is and where the information is than it does on where the medications are located. One could make a strong case that the most fertile setting in which to provide pharmaceutical care is wherever the patient is, including long term care facilities, hospices, acute-care institutions, patient's homes, and staff-model Health Maintenance Organizations.

Organization

Once pharmacists' attitudes have embraced the notion of pharmaceutical care, pharmacists attempt to take the next step—to appropriate the notion into practice. That next step has to do with organizational issues and systems issues.

The well-known management writer and teacher Peter Drucker notes that ours is an era of change in organizations and in functions. We have passed through the stages of manufacturing productivity (making things) to service productivity (moving things) to the age of knowledge productivity (teaching about things) (Drucker 1991). In this societal transformation, knowledge is the primary resource for individuals and for the economy overall (Drucker 1992). Since pharmaceutical care is a relationship built on empowerment (that is, communicating knowledge and assisting in its understanding and application), it is not surprising that to facilitate communication, structural and policy changes often need to occur in the pharmacy—whether community/ambulatory or institutional.

Originally pharmacies were designed to enable product preparation and distribution, not information sharing or caring. Thus, hospital pharmacies were often relegated to a basement area—out of the way—and the "lab" of the community pharmacy was hidden away in the back of a store. The assimilation of pharmaceutical care into practice necessitates an organizational reengineering, from a patient's perspective. In the hospital or long-term care facility it might mean leaving the pharmacy as is—meaning, both leaving the product-distribution layout as is and having the pharmacist leave the product-distribution area, at times, to move in proximity to the patient. In the community/ambulatory facility, where the patient visits, the assimilation of pharmaceutical care often requires physical alteration of layout of the facility to make it conducive to provide one-on-one semi-private meeting space.

Many ambulatory pharmacies, including the Veterans' Administration outpatient sites and many chain and independent pharmacies, have realized that the conveyance of knowledge cannot occur in a cluttered, noisy area. Computer terminals and pharmacists have been relocated to patient interview areas, away from the activities of the dispensing lab. These separate sit-down areas for patient/ pharmacist contact support the development of the human side (i.e., the art) of pharmacy. This issue of the importance of attending to structural variables in order to optimize care has been reviewed in depth (Meichenbaum and Turk 1987).

Technology has given pharmacists mobility. Unlike the typewriter, the computer can print a label in an area physically separate from the keyboard. Pharmacists can meet with patients in an area remote from the dispensing process by feet or miles and still access patient information, process customized prescription orders that concur with a patient's lifestyle (and automatically print out in the dispensing lab—either in-house or off-site), and provide pharmaceutical care in a professionally friendly, non-store type of environment. Extensive cognitive-service computer systems and prototypical policies, procedures, and layout redesigns have been developed and marketed to assist pharmacists in adopting a practice structure receptive to pharmaceutical care (American Pharmaceutical Association 1994).

Functions

In addition to transforming their attitudes and organizational settings, pharmacists who practice pharmaceutical care have transformed their functions. What pharmacists who are practicing pharmaceutical care do is laid out in several conceptual models. The ABCs of pharmacy practice serve as one framework.

A—assessment

B—bottling

C—counseling

S—surveillance

Assessment

The assessment phase of the drug use process is the most critical. In the nursing home or hospital, this means that pharmacists are making rounds, both independently and with other health care providers, and providing proactive input prior to the writing of medication orders. For instance, retrospective thirty-day chart reviews would be insufficient, by themselves, to fulfill the meaning of pharmaceutical care. In the community setting, pharmaceutical care means that pharmacists are the first contact with patients who enter the pharmacy. It means that pharmacists, with the computer at hand, meet the patients before a prescription medication label is generated to focus on the three domains of current concern to public health: preventable adverse medication reactions, treatment adherence or compliance, and informed consent.

It is during the assessment phase that the pharmacist "obtains, records and maintains" patient information. After proper data gathering and evaluation, pharmacists determine the appropriateness of the regimen, considering such aspects as medication; dosage parameters; and drug-drug, drug-food, drug-condition, and drug-lifestyle interactions, and ensure that no obvious adverse sequelae are likely.

It is also during this assessment phase that pharmacists ascertain patients' understanding of the treatment. Facilitating treatment adherence occurs at this time when, before processing the prescription, the pharmacist establishes and reinforces a relationship of understanding with the patient. Meichenbaum and Turk (1987, 63) note that, "once a workable relationship has been established between the health care practitioner and the patient, a variety of adherence enhancement strategies can be employed."

Finally, it is during this assessment phase that pharmacists enable the patient to give informed consent by providing them with sufficient knowledge to make autonomous decisions regarding generic substitution, pharmaceutical alternates, starter doses, quantities, and therapeutic interchange, at the least. On a fiscal and an ethical basis, the paternalism of the past, when physicians, manufacturers, or pharmacists made virtually all medication decisions, has dissipated. Part of pharmaceutical care is empowering patients with knowledge (i.e., teaching people about things) to make decisions.

One could argue that the assessment is the most crucial function performed by pharmacists. One could also argue that without the assessment phase, society would not need pharmacists. FDA Commissioner Kessler (1993) noted that society does not need pharmacists merely to distribute drugs.

Bottling

The B in ABCs stands for bottling, which means repacking and labeling the medication. As unit-of-use packaging takes hold in this country, the need for repacking will diminish. As dispensing machines become vogue, the need for both repacking and labeling will diminish. There will be a need for oversight and checking but that need may not require pharmacists' eyes to ensure fastidiousness.

Counseling

After the assessment and bottling (repacking and labeling) are complete pharmacists check the final deliverable before it goes to the patient. At this time, pharmacists again meet with patients to discuss and/or demonstrate, if appropriate, the proper use of the medication and/or device (eg., peak flow meters, home blood pressure monitoring manometers, home blood glucose monitors, etc). Two-way conversation also covers topics such as missed doses, storage options, when and how to start the therapy, duration of the therapy, educational materials, compliance guides, side effects, and precautions.

Surveillance

Patient-specific monitoring is part of the pharmaceutical care process. This can take the form of 24–48 hour post-dispensing telephone follow up of at-risk patients; mandatory first-refill counseling by pharmacists; ordering or performing therapeutic drug monitoring or other indicated laboratory tests; and general health status inquiries. This aspect of pharmaceutical care moves pharmacists away from the episodic filling/commodity procedures and makes them active participants in the drug use process who are being concerned about what transpires between prescription refilling episodes.

Health education for disease self-management is also a cognitive service opportunity associated with pharmaceutical care monitoring efforts. This type of patient empowerment occurs in pharmacies, hospital clinics, or wherever the patients are, by appointment, and focuses on creating and implementing patient-specific educational plans. This type of education is usually disease-specific, typically focusing on areas such as diabetes (general education, insulin injection training, blood glucose meter training, nutrition); hypertension (general education, self-monitoring of blood pressure); asthma (proper usage of medication devices, self-monitoring of peak-flow); anticoagulation positive outcome strategies; and areas such as women's health or smoking cessation.

Professional Communications

We have discussed how the appropriation of pharmaceutical care necessitates changes in pharmacists' attitudes, pharmacy organization and structure, and pharmacists' relationships and functions. Pharmaceutical care also requires new forms of communication for pharmacists. Under the older value chain distributional paradigm, pharmacists were required only to document by exception. That is, it was assumed that a prescription would be processed exactly as written. Documentation of processing the order was on file in the pharmacy. If a presented prescription were not filled exactly as written, for whatever reason, then the pharmacist would be obligated to telephone the prescriber. No further documentation was useful.

In the pharmaceutical care paradigm, communication and documentation roles have expanded. What some have called seamless care (or continuity of care) compels pharmacists to graft pharmaceutical care documentation into the medical care picture. Both legal mandates (e.g., OBRA 1990) and professional standards require ongoing pharmaceutical care plan documentation. Contemporary sharing of judgments and strategies, from pharmacists to other providers, fosters continuity of care. (See attached example.)

Closing: Toward New Measures of Success

The profession of pharmacy found itself at a strategic decision point in the early 1990s. The prescription had become a replicable commodity. While prescriptions were once a mysterious creation brought forth by artful compounding, pharmaceutical manufacturing and marketing had muted the demand for individualized titrations. Thus, on one hand the profession could continue to try to control the dispensing of what had become a commodity, with winners, losers, and success determined by location, corporate alliances, and price. On the other hand, pharmacy could underscore the vast, mounting literature detailing iatrogenesis from medication mishaps and could reposition itself. Pharmacy could present itself as profession eager to accept new responsibilities and as health care providers who could provide meaningful enhancement to the drug use process, resulting in positive impacts on cost, quality, and outcomes.

Pharmaceutical care, as discussed in Chapter 7 and held forth in this chapter, purposefully repositions the pharmacist as an active player and stakeholder in the drug use process. Under the rubric of pharmaceutical care, the pharmacist's motivation for asking the patient, "How are you?," goes beyond social nicety to the realm of patient assessment and/or monitoring for the purpose of enhancing caring and fostering patient empowerment.

Furthermore, pharmaceutical care is also changing the measures of success for pharmacists. Product output parameters, such as the number of prescriptions processed per day, and the acclaims of creative product purchasing negotiations with wholesales are muted by pharmaceutical care, technology, and political reforms in health care. Newer measures of success for pharmacists include comparative outcomes such as per-person per-month average medication ingredient costs; compliance indices; patient satisfaction with pharmacy services indices; mortality proxies (eg., incidence of medication-related adverse drug reactions); and patient self-efficacy ratings (eg., Does the patient feel that they know how to use a metered dose inhaler properly?). Without such an economic validation of the new roles for pharmacists, the change to pharmaceutical care would be fleeting.

References

AACP Commission to Implement Change in Pharmaceutical Education. 1992. *The Responsibility of Pharmaceutical Education for Scholarship, Graduate Education, Fellowships and Postgraduate Professional Education and Training*. Alexandria, VA: American Association of Colleges of Pharmacy.

American Pharmaceutical Association. 1994. *Pharmaceutical Care Profiles*. Washington, DC: American Pharmaceutical Association Foundation Newsletter.

Andrews, A. (1992, June). Community pharmacists cognitive services: Interventions and their economic value that result from prescription-related problems in Washington state. Renton, WA: The Washington State Pharmacists Association.

Berger, B. A., et al. 1990. Effectiveness of an Educational Program to Teach Pharmacists to Counsel Hypertensive Patients and Influence Treatment Adherence. *Journal of Pharmacology, Marketing & Management* 5:27–41.

Bloom, M. Z. 1991. FDA's Kessler: A Prescription for Change. *American Pharmacy*. NS31:134–7.

Bridges, W. 1991. *Managing Transitions: Making the Most of Change, 58–9. NY: Addison-Wesley.*

Col, N., J. E. Fanale, and P. Kronholm. 1990. *The Role of Medication Noncompliance and Adverse Drug Reactions in Hospitalizations of the Elderly. Archives of Internal Medicine.* 150 (April):841–2.

Davidsen, F., et al. 1988. Adverse Drug Reactions and Drug Non-compliance as Primary Causes of Admission to a Cardiology Department. *European Journal of Clinical Pharmacology.* 34:83–6.

Department of Health and Human Services, Health Care Financing Administration. 1992. Medicaid Program: Drug Use Review Program and Electronic Claims Management System of Outpatient Drug Claims. Interim final rule with comment period. *Federal Register.* 57(212):49397–405.

Drucker, P. F. 1991. The New Productivity Challenge. *Harvard Business Review*. December:69–79.

Drucker, P. F. 1992. The New Society of Organizations. *Harvard Business Review.* October:95.

Forstrom, M. J. et al. 1990. Effect of a Clinical Pharmacist Program on the Cost of Hypertension Treatment in an HMO Family Practice Clinic. *DICP.* 24:304–309.

Grymonpre, R. E., et al. 1988. Drug-associated Hospital Admissions in Older Medical Patients. *Journal of American Geriatric Sociology.* 36:1092–8.

Huffmann, D. C. 1993. November 15. Personal Communication. Alexandria VA: NARD Management Institute.

Kessler, D. A. 1991. Communicating with Patients about Their Medications. *New England Journal of Medicine.* 325:1650.

Kessler, D. A. 1993. Commencement Address. Philadelphia College of Pharmacy & Science. May 15.

Knowlton, C. H. 1993. Pharmaceutical Care: Getting There from Here. *Pharmacy Business* 4(3):6–10.

Knowlton, C. H. and D. A. Knapp. 1994. Community Pharmacists Help HMO Cut Drug Costs. *American Pharmacy.* NS34:36–42.

Kusserow, R. P. 1990a. Medication Regimens: Causes of Noncompliance. Washington DC: Office of the Inspector General. OEI–04–89–89121.

Kusserow, R. P. 1990b. The Clinical Role of the Community Pharmacist, Washington DC: Office of the Inspector General. OAI–01–89–89160.

McGhan, W. F., T. R. Einarson, and D. L. Savers. 1987. A Meta-analysis of the Impact of Pharmacists Drug Regimen Reviews in Long Term Care Facilities. *Journal of Geriatric Drug Therapy*. 1:23–34.

McKenney, J. M., and A. J. Wasserman. 1979. Effect of Advanced Pharmaceutical Services on the Incidence of Adverse Drug Reactions. *American Journal of Hospital Pharmacy*. 36:1692–7.

Meichenbaum, D. and D. C. Turk. 1987. *Facilitating Treatment Adherence: A Practitioner's Guidebook*. New York, NY: Plenum Press.

Miller, L. 1994. October 5. Personal Communication. Chicago: American Association of Diabetes Educators.

Morrisey, M. R., J. B. Plein, and E. M. Plein. 1991. Prospective Review of Dosing of Renally Eliminated Medications for Nursing Home Residents. *Consultant Pharmacist*. 6:623–38.

National Association of Boards of Pharmacy. 1992. Model State Pharmacy Practice Act, Final Draft, 2. Park Ridge, IL: National Association of Boards of Pharmacy.

Normann, R., and R. Ramirez. 1993. From Value Chain to Value Constellation: Designing Interactive Strategy. *Harvard Business Review*. 71(4):65–77.

Omnibus Budget Reconciliation Act of 1990 (OBRA 1990). Section 4401, 42 U.S.C., 483.60. Washington DC.

Rupp, M. T. 1990. Documenting Prescribing Errors and Pharmacist Interventions in Community Pharmacy Practice. *American Pharmacy*. NS28:30–7.

Sullivan, D. D., D. H. Kreling, and T. K. Hazlet. 1990. Noncompliance with Medication Regimens and Subsequent Hospitalizations: A Literature Analysis and Cost of Hospitalization Estimate. *J Res Pharm Econ*. 2:19–33.

13

Compensation for Pharmaceutical Care
Michael T. Rupp, Ph.D.

Overview

For pharmaceutical care to advance from practice philosophy to practice reality, a number of formidable obstacles must first be overcome. Some of these are discussed in other chapters. They include pharmacists' competence, barriers in the physical environment, and inadequate access to patient information. Clearly, overcoming these obstacles represents an essential step toward ensuring that pharmaceutical care *can* become the standard of pharmacy practice. But removing these barriers alone will not ensure that pharmaceutical care *will* become the standard of practice. For this to occur there is yet another critical condition: compensation.

This chapter will present an overview of compensation in pharmacy with particular emphasis on the implications of pharmacy's transition from product-centered, task-oriented activities to a more patient-centered, outcome-oriented professional role. The meaning of the term "value" will then be explored within the context of pharmaceutical care. What is value? How is it measured? What is the relationship between value and pharmaceutical care? Why are these questions important for securing equitable compensation from payers for pharmacists' professional services? Recent advances in the definition and measurement of the value of physicians' services will be described and their potential application to pharmacy will be discussed.

The chapter will continue with a comparison of alternative approaches to structuring payment for pharmacists' services. The components of an "ideal" compensation system will also be outlined. Among the questions that must be answered in developing the ideal compensation system are:

- *What* services will be compensated and how will they be selected?
- *Who* will be compensated, and how can patients and payers be assured that pharmacists meet the professional qualifications necessary to ensure competent and consistent performance of professional services?
- *How* will services be compensated?
- *What* are the operational requirements of an efficient payment system?

The chapter will conclude with an example of one community pharmacy organization's approach to securing compensation for the delivery of pharmaceutical care.

History

The professional services that pharmacists historically performed were linked exclusively to the drug products they prepared and dispensed. Indeed, until the latter part of this century, pharmacy practice was virtually synonymous with drug dosage formulation and delivery. While pharmacists have always recognized that assuring proper use of the products they dispense is essential for achieving desired therapeutic outcomes in patients, the pharmacy profession has not historically embraced this role as a professional responsibility of the *pharmacist*.

During the past quarter century, a fundamental change has occurred in the definition of pharmacy practice and the recognized professional role of the pharmacist. While it is impossible to say precisely when or where this transformation began, Brodie's advancement of "drug-use control" as the primary mission of pharmacy in 1967 represents a particularly noteworthy milestone (Brodie 1967). The continuing evolution of pharmacy practice was further reflected in the 1975 report of the Study Commission on Pharmacy, headed by Dr. John Millis, which concluded:

> *Pharmacy is a health service.* The only justification for inventing, manufacturing, distributing, prescribing, or dispensing drugs is that they can and do have a beneficial effect upon people who are ill and that drugs can cure disease, control disease, prevent disease, or ameliorate the sufferings of the victims of disease (Study Commission of Pharmacy 1975).

The Millis Commission stated unequivocally that delivering pharmaceutical products to patients is not—or should not be—an end in and of itself. Rather, drug distribution is but a means to an end, with the end being the enhanced health and well-being of the patient. While the distributive activities that are involved in delivering drug products to patients remain important elements of pharmacy practice, as the profession has evolved these activities no longer *define* pharmacy practice. That is, the drug product per se is no longer the social object around which pharmacy practice is organized. Rather, it is the patient, or perhaps more precisely, the *interaction* that occurs between the patient and the drug product, that is the central focus of contemporary pharmacy practice.

In recent years, the concept of a patient-centered approach to pharmacy practice has been further advanced in a philosophy known as "pharmaceutical care (Hepler and Strand 1990)." While this emerging concept has yet to be fully operationalized, one aspect is clear: implementing pharmaceutical care requires the pharmacist to adopt a patient-centered approach to practice that focuses on ensuring the achievement of desired patient outcomes.

The impact that this concept has had on pharmacy practice is evidenced in the revised mission statement for the profession that was recently adopted by the American Pharmaceutical Association's Board of Trustees. It states:

> The mission of Pharmacy is to serve society as the profession responsible for the appropriate use of medications, devices and services to achieve optimal therapeutic outcomes (American Pharmaceutical Association Board of Trustees 1991).

However, as many professional organizations and educational institutions have rushed to embrace pharmaceutical care as the new mission of practice, it has become increasingly clear that practicing pharmacists face formidable barriers to consistently providing this level of care, particularly in the community setting.

In November 1990, the Office of HHS Inspector General, Richard P. Kusserow, released a report titled The Clinical Role of the Community Pharmacist (U.S. Department of Health and Human Services 1990). Several conclusions of the Inspector General's report are particularly relevant to this discussion. First, the report stated, "there is strong evidence that clinical pharmacy services add value to patient care," and that the value created by these services "includes not only improvements in clinical outcomes and enhanced patient compliance, but also reductions in health care utilization costs associated with adverse drug reactions." Second, despite the recognized potential value of clinical services, the report concluded that these services "are not widely provided in community pharmacy settings." Finally, the report stated that "in the community pharmacy setting, significant barriers exist that limit the range of clinical services generally provided." One of the most formidable of these barriers is "a transaction-based reimbursement structure [which] links pharmacists' reimbursement to the sale of a product rather than provision of services."

All of the barriers identified in the Inspector General's report are deserving of attention from the pharmacy profession. However, the relative absence of equitable compensation policies among payers may represent the single greatest barrier to ensuring the consistent provision of pharmaceutical care by pharmacists. For this reason, the development of compensation strategies that recognize the value of professional services and equitably reward pharmacists who competently and consistently provide these services, represents a clear and urgent priority for the profession.

Professional Services: The Essence of Pharmaceutical Care

In recent years, there has been a surge of interest in professional services within the pharmacy profession. Undoubtedly, pharmacists' growing acceptance of a new and expanded professional mission (i.e., "pharmaceutical care") is partly responsible for this increased interest. However, there can be little doubt that it has also been fueled by a recognition on the part of pharmacists and pharmacy organizations that reimbursement for the product component of care will be increasingly restricted in the future.

As interest in professional services has grown, a new vocabulary has emerged that seeks to better define and describe the contemporary professional role of the pharmacist. The pharmacy literature during the past decade is replete with references to pharmacists' "clinical," "professional," "cognitive," and "value added" services. Despite this burgeoning jargon, a consensus has yet to be reached as to just what constitutes a "professional pharmacy service." Since these are the very activities for which pharmacists are seeking compensation, it is important to clarify this term for purposes of our discussion here.

Clearly, many services are provided in pharmacies that may be legitimately argued to "add value" to the bundle of goods and services delivered to consumers. For example, the familiar distributive tasks that are performed during the processing of a prescription order add value to the bulk drug product. Likewise, the various auxiliary services that many pharmacies offer, such as home delivery and mail service, also add value.

But many of these *pharmacy* services do not require the specialized knowledge, expertise, or professional judgement of a *pharmacist*. Many of these services can be—and now are—performed quite adequately by mechanical devices or support personnel, albeit with some supervision. While these services do technically "add value," they cannot be considered value-added services in the professional sense.

Instead, the term "professional services" refers to the non-distributive cognitive (i.e., judgmental) activities that pharmacists are able to perform by virtue of their specialized knowledge, training, and expertise. Indeed, it is this inseparability of the service from the individual who performs it that represents one of the hallmarks of any professional service (Kotler and Bloom 1984). In pharmacy, these services include such things as compounding (as distinguished from simple reconstitution), prescription screening and intervention, self-care consultation, therapeutic drug monitoring, pharmacokinetics dosing, drug utilization review and evaluation, and patient counseling and education. Although they differ in their immediate objectives, each of these services share a requirement for the specialized knowledge and skill of the pharmacist to gather and interpret patient-relevant information and to make decisions or take actions to positively influence patient health outcomes.

It must be concluded then that it is the degree of *professional judgement* involved in the performance of a particular activity that merits for some the label "professional service." Since it is the profession that defines what constitutes professional judgement, it is pharmacy and pharmacists who are in the best position to determine whether or not a particular activity requires the specialized knowledge and skill of a pharmacist to ensure consistently competent performance.

Value, however, is another matter entirely. The value of a professional service—and indeed of *any* good or service—is determined not by the producer but by the consumer. Moreover, it is important to recognize that value is not intrinsic to any product or service. That is, products and services have no intrinsic value. Rather, they are assigned or imbued with value by the consumer, based on the extent to which the consumer believes the use of the product or service will achieve desired outcomes.

Value, Exchange, and Compensation

The relationship between the concept of value and economic compensation can be found in any marketing text. Central to the definition of marketing is the notion of the "exchange relationship (Kotler 1984)." In a very real sense, the ultimate goal of all marketing activities is to enhance the voluntary exchange of values between producers and consumers of goods or services. This exchange is typically in the form of money from the consumer in return for a product or service from the producer.

For this voluntary exchange of values to occur, certain conditions must first be satisfied. Perhaps the most important of these conditions is that both the producer and the consumer must recognize the value of what the other brings to the exchange. Moreover, both parties must believe that in the exchange they will receive something of equal or greater value than the thing they are giving up. Without this shared recognition of value given and value received, voluntary exchange simply cannot take place.

At one time, economists debated about whether the concept of value really had two distinct meanings. The debate centered around the question of whether things could have high value *in use,* and yet have little or no value *in exchange* and vice versa. A similar type of reasoning has been used by pharmacists for many years to explain their inability to secure compensation for their professional services. That is, pharmacists have long argued that their professional services have high value in use, but little value in exchange as demonstrated by the relative absence of compensation.

While some theoretical economists may still be debating the definition of value, from a more pragmatic marketing perspective the answer to this question is clear. **If there is not a willingness on the part of consumers to exchange value (i.e., to pay) for a product or service, then that product or service**

has no value, at least not in the economic sense of the term. So from a marketing perspective, the fundamental barrier to securing compensation for professional services in pharmacy is simply that the value of pharmacists' professional services is still not widely recognized by the *economic* consumers of these services, that is, the people who pay for them. At the very least, this value has not been sufficiently quantified to serve as the basis for *exchanging* value (i.e., paying) for these services.

While simple to state, the solution to this dilemma is much more difficult to achieve. Pharmacy providers must demonstrate to payers, in specific, measurable, and relevant terms, the valued outcomes that are created by their professional services. For this reason, defining and measuring the value of pharmacists' professional services is arguably the single greatest challenge that the profession will face in the coming years. It is *only* from this shared understanding of value created and value received that meaningful dialogue aimed at creating standard payment systems for pharmacists' professional services can begin between pharmacists and payers.

What is the Value of Professional Services?

Simply stated, the goal of pharmaceutical care is to maximize the positive outcomes that patients realize while minimizing the negative outcomes they experience. In recent years, a number of excellent articles have appeared in the literature that reviewed the published studies on the value of professional pharmacy services (Willett et al. 1989; Hatoum et al. 1986; Manasse 1989a; Manasse 1989b; American Pharmaceutical Association Academy of Pharmacy Practice and Management 1989;). In general, these studies support Inspector General Kusserow's conclusion that these services add value to patient care by enhancing the achievement of therapeutic and economic outcomes. However, the usefulness of much of the available research in the development of compensation policies is limited by two factors. First, most of these studies were conducted in institutional settings. Particularly prominent in the literature are studies of pharmacy services delivered to patients in a single hospital. As a result, the applicability of many of these studies to community practice is often limited.

A second limitation of much past research is that calculation of the value of professional services was often restricted to measuring the effect of services on the costs of care only, particularly those costs directly associated with the drug product. To date, relatively few studies have attempted to measure the impact of professional pharmacy services on a more comprehensive battery of relevant patient health and economic outcomes. Fewer still have done so in the community practice setting.

An example of a study that overcame some of these limitations involved the prospective drug utilization review activities of pharmacists in 89 independent and chain community pharmacies in five states (Rupp, DeYoung, and Schondelmeyer

1992). In this study, researchers found that pharmacists intervened to correct prescribing errors on 1.9 percent of all new prescription orders they screened during the routine dispensing process. When these interventions were evaluated by a panel of experts, it was concluded that over 28 percent of the errors that pharmacists identified and corrected could have harmed the patient.

In a subsequent analysis of data collected during this study, the value of the pharmacists' screening and intervention activities was estimated by calculating the direct cost of medical care that was avoided as a result of these activities (Rupp 1992b). Using this approach, the mean estimated value of pharmacists' interventions was found to be $123 per intervention in 1990 dollars. When distributed across all new prescriptions that were screened and dispensed during the study, the mean value that pharmacists added to each new prescription by screening for prescribing problems was estimated to be $2.32. Thus, in this study an attempt was made to estimate the effect of a professional pharmacy service on the total cost of health care.

Despite the relative lack of published research that fully characterizes and quantifies the impact of professional pharmacy services on relevant patient outcomes in the ambulatory practice setting, a number of promising research initiatives are currently ongoing. As results from these projects are released, the case for compensating pharmacists for their professional services may be further strengthened.

The Ideal Compensation Model

What are the characteristics of an "ideal" compensation system for professional pharmacy services? While it is beyond the scope of this chapter to describe such a system completely, several desirable qualities of such a system can be identified.

First and foremost, the system must be fair; it must recognize that pharmacists and other providers of prescription drug products who perform different levels of service also create different values to patients. The system should equitably reward providers who competently and consistently perform professional services that can be demonstrated to have a measurable effect on relevant patient outcomes. Importantly, the system must also have the capacity to distinguish those providers who do competently and consistently perform these services from those who do not. This means that the system must also be supported by a comprehensive quality assurance program.

A second characteristic of the ideal compensation system is that it should be simple; conditions and criteria for payment must be clearly defined and easily understood by both providers and payers. Additionally, the process for submitting claims and receiving payment would ideally be consistent with current electronic claims processing systems and not add unduly to an already burdensome administrative process.

Third, the ideal payment system must be dynamic; it must accommodate frequent adjustments to reflect the contemporary realities of a rapidly changing health care environment.

Developing a compensation system with all of these qualities will require providers, payers, and policy makers working together to answer a number of difficult questions. Among the thorniest of these questions are the three addressed below.

What Will Be Compensated?

The delivery of pharmaceutical care is a complex process consisting of many individual activities and responsibilities. To facilitate equitable compensation to pharmacists for the value their services create, it is necessary to "unbundle" pharmaceutical care so as to recognize the value of its separate component parts. While this unbundling can be approached in a variety of ways, separating payment for the pharmaceutical product (i.e., reimbursement) from that for the professional service (i.e., compensation) would appear to be an essential first step. This then may be followed by further unbundling pharmacy services and classifying them according to various criteria.

Figure 13-1 illustrates the concept of unbundling pharmaceutical care by separating out the components of an outpatient pharmacy services benefit. As illustrated here, professional pharmacy services can be further divided into two broad classes: administrative services and patient care services. Administrative services, such as generic substitution, therapeutic interchange, and formulary enforcement, are typically performed by a pharmacist in compliance with the requirements of a pharmacy benefit program. It has been well documented that these tasks add significantly to the cost of dispensing and create significant hard-dollar savings to third-party payers (Schafermeyer, Schondelmeyer, and Thomas 1990; Carroll 1991). Thus, a system whose fee schedules recognize and reward providers for the provision of these administrative services is desirable.

The final class, true patient care services, may be further sub-divided into primary care services, such as self-care consultation, and services that are performed by a pharmacist pursuant to implementation of the therapeutic plan of a primary care provider, such as prospective drug utilization review, drug therapy monitoring, and patient counseling. To ensure their consistent performance, payment policies must recognize the incremental value contributed by the routine provision of these services. This implies the need for a separate professional fee that is tied to the competent and consistent performance of these services.

Regardless of how it is done, the unbundling of pharmaceutical care is important for communicating to third-party payers and pharmacy benefits managers that an outpatient pharmacy services benefit is—or should be—much more than just a prescription drug benefit. At the same time, it is important that the economic consumer of pharmaceutical care recognize that drug products do not confer

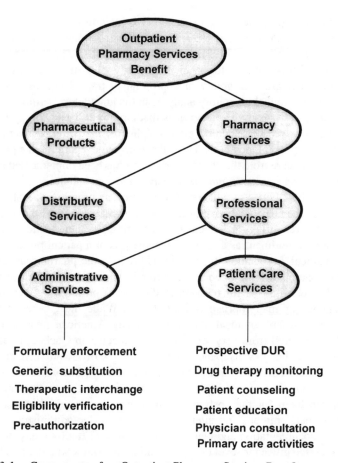

Figure 13.1. Components of an Outpatient Pharmacy Services Benefit.

therapeutic benefits to patients. Rather, it is the appropriate *use* of these products from which patient benefits, and risks, accrue. The pharmaceutical product is merely a potential vehicle for the delivery of desired therapeutic benefits to patients. The degree to which these benefits are actually realized by patients depends greatly on the delivery system that surrounds these products. The delivery system should be designed to ensure the optimal use of pharmaceutical products by patients. This is the *pharmaceutical care* role of the pharmacist.

In addition to services that are routinely performed during prescription drug delivery, a true unbundling approach to pharmaceutical care would also include recognition of professional activities that pharmacists perform outside of the traditional prescription dispensing role. For example, a comprehensive system would also be able to accommodate classes of services related to patient self-care consultation (Srnka 1993), as well as a growing list of pharmacy-based services that target patients with special needs including diabetic patients (Marcrom, Horton, and Shepherd 1993; Campbell 1986), those requiring home IV infusion therapy (Bennett 1993), patients requiring therapeutic drug monitoring (Knowlton, Zarus, and Voltus 1993; McCurdy 1993) and a host of others. As technology increases the ability of appropriately trained personnel to reliably perform many clinical laboratory analyses in the ambulatory setting, the number of specialized pharmacy-based services that employ this technology to monitor the progression of disease and the effects of therapy may be expected to increase.

While still in its infancy in the U.S., the concept of separating the professional components of care from the distributive aspects has been implemented in perhaps its broadest sense in *l' opinion pharmaceutique,* or "pharmaceutical opinion" program in the Quebec province of Canada. In this program, the pharmacist is paid a fee by the provincial government—currently about three times the dispensing fee—for rendering "a judgement concerning the therapeutic value of one drug or a drug regimen, as a result of the analysis of a patient profile (Canadian Pharmaceutical Association 1991)." In addition to the pharmaceutical opinion program, pharmacists in Quebec are currently paid the equivalent of twice the standard dispensing fee for refusing to dispense a prescription they believe to be erroneous or inappropriate (Poston 1992). While the Quebec model may appear to represent an ideal approach to many American pharmacists, until recently it suffered from very low use by pharmacists in Quebec. In attempting to understand this low use, the Quebec Ministry of Health investigated and concluded that there were three primary causes. First, while the level of payment that was available was not trivial, many pharmacists felt that it did not fully compensate them for the costs of the time that was required to perform and document their opinions and interventions. Second, the administrative requirements for documentation and claims submission were felt by many pharmacists to be excessive given the level of compensation that was available. Finally, many pharmacists were concerned about harming their relationships with physicians by calling their prescribing decisions into question.

Responding to the first two concerns, in June of 1992 the provincial government of Quebec increased fees for both the pharmaceutical opinion and refusal to dispense programs and streamlined the administrative requirements for payment. As a result of these changes, pharmacist participation in both programs has increased dramatically. Whereas only 546 claims were made by pharmacists in 1991 for refusing to dispense a medication, the annual rate in 1992 was 7,964. Likewise, the annual number of claims for pharmaceutical opinions rose from 396 in 1991 to 5,679 in 1992 (Gariepy 1993).

The need to define and communicate services for which payment is being requested has been met in other medical professions by creating standard terminology systems for the efficient communication of professional services that are performed by its members. These systems facilitate precise and efficient communication between provider and payer regarding the service that was performed and for which payment is being requested. An example is the Current Procedural Terminology (CPT) coding system employed by physicians (American Medical Assocation 1993). The development of such a system in pharmacy is an important priority for the profession as the profession seeks to structure standard compensation systems for pharmaceutical care. Important recent initiatives in this area will be discussed later in the chapter.

As a final consideration of *what* will be reimbursed, consideration must be given to selecting appropriate indicators of service performance upon which to base payment. For example, a seemingly logical basis for compensating pharmacists who consistently screen for prescribing errors would be to pay pharmacists on a per-intervention basis. That is, the more errors that a pharmacist caught and corrected, the more he or she would be paid.

However, further examination suggests that such a payment strategy, while intuitive and seemingly logical, may not reward pharmacists for the right thing. For example, if the pharmacist is practicing in a relatively closed system where the majority of prescriptions are routinely written by a small and stable set of physicians, one would expect the pharmacists' interventions to produce a learning curve effect in which prescribers with whom the pharmacist has intervened would make progressively fewer and fewer errors over time. Thus, the overall quality of prescribing by physicians in the area would improve over time as a result of the pharmacist's consistent monitoring and intervention activities. If, however, payment for pharmacists' prospective DUR activity were based entirely on the number of errors they caught and corrected, the pharmacist would essentially be penalized for having positively influenced the prescribing behavior of area physicians. So in this case, and perhaps many others, it may be more appropriate to base payment on some reliable measure of performance of the service itself, rather than on some output or outcome indicator in whose creation this service may, or may not, result.

Who Will Be Compensated?

Two related questions that must be answered here are, "what professional qualifications are necessary to ensure competent performance of professional pharmacy services," and "how can patients and payers be assured that providers meet these qualifications?" Essentially, both of these questions relate to the broad issue of quality assurance.

It is generally assumed that any licensed pharmacist should be capable of ensuring the competent performance of the basic distributive activities required for routine prescription drug delivery, whether they personally perform these services or merely oversee their performance. Likewise, most licensed pharmacists should be capable of performing routine administrative services such as drug product selection (i.e., generic substitution) and structured formulary management activities. It is therefore unlikely that payers would require additional evidence of proficiency beyond professional licensure as a precondition for compensation for these types of services.

In contrast, the professional qualifications that are necessary to ensure the consistently proficient performance of some other professional services may not be as clear-cut. By definition, these services should not be performed by non-pharmacists, however, whether professional licensure alone is a sufficient indicator of proficiency depends on the nature of the service, the knowledge and expertise that is required to perform it, and the extent to which the knowledge and expertise required can not be assumed to have been gained during a typical entry-level degree program.

It is not unrealistic to expect that for some professional services, additional evidence of proficiency, such as advanced training or experience, may be required as a condition of compensation. One mechanism by which these additional proficiencies might be assured is through the certificate programs that have been created by schools of pharmacy to enhance practitioner competencies in such areas as long-term care, drug therapy monitoring, pharmacokinetics dosing and a number of disease-specific services (Chalmers 1990; Suveges and Blank 1992).

In addition to personnel considerations, past research has also identified a variety of structural, environmental, and organizational barriers to the consistent performance of professional services. So beyond the eligibility requirements associated with *who* may perform a compensatable professional service, it is not unlikely that certain conditions associated with *where* and *how* these services are performed will be required by some payers.

An example of one organizational barrier to the consistent provision of professional services appears in Figure 13-2 which illustrates the relationship between hourly prescription volume and pharmacists' rate of intervention to correct prescribing errors (Rupp, DeYoung, and Schondelmeyer 1992). If distributive workload were not related to the performance of this activity, the observed distribution of intervention rates across pharmacies would be expected to exhibit a constant rate of approximately the median value of 1.9 percent, which is represented by the horizontal dashed line. However, as the downward sloping regression line clearly demonstrates, a marked *negative* relationship was found between the performance of this professional service by pharmacists and the distributive workload imposed upon them by the organization. The authors concluded:

> The results of this study suggest that some pharmacists may be exceeding their personal dispensing threshold. In doing so, they are placing patients at an increased risk of harm from medication errors and related problems. Clearly, pharmacists themselves are responsible for taking sufficient time to fulfill their patient care role. However, correcting this situation will also require action by the payors of prescription care to recognize the value of pharmacists' extra-distributive professional services and to develop mechanisms to ensure that these services are routinely performed (Rupp, DeYoung, and Schondelmeyer 1992).

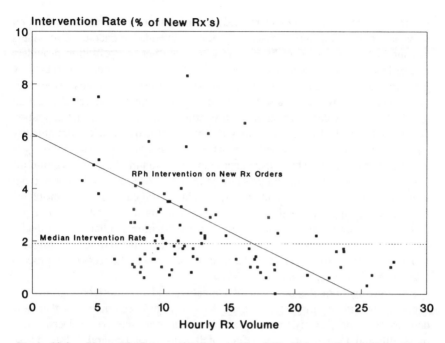

Figure 13.2. Pharmacist Intervention Rate vs. Hourly Rx Volume. *Source*: Rupp M. T., M. DeYoung, and S. W. Schondelmeyer. 1992. Prescribing Problems and Pharmacist Interventions in Community Practice. *Med Care*, 30:931.

A final consideration regarding the issue of who will be paid is whether payment should be directed to the *pharmacy* or to the *pharmacist*. This issue is particularly relevant in the majority of practice settings where the pharmacist is a non-owner employee. Clearly, pharmacy organizations provide the resources necessary for the provision of care by their pharmacist employees. However, organizations do not provide pharmaceutical care, *pharmacists* do. If the reward system is directed exclusively toward the organization, practitioners may have no direct incentive to routinely perform professional services. Indeed, in busy community practices with high distributive workloads, the practicing pharmacist often faces significant barriers and even *dis*-incentives to performing these time-consuming services. The ideal compensation system, therefore, would recognize the need to encourage and reward both the pharmacy organization and the individual pharmacist for delivering pharmaceutical care.

How Will Services Be Compensated?

This issue encompasses at least two separate questions. First, how should fees be determined? Second, how will the operational mechanics of payment function?

Although various permutations exist, there are really only two approaches to establishing fees that are commonly used in health care; capitation and fee-for-service. Capitation is a pre-determined, fixed-fee that reimburses providers on a per-patient per-time period basis. Capitation is intended to encourage providers to contain the costs of care by placing at risk the net compensation providers realize from the services they perform. As a result, the provider is theoretically given incentive to perform high quality care at the lowest possible cost. However, some questions have been raised as to whether this effect is observed in actual practice. Some evidence exists in both pharmacy and medicine that capitation and other fixed-fee arrangements may sometimes negatively affect the quantity and quality of services provided to patients (Raisch 1992; Hillman 1990).

Perhaps the most notable experiment with capitation in pharmacy was the ill-fated Iowa Medicaid capitation program of the late 1970s. Although not without some early successes, this ambitious experiment identified a variety of problems with implementing a capitation-based system. Among these problems were patient and provider resistance, lack of adequate risk-sharing by pharmacists, inadequate mechanisms for periodic readjustment of fees, and the failure to distinguish between the drug product and the pharmacist's services in the fee-setting process (Yesalis et al. 1984a; Yesalis et al. 1984b)

Recognizing both the potential of capitation and the shortcomings of past experiences with it, Inspector General Kusserow has recommended that new demonstration projects using capitated payment be conducted (U.S. Department of Health and Human Services Office of the Inspector General 1990). These projects would include economic rewards and penalties tied to the achievement of defined patient outcomes.

The alternative approach to capitation for setting provider fees is broadly subsumed under the term "fee-for-service." Because physicians have the longest and most successful history of compensation for their professional services, it is instructive to examine the medical model for insight into alternative approaches to establishing fees for professional services that might be considered by pharmacy providers.

Historically, the professional fees physicians charged resulted from free market transactions between individual physicians and their patients. Physicians would adjust the fees they charged individual patients based, in part, on the willingness and ability of their patients to pay these fees. With the advent of public and private health insurance, a "third party" was permanently and irrevocably inserted into the physician-patient relationship. While the mechanics of payment changed, the underlying basis of payment did not, at least not immediately. Rather, physicians were initially able to successfully influence health policy makers to ensure that payment would continue to reflect the fees that physicians wished to charge for their services. Thus began the era of third-party payment based on the *usual, customary, and reasonable* (UCR) method of fee setting (Roe 1981).

By the early 1980s, the UCR method of compensation was widely considered to be a financially unsound approach that tended to encourage abuse by providers (Glaser 1990). Simply stated, the fundamental problem was that what physicians considered to be a usual and customary charge was often not considered reasonable by payers. It was generally agreed among government payers that a new basis for determining fees for physicians' services was needed. This opinion was particularly prevalent in the Medicare program where it was concluded that a standard fee schedule was needed for physician services. The result of this decision was the Harvard Resource-Based Relative Value Scale (RBRVS) project (Hsiao et al. 1988).

Funded in part by the Health Care Financing Administration (HCFA), the RBRVS is an ongoing attempt by a group of health care economists to create a rational and systematic alternative to the prevailing methods of reimbursing physician services that is based on the estimated resource input costs required to perform the services. The goal of this project is to create a system of resource-based formulas for establishing equitable physician fees for services rendered to patients.

Essentially, the RBRVS defines the resource inputs to physicians' services as consisting of three separate components: work expended by the physician in terms of time required before, during, and after the service, and the intensity with which the time is spent; the practice costs necessary to supply the service; and the opportunity costs of training, including recognition of the income that physicians forego when they pursue additional training in order to qualify for specialty practice (Becker et al. 1990). The RBRVS combines these resource inputs into a model that is intended to reflect the relative costs that efficient physicians would incur in providing a given medical service if a perfectly competitive market existed.

To create the RBRVS, the Harvard researchers surveyed 3,000 physicians in 18 specialties to determine the work necessary to perform over 400 medical services. Adjustments were made for between-specialty differences by having physicians in the 18 specialties identify pairs of services that required similar amounts of work. Since it was impossible to gather data on all 7,000 Medicare procedure (i.e., billing) codes, the researchers instead grouped procedures into broad classes of services that were assumed to be relatively similar in terms of resource inputs. They then extrapolated results from the 400 surveyed services to procedures in their respective classes that were not surveyed. When they compared the resulting fee scale to actual physician charges, the researchers concluded, perhaps not surprisingly, that, "current physician charges are not closely related to resource costs (Becker et al. 1990)."

The general approach used in the RBRVS has received widespread support from policy makers including the Health Care Financing Administration, and even some physician organizations including the American Medical Association. Moreover, similar input-based approaches to fee setting have been explored in other health professions, including dentistry (Marcus et al. 1990). In spite of the support that has been expressed for the RBRVS as a method of determining compensation for physician services, this approach has been criticized on a variety of conceptual and practical grounds (McMahon 1990).

Clearly, the RBRVS has a number of significant limitations as a measure of value, at least for purposes of serving as the basis for voluntary exchange. First, the RBRVS considers only the inputs of medical services, not the outcomes. This is inconsistent with the realities of a free market. While the costs of inputs represents a rational basis for determining the *price* of a service from a producer's perspective, it is clearly not a reliable method of determining the *value* of a service from a consumer's perspective. In a competitive market, services whose prices exceeded consumers valuation of them would simply not be demanded, irrespective of the costs that producers incurred in producing these services.

A second and related limitation of the RBRVS is that it does not directly consider differences in the *quality* of services provided. Thus, providers of low quality services are paid at the same rate as those providing high quality services.

The Office of Technology Assessment has defined the quality of health care as "the degree to which the process of care increases the probability of outcomes desired by patients and reduces the probability of undesired outcomes given the current state of knowledge (U.S. Congress Office of Technology Assessment 1988)." This definition of quality suggests that while the process of care (i.e., services of providers) is the primary *object* of quality and quality assessment, the *basis* or rationale for this approach is what is known, or what is thought to be known, about the causal relationship between health care services and the outcomes desired by patients.

To many, the implications of their relationship is clear: if quality is to be assured in the provision of health care services, then it is necessary to link the activities of providers to the achievement of desired patient outcomes. Such a rationale would seem to present a compelling argument for considering outcomes in the design of compensation systems for the services of health care providers, including those of pharmacists. If so, a compensation model that considers both resource inputs and patient outcomes, i.e., a resource-*based* but outcomes-*adjusted* approach to valuing pharmaceutical care, may be the ideal model.

As a final consideration on the subject of establishing rational and acceptable fee schedules for professional services, some have questioned whether it is realistic to expect that an entirely workable system can ever be created through a purely research-based approach. In this vein, arguments have been advanced for maintaining some element of negotiation in the development of future fee schedules, regardless of the systematic basis that is employed to assign value. As one critic has stated,

> Writing a fee schedule is the simplest part. The most urgent task is to design a decision-making system to allocate the money and resolve disputes . . . A standing negotiating system is indispensable for revising the fee schedules that are ultimately adopted, by reducing weights as work becomes simpler and by adding and pricing new procedures (Glaser 1990).

Operational Mechanics of Compensation

In addition to a rational basis for setting fees, a workable compensation system for professional pharmacy services must also be operationally efficient. Some of the issues discussed above, such as the creation of standardized service codes and fees, the development of provider eligibility requirements, and the establishment of mechanisms to resolve disputes, will contribute to the creation of such a system. However, a workable system must also have an efficient means of processing claims and providing payment to providers.

In 1980, the National Council for Prescription Drug Programs (NCPDP) introduced the Universal Claim Form to facilitate the efficient submission, processing and payment of pharmacy claims. In 1988, direct electronic submission and adjudication of claims in an on-line, real-time environment became possible. Since then, the Standardization Committee of NCPDP has assumed responsibility for developing and maintaining a standard format for the electronic submission of third-party drug claims. This standard defines data format, transmission protocol and other telecommunication requirements, and is periodically revised by NCPDP to reflect changes in technology and the health care environment.

NCPDP recommends the use of their standardized format for electronic communication of claims between pharmacy providers, insurance carriers, third-party administrators, and others involved in the submission, processing and payment of claims.

As this chapter was being written, an ambitious new initiative had recently been launched in the NCPDP. Spearheaded by the new Professional Pharmacy Services work group, the objective of this initiative is to create, "a standardized, practical framework that will allow the electronic documentation, storage and transmission of clinical and billing data that describe the delivery of professional pharmacy services (NCPDP Professional Pharmacy Services Work Group WG-10 1994). As part of this objective, a task group had been formed and charged with creating "a systematic listing of terms, definitions and identifying codes that describe the delivery of professional pharmacy services (NCPDP Professional Pharmacy Services Work Group WG-10 1994)."

As the primary pharmacy organization involved in the development of electronic claims standards, this initiative at the NCPDP holds great promise for facilitating the routine billing of professional pharmacy services. While the mere existence of such a standard will not necessarily ensure that pharmacists will be paid for their services, it will significantly enhance the speed and efficiency of claims submissions and processing where providers and payers can reach agreement on the value of these services.

In addition to providing a record of the transaction upon which payment is based, a comprehensive system must also provide payers with the capacity to verify the provision of services and, if necessary, to secure additional information. This would suggest the need for detailed pharmacy-based systems for documenting the provision of professional services. Such systems could provide payers with access to an auditing capacity that would be useful for preventing fraudulent claims. In addition, a pharmacy-based system in which documentation of professional services is performed contemporaneously with the patient encounter could provide a useful mechanism for resolving the disputes that inevitably arise between providers and payers. In addition, consistent documentation by pharmacists of their clinical observations, decisions, and actions could enhance the continuity and quality of care delivered to patients. Such pharmacy systems are currently in development at many of the major pharmacy computer vendor companies.

The previous discussion outlined desirable elements of an ideal system that would compensate pharmacists for the services they routinely perform in the delivery of pharmaceutical care. However, pharmacists who wish to pursue compensation for their professional services must recognize that they are still entering largely uncharted waters. Most government and private third-party payers still do not have well-defined policies for paying pharmacists for their professional services. This is not to say that payers have no interest in pharmacists' services. Rather, for the most part they simply do not understand what these services are or how the services will benefit them and their beneficiaries. That is, they do not understand how these services do, in fact, add value to the bundle of health care goods and services for which they already pay. Overcoming this barrier and demonstrating to payers the value of pharmacists' services represents a priority—perhaps *the* priority—for pharmacy-practice-related research in the years ahead.

Until generally accepted policies exist, payment for pharmacists' cognitive services will continue to be achieved one service, and one payer, at a time. But despite the absence of standard compensation policies, a growing number of pharmacists have been successful at getting paid for the non-distributive professional services they provide to patients. As a result of their collective experiences, an effective—if still somewhat cumbersome—system for getting paid for professional services has been emerged.

An Example: The Family Pharmacare Experience

One example of a pharmacist who has been successful at obtaining third-party payment for his professional services is Dennis J. McCallian, Pharm. D., owner of The Family PharmaCare Center, Inc., an independent community pharmacy in West Lafayette, Indiana. Following is a discussion of the approach that is used at Family PharmaCare to deliver and be compensated for professional services. The reader is encouraged to supplement this discussion with some of the other excellent resources in this area. One of the most detailed of these resources is Klotz and Andrusko-Furphy's *Cognitive Services Manual* (Klotz and Andrusko-Furphy 1992). This useful text, which includes examples of many of the forms and related documents that payers routinely require, was the primary source document in the creation of Family PharmaCare's compensation system.

As illustrated in Figure 13-3, Family PharmaCare's approach to delivering and obtaining compensation for professional services is organized into a six-step process.

```
┌─────────────────────────────────────────────┐
│                   STEP 1                      │
│         Patient Identified or Referred to FPC │
└─────────────────────────────────────────────┘
```

► 'Request for Special Pharmacy Services' form
                        ↓

```
┌─────────────────────────────────────────────┐
│                   STEP 2                      │
│     Assess Patient Need and Eligibility for Service │
└─────────────────────────────────────────────┘
```

► 'Patient Information' form
► 'Statement of Medical Need' or 'Request for Special Pharmacy Services' form
► 'Intake Referral for Special Services' form
► Determine method of payment and verify insurance (if applicable)

                    Not accepted
        Accepted ↓   → Patient and Physician notified within 24 hours

```
┌─────────────────────────────────────────────┐
│                   STEP 3                      │
│      Obtain Patient Consent and Assignment of Benefits │
└─────────────────────────────────────────────┘
```

► 'Consent for Pharmacy Services and Assignment of Benefits' form
                        ↓

```
┌─────────────────────────────────────────────┐
│                   STEP 4                      │
│            Deliver and Evaluate Service       │
└─────────────────────────────────────────────┘
```

► Patient Outcome measures (as appropriate)
► Written feedback to referring physician
                        ↓

```
┌─────────────────────────────────────────────┐
│                   STEP 5                      │
│          Generate Invoice and Submit Claim    │
└─────────────────────────────────────────────┘
```

► Completed 'Request for Special Pharmacy Services' OR 'Statement of Medical Need'
► FPC Pharmacy Services Invoice
► Completed 'Patient Consent and Assignment of Benefits'
► Insurance Claim Form (HCFA 1500 or equivalent)
► Completed 'Special Pharmacy Services Justification' (if necessary)
                        ↓

```
┌─────────────────────────────────────────────┐
│                   STEP 6                      │
│               Collection Process              │
└─────────────────────────────────────────────┘
```

► Accounts Receivable Claims Log
► Claim Inquiry (if necessary)
► Claim Resubmission (if necessary)

Figure 13.3. Professional Pharmacy Services Delivery and Compensation Process. *Source*: Dennis J. McCallian; Pharm.D., The Family PharmaCare Center, Inc., 500 Sagamore Parkway West, Suite 5W, West Lafayette, IN.

Request For Special Pharmacy Services

Patient: _____ Date: _____
Address: _____

℞

☐ Patient Counseling/Education ☐ Prescription Compounding
☐ Medication Review and Evaluation ☐ Injection/Device Training
☐ Compliance Assessment ☐ Other

Explanation: _____
_____
_____

Family PharmaCare
Your health is our business.
500 Sagamore Parkway West, Suite 5W
West Lafayette, IN 47906
(317) 497-7000
FED. I.D. #35-1886202

Physician's Signature
or
Referral Source

Figure 13.4. Request for Special Pharmacy Services. *Source*: Dennis J. McCallian, Pharm.D., The Family PharmaCare Center, Inc., 500 Sagamore Parkway West, Suite 5W, West Lafayette, IN.

Step 1: Patient Identification or Referral

Establishing the existence of medical need is the first step in obtaining third party payment for any health care service (Rupp 1992a). At Family PharmaCare this is accomplished by requesting that physicians provide a signed "Request for Special Pharmacy Services". This form, which appears in Figure 13-4 represents a formal requisition by a physician for the delivery of a professional pharmacy service to a patient and is analogous to a traditional prescription order. For patients referred to the practice without a signed request, a "Statement of Medical Need" is generated by the pharmacy and sent to the physician for signature. The essential components of a "Statement of Medical Need" appear in Table 13-1.

Table 13-1. Components of a Statement of Medical Need

Components of a Statement of Medical Need
• Patient Identification
• Patient Diagnosis (ICD-9-CM)
• Description of Recommended Therapy/Service
—Medical Rationale for Service
—Objectives of Service
—Anticipated Duration of Service
• Referring Physician Signature

Supplies of the "Request for Special Pharmacy Services" form are distributed to area physicians' offices during personal visits by Family PharmaCare staff to detail the services that are available. Physicians are encouraged to refer to Family PharmaCare patients who they believe may be appropriate candidates for one or more of the services offered and to allow staff in the practice to determine whether the patient is an acceptable candidate.

Step 2: Assess Patient Need and Eligibility for Service

As the label implies, the purpose of this step is to assess the referred patient to determine whether he or she represents an appropriate candidate for the service requested. This qualification process is performed in two stages. Stage one involves the pharmacist's determination as to whether a reasonable likelihood exists that the patient's health status will be improved by the service for which the patient is being considered. If the referred patient is new to the practice, a complete medical history is taken. An "Intake Referral for Special Services" form is also completed to ensure that all pertinent medical and insurance information is documented prior to the initiation of pharmacy services.

If the patient is considered to be an acceptable candidate on the basis of this information, he or she is then qualified as to method of payment. If the patient is not private pay this often involves a lengthy process of verifying the type and amount of the patient's health insurance coverage and the documentation needs of the carrier for payment.

Where both the medical need and financial qualification criteria are met, the patient is accepted as a patient for the service under consideration. Otherwise, the patient is not accepted as a patient. In either case, both the patient and the referring physician are notified of the decision in writing within 24 hours of the patient's presentation to the pharmacy.

Step 3: Obtain Patient Consent and Assignment of Benefits

Independent of the decision regarding whether the patient is an acceptable candidate for the service under consideration, it is necessary that the patient give his or her consent and agreement for services to be performed. In cases where payment will be sought from the patient's insurance carrier, it is usually necessary to have the patient assign their insurance benefit to Family PharmaCare. Following the procedure described by Klotz and Andrusko-Furphy (1992), this is accomplished at Family PharmaCare via the completion of a "Patient Consent for Pharmacy Services and Assignment of Benefits" form. This form also grants authorization to the referring physician to furnish Family PharmaCare with all necessary medical information and ensures the patient understands that he or she is ultimately liable for any charges that are not covered by insurance.

Step 4: Deliver and Evaluate Service

The next step in the process is to actually deliver the service to the patient. Concurrent with the delivery of services at Family PharmaCare is the routine completion of patient care plans and progress notes. As discussed earlier in the chapter, this type of documentation is useful both for ensuring continuity of patient care from encounter to encounter and for providing a permanent record of services rendered should a dispute arise with an insurance carrier. Appropriate patient outcome measures related to the service being provided and/or the condition being treated are also routinely recorded. Written feedback on the patient is also provided on a routine basis to the referring physician.

Step 5: Generate Invoice and Submit Claim

The materials that are included in the claim packet sent to the patient's insurance carrier differs from payer to payer. However, a typical claims packet might include: a signed request from the physician, in the form of a completed "Request for Special Pharmacy Services" or "Statement of Medical Need;" an itemized invoice of charges for the services rendered; a completed "Patient Consent and Assignment of Benefits" form; and a completed HCFA 1500 claims form or equivalent form required by the insurer. In addition, carriers may require copies of care plans, progress notes, or a variety of other materials to justify the services performed and/or the amounts charged.

Step 6: Manage the Collection Process

As in most physician offices, Family PharmaCare has a dedicated staff member who administers the collections process to ensure that claims packets are complete and in full compliance with the requirements of the carrier and to track accounts receivable for the practice. Clearly, devoting significant personnel time to this activity can only be justified in the long term if professional services in the practice are able to recover the costs of providing and billing for them and contribute to pharmacy profit. In the short term, however, pharmacy organizations using this approach must be willing to suffer through an initial learning curve in developing an approach to seeking compensation for pharmaceutical care that best fits their own practice.

Conclusion

In his economic treatise, *Wealth of Nations,* Adam Smith commented on pharmacists and the value of their professional services:

> Apothecaries' profit is become a bye-word, denoting something uncommonly extravagant. This great apparent profit, however, is frequently no more than

the reasonable wages of labour. The skill of an apothecary is much nicer and more delicate matter than that of any artificer whatever; and trust which is reposed in him is of much greater importance. He is the physician of the poor in all cases, and of the rich when the distress or danger is not very great. His reward, therefore, ought to be suitable to his skill and his trust, and it arises generally from the price at which he sells his drugs. But the whole drugs which the best employed apothecary, in a large market town, will sell in a year, may not perhaps cost him above thirty or forty pounds. Though he should sell them, therefore, for three or four hundred, or at a thousand per cent. profit, this may frequently be no more than the reasonable wages of his labour charged, in the only way in which he can charge them, upon the price of his drugs. The greater part of the apparent profit is real wages disguised in the garb of profit (Smith 1776).

Although the practice of pharmacy has changed dramatically in the two centuries since those words were written, the basis for compensating pharmacists has not. In general, the value of pharmacists' professional services is still interwoven with, and obscured by, the price of the products they sell. The future of compensation for cognitive services must break from this tradition. If pharmaceutical care is to expand beyond the halls of academia and the great medical centers to the level of the typical community (and hospital) pharmacy, standard compensation systems must evolve that encourage and reward pharmacists and pharmacy organizations for the time and effort required to provide this level of care. For the reasons described earlier, it is essential that payment for pharmacists' professional services be based on the value of the services themselves and not on a drug product that may or may not have been delivered during performance of the service.

The creation of pharmacy services terminology and related electronic claims transmissions standards will help speed the evolution of new payment systems. Likewise, the growing body of research in outcomes assessment and pharmacoeconomics will allow the pharmacy profession to better understand the economic value of pharmaceutical care and better communicate this value to payers.

Until standard compensation systems become widely used, procedures like those used at Family PharmaCare, while somewhat time consuming and labor intensive, are available to support pharmacists who wish to pursue payment for pharmaceutical care and related professional services.

But while standard third party compensation policies for professional pharmacy services are still evolving, pharmacists would be wise not to await the resolution of this process before seriously examining how their practices must change to take advantage of the new business relationship and compensation systems that are developing. Moreover, in something of a chicken-or-egg dilemma, pharmacists must recognize that the number of pharmacists who consistently and routinely provide pharmaceutical care to their patients is likely to have an influence on the speed at which new payment systems develop. So, while not a self-fulfilling prophecy, pharmacists are in a position to significantly influence their own destiny when it comes to securing compensation for pharmaceutical care.

References

American Medical Association. 1993. *Physicians' Current Procedural Terminology*. Chicago: American Medical Association.

APhA Academy of Pharmacy Practice and Management, Cognitive Services Working Group. 1989. Payment for Cognitive Services: The Future of the Profession. *American Pharmacy* NS29:34–8.

APhA Board of Trustees. 1991. *American Pharmacy* NS31:29.

Becker, E. R., et al. 1990. Refinement and Expansion of the Harvard Resource-Based Relative Value Scale: The Second phase. *American Journal of Public Health* 80:799–803.

Bennett, J. A. 1993. Developing a Successful Home Infusion Practice. *Drug Topics* June 7, 1993:62–73.

Brodie, D. C. 1967. Drug-use Control: Keystone to Pharmaceutical Service. *Drug Intelligence and Clinical Pharmacy* 1:63–5.

Campbell, R. K. 1986. Pharmaceutical Services for Patients with Diabetes: Developing a Diabetes Program for Your Pharmacy, Module 2. *American Pharmacy* NS26 (supplement 2):1–11.

Canadian Pharmaceutical Association. 1991. Alternative Reimbursement Schemes for Pharmacy Services: A Discussion Paper. Ottawa: CPhA.

Carroll, N. V. 1991. Costs of Dispensing Private-pay and Third-party Prescriptions in Independent Pharmacies. *Journal of Research in Pharmaceutical Economics* 3:3–16.

Chalmers, R. K. 1990. Chair Report of the AACP/ACPE Conference on Certificate Programs. *American Journal of Pharmacy Education* 54:80–3.

Gariepy, Y. 1993. Quebec Turnaround (letter). *American Pharmacy* NS33:5.

Glaser, W. A. 1990. Designing Fee Schedules by Formulae, Politics, and Negotiations. *American Journal of Public Health* 80:804–9.

Hatoum, H. T., et al. 1986. An Eleven-year Review of the Pharmacy Literature: Documentation of the Value and Acceptance of Clinical Pharmacy. *Drug Intelligence and Clinical Pharmacy* 20:33–48.

Hepler, C. D., and L. M. Strand. 1990. Opportunities and Responsibilities in Pharmaceutical Care. *American Journal of Hospital Pharmacy* 47:533–43.

Hillman, A. L. 1990. Health Maintenance Organizations, Financial Incentives, and Physicians' Judgements. *Annals of Internal Medicine* 112:891–3.

Hsiao, W. C. et al. 1988. A National Study of Resource-Based Relative Value Scales for Physician Services: Final Report. September 27, 1988. Boston: Harvard University.

Kidder, S. W. 1987. Cost-benefit of Pharmacist-conducted Regiment Reviews. *The Consultant Pharmacist* Sept/Oct:394.

Klotz, R. S., and K. T. Andrusko-Furphy. 1992. *Cognitive Services Manual.* Tustin: Specialized Clinical Services.

Knowlton, C. H., S. A. Zarus, and O. Voltis. 1993. Implementing a Pharmacy-based Therapeutic Drug Monitoring Service. *American Pharmacy* NS33:7:57–63.

Kotler, P. 1984. *Marketing Management: Analysis, Planning and Control.* Englewood Cliffs: Prentice-Hall.

Kotler, P., and P. N. Bloom. 1984. *Marketing Professional Services.* Englewood Cliffs: Prentice-Hall.

Manasse, H. R. 1989a. Medication Use in an Imperfect World: Drug Misadventuring as an Issue of Public Policy, Part 1. *American Journal of Hospital Pharmacy* 46:929–44.

Manasse, H. R. 1989b. Medication Use in an Imperfect World: Drug Misadventuring as an Issue of Public Policy, Part 2. *American Journal of Hospital Pharmacy* 46:1141–52.

Marcrom, R. E., R. M. Horton, and M. D. Shepherd. 1992. Create Value-Added Services to Meet Patient Needs. *American Pharmacy* NS32:48–59.

Marcus, M., et al. 1990. A Proposed New System for Valuing Dental Procedures: The Relative Time-cost Unit. *Medical Care* 28:943–51.

McCurdy, M. 1993. Oral Anticoagulation Monitoring in a Community Pharmacy. *American Pharmacy* NS33:61–72.

McMahon, L. F. 1990. A Critique of the Harvard Resource-based Relative Value Scale. *American Journal of Public Health* 80:793–8.

NCPDP Professional Pharmacy Services Work Group WG-10. 1994. Scope Statement for Pharmacy Services Terminology task group TG-1 approved 2/7/94 at the Annual Meeting in Scottsdale, Arizona.

Poston, J. W. 1992. Quebec Provincial Drug Benefit Program Update. Personal communication. Canadian Pharmaceutical Association.

Raisch, D. W. 1992. Relationships Among Prescription Payment Methods and Interactions Between Community Pharmacists and Prescribers. *Annals of Pharmacotherapy* 26:902–6.

Roe, B. B. 1981. The UCR Boondoggle: A Death Knell for Private Practice? *New England Journal of Medicine* 305:41–5.

Rupp, M. T. 1992a. Strategies for Reimbursement. *American Pharmacy* NS32:79–86.

Rupp, M. T. 1992b. The Value of Community Pharmacists' Interventions to Correct Prescribing Errors. *Annals of Pharmacotherapy* 26:1580–4.

Rupp, M. T., M. DeYoung, and S. W. Schondelmeyer. 1992. Prescribing Problems and Pharmacists Interventions in Community Practice. *Medical Care* 30:926–40.

Schafermeyer, K. W., S. W. Schondelmeyer, and J. Thomas. 1990. *An Assessment of Chain Pharmacies Costs of Dispensing a Third Party Prescription.* West Lafayette: Purdue University Pharmaceutical Economics Research Center.

Smith, A. [1776] 1981. In *Adam Smith: Inquiry into the Nature and Causes of the Wealth of Nations*, Reprint, ed. R. H. Campbell and A. S. Skinner, 128–9. Indianapolis: Liberty Classic Press.

Srnka, O. M. 1993. Implementing a Self-Care Consulting Practice. *American Pharmacy* NS33:61–71.

Study Commission of Pharmacy. 1975. *Pharmacists for the Future*. Ann Arbor: Health Administration Press.

Suveges, L. G., and J. W. Blank. 1992. Development of a Conceptual Model for Certificate Programs in Pharmacy. *American Journal of Pharmacy Education:* 56:109–13.

U.S. Congress Office of Technology Assessment. 1988. *Quality of Medical Care: Information for Consumers*. Washington DC: Government Printing Office. Publication OTA–H–386.

U.S. Department of Health and Human Services Office of the Inspector General. 1990. *The Clinical Role of the Community Pharmacist*.

Willett, M. S., et al. 1989. Prospectus on the Economic Value of Clinical Pharmacy Services. *Pharmacotherapy* 9:45–56.

Yesalis, C. E., et al. 1984a. Capitation Payment for Pharmacy Services, Part 1: Impact on Drug Use and Pharmacist Dispensing Behavior. *Medical Care* 22:737–45.

Yesalis, C. E., et al. 1984b. Capitation Payment for Pharmacy Services, Part 2. *Medical Care* 22:746–54.

14

Competence for Pharmaceutical Care

Susan M. Meyer, Ph.D.
Carl E. Trinca, Ph.D.

What Should Competence Mean to You?

By definition, competence is the capability to perform a particular function. Demonstrating competence to practice pharmacy means demonstrating that, as a practitioner, one has command of the requisite knowledge base and possesses the skills, values, and attitudes necessary to provide contemporarily defined pharmaceutical care. The desired outcomes of an educational program designed to prepare practitioners for the contemporary practice of pharmacy then, necessarily, include the knowledge base and those skills, values, and attitudes required of practitioners.

Because competence is more than knowledge of facts, assessment of contemporary competence—that is, determining whether or not a practitioner (beginning or experienced) has the requisite knowledge, skills, values, and attitudes—must require the individual to do more than recall memorized facts. Assessment of competence must be valid and reliable. The term validity refers to how well a particular measure or instrument assesses what it is intended to assess. For example, if a particular outcome or competency statement in a unit on cardiovascular disorders calls for the learner to be able to evaluate a given patient chart, data, and history and to identify the probable primary problem, then an assessment item requiring the learner to select the beta-blocker from a list of five cardiovascular medications would not be a valid assessment. A valid assessment of that outcome could involve giving the learner a written patient case with supporting materials from the patient's chart and asking him or her to identify the probable primary problem. Valid assessments require the learner to demonstrate the desired behavior stated in the outcome/competency in a context that, as closely as possible, simulates actual practice. Reliable assessments yield similar, consistent results over a period of time.

Assessment may be performed for a variety of purposes. One such purpose is to determine the degree of competence exhibited by a practitioner or student to facilitate appropriate placement in an educational program. If a student or practitioner is able to demonstrate certain competencies, then he or she might be placed in a more advanced educational program than the one in which those competencies are addressed and developed. Assessments may be categorized as summative or formative, based on when the assessment occurs during the instructional process and/or the purpose of performing the assessment. Summative assessment is used to measure the degree of learner achievement at the end of an instructional process. Examples of summative assessments include a final exam for assigning a course grade and a licensing exam to determine capability to practice pharmacy in a given state. The results of formative assessments influence and serve as a motivation for constructive change. Formative assessment results are, or should be, used to facilitate student improvement by "diagnosing" areas of weakness. Assessments for this purpose should be conducted frequently during the instructional process to facilitate continuous improvement of the student's learning.

There are various types of assessment instruments and methods, each with advantages and disadvantages as well as appropriate and inappropriate uses. In pharmaceutical education, most practitioners and students are familiar with multiple-choice examination items. These items provide the learner with up to five alternatives from which the best or most correct response to a question must be selected. This type of item is easy to administer, provides an objective assessment, and is easy to score, making it attractive for use with large groups. It is appropriate for assessing the learner's ability to recall certain facts or identify or recognize items from among less attractive alternatives. When following a case description or scenario, other types of abilities, such as comprehension, application, and analysis may be assessed using multiple-choice items. However, multiple-choice assessment items may not be the most valid or appropriate to assess contemporary practice competence.

Another assessment tool commonly used in pharmaceutical education is the case study. This method attempts to simulate the patient-pharmacist interaction with the use of written information and descriptions or computerized scenarios. In a case study, the learner is often asked to think and respond as the pharmacist should in the situation described. The use of case studies may be a more valid method than the multiple-choice item for assessing many practice competencies because the cases, when appropriately developed and presented, can more closely resemble actual practice. Another more valid approach to assessing contemporary practice competency is to have the learner demonstrate the desired behavior or skill in a practice setting. The instructor or other observer measures the behavior of the learner against preset criteria to determine the level of achievement reached by the learner. While demonstration has the potential to be a more valid measure of practice competence, such an approach is more time consuming, requiring one-to-one interaction between the observer and learner, and carries the possibility of variations in interpretation of the criteria across observers.

Another method of assessment with potential for use in pharmaceutical education involves the use of portfolios. A portfolio is a collection of "evidence" of the experience and competence of a student or practitioner. A student's portfolio might consist of samples of classwork completed, instructor feedback and recommendations for improvement, and reflections prepared by the student on the quality of his or her work, plans to improve that quality, career plans, and other related materials. A practitioner's portfolio might consist of job descriptions, continuing professional education activities, examples of special projects or presentations given, supervisor feedback, and reflections prepared by the practitioner related to his or her practice, plans for professional improvement, thoughts about issues facing the profession, and other related materials. It is the practitioner's responsibility to evolve with the profession and maintain his or her competence at contemporary levels.

Who Must be Competent and Why?

In an era of health care reform and preventative health care, pharmacists must be competent members of the primary health care team. In this context, they must possess the knowledge, skills, values, and attitudes necessary to provide pharmaceutical care.

Pharmacy practitioners can be loosely organized into three, interrelated categories based on their relationship to the educational process: practice faculty (educator/practitioner), pharmacist (practitioner/educator) and student. Each requires both shared and unique competencies in order to achieve their role expectations and render pharmaceutical care.

Practice Faculty

Practice faculty, or educator/practitioners, are generally:

- Experienced—they possess confidence in their skills and abilities to make better decisions
- Efficient—they possess an array of possible problem-solving options because of their experience
- Proficient—they are highly skilled or expert

Educator/practitioners are often specialists; that is they possess education and training beyond that of the generalist, often in focused areas of practice. Specialists also gain efficiency and proficiency with experience, but may loose their breadth or generalist skills. Educator/practitioners are teachers and scholars who maintain a viable practice, usually in their specialty areas, as part of their academic responsibilities.

Pharmacist

The pharmacist, or practitioner/educator, may also share experience, efficiency, and proficiency with his or her practice faculty colleagues. A key component to the practitioner/educator's role is the commitment to assisting with the preparation of future pharmacists. A pharmacist's competence to teach others about rendering pharmaceutical care is grounded in greater depth (e.g., the degree of complexity of their problem-solving efficiency and proficiency) and breadth (e.g., the scope or range of services which are required) of competence.

Student

Students are preparing to become entry-level practitioners; that is, upon graduation they will be beginners who possess a specific, well-defined set of knowledge, attitudes, skills, behaviors, and values. Students do not share either experience, efficiency, or proficiency with practice faculty and pharmacists. Yet students will gain experience, and hence efficiency and proficiency, in being a student pharmacist. Therefore, relative to other students, a more senior student will have a more developed set of knowledge and skills. Further, students are entering on a continuum of lifelong learning. As a result, with time they can look forward to gaining experience, efficiency, and proficiency.

While gaining experience, the practice faculty and the pharmacist may fail to maintain contemporary competence. In other words, students or entry-level practitioners may posses greater knowledge or skill in certain areas than practitioners with considerably more experience. It is essential that these experienced practitioners, whether practice faculty or pharmacists, grow in their ability to meet contemporary practice needs and demands.

From these examples, it is clear that the profession and society must place greater value on both contemporary competence and experience. Practice faculty have a responsibility to work both with practitioner/educators and with students; pharmacists must be teachers as well, focusing primarily on students, but also assisting faculty in understanding contemporary practice needs and demands. Students not only learn from both practice faculty and pharmacists but also have a responsibility to teach each other, underclassmen, and students of other health professions. When these relationships are understood and fostered, human resources for pharmacy will be optimized.

What Competencies are Required for You to Render Pharmaceutical Care?

Contemporary competence for pharmacists can be defined in different contexts. Pharmacists must be competent as health care professionals. The Pew Health

Professions Commission (1991) has suggested in its Agenda for Action that the following 17 competencies will be required of all health care professionals, within the context of their particular professions, by the year 2005:

Care for the community's health: includes understanding factors that determine and influence health and the working with others to improve health

Expand access to effective care

Provide contemporary clinical care: includes maintaining contemporary clinical skills

Emphasize primary care: includes practicing in new care delivery settings

Participate in coordinated care: includes functioning as part of a primary health care team to provide coordinated health care services

Ensure cost-effective and appropriate care: includes making health care decisions based on quality and cost considerations

Practice prevention

Involve patients and families in the decision-making process

Promote healthy lifestyles

Assess and use technology appropriately

Improve the health care system: includes understanding the health care system from political, economic, social, and legal perspectives

Manage information: includes use of medical science information, and patient-specific data

Understand the role of the physical environment: includes understanding the impact of environmental hazards on health

Provide counseling on ethical issues: includes participation in discussions of ethical issues in health care

Accommodate expanded accountability: includes responding to increasing levels of public, governmental, and third party participation in and scrutiny of the health care delivery system;

Participate in a racially and culturally diverse society: includes understanding different cultural values related to health and health care delivery

Continue to learn: includes maintaining professional competency throughout practice life

The Commission to Implement Change in Pharmaceutical Education (American Association of Colleges of Pharmacy 1992) defined two types of competencies: underlying general competencies and professional competencies. In order to perform necessary pharmacy practice functions, practitioners must possess both types.

General competencies include thinking, communicating, having values and applying ethical principles, self-awareness, self-learning, and citizenship. These competencies, which exemplify an educated professional, may be viewed as follows:

Thinking abilities include logical and analytical thinking, problem solving, and decision making. In order to function as a citizen and professional, the practitioner must:

- understand the scientific method and its application in discovering and assessing new knowledge
- use mathematics to understand processes and evaluate risk
- think critically in order to examine issues rationally, logically, and coherently

Communication abilities include writing, reading, speaking, listening, and using data, media, and computers. The practitioner must not only master communication skills but also must appreciate the differences between cultures and languages and possess an awareness of how art, music, and literature contribute to understanding.

Values and ethics guide professional behavior and, therefore, have a direct impact on rendering pharmaceutical care. The practitioner must posses personal values and demonstrate professional ethics in applying pharmaceutical care principles to individual patients in everyday practice.

Self-awareness is contextual competence including appreciation for self, diversity, and profession. Self-awareness leads to improvement of self and of others.

Self-learning fosters the ability to adapt to and promote change. As a result, improvement and continued learning enhances the profession's ability to serve the public.

Citizenship is a recognition of the practitioner's responsibility to contribute to society, to the profession, and to the individual. Citizenship also means professional and social leadership; society offers trust to the practitioner and the practitioner provides leadership in return.

Professional competencies drive the competencies of thinking, communicating, having values and applying ethical principles, having self-awareness, being a self-learner, and being a good citizen.

The practice of pharmacy demands that practitioners draw upon professional competencies that enable them to perform the functions that support practice. Some of these professional competencies are listed below.

Problem solving and decision making is what pharmaceutical care is all about. Practitioners must be able to gather, organize, and interpret data in order to make judgments and decisions which benefit individual patients and populations.

Managing patients, personnel, fiscal and physical resources, and supplies requires the application of management theory and the ability to organize, plan, direct, and control pharmaceutical care systems.

Learning, whether textbook or experiential, occurs through practice. Practitioners must view practice as a learning experience.

Communicating, teaching, educating, and collaborating follow learning. Practitioners have a responsibility to share knowledge with others—students, colleagues, other health professionals, and patients.

Preparing for the future through policy development and professional governance offers the practitioner opportunities for shaping change.

This rich mix of competencies which define a professional is essential for contemporary pharmacy practice. These competencies do not define the content—the specific conceptual or technical knowledge—necessary to create, maintain, or retrain the contemporary practitioner. The content varies depending on whether the individual is a student, a pharmacist, or a practice faculty member; whether the individual is at the entry level or experienced; and whether the individual is a generalist or specialist.

How Do You Become Competent?

The Mission of Pharmaceutical Education (American Association of Colleges of Pharmacy 1992) states that educators are responsible for preparing students to enter into the practice of pharmacy and that the mission of pharmacy practice is to render pharmaceutical care. It is therefore concluded that to enter practice is to render pharmaceutical care.

Professional Education

An individual can become competent to render pharmaceutical care in several ways. For the novice, a professional education in an accredited pharmacy program provides the accepted pathway in the United States. It is beyond the scope of this chapter to provide a discussion on selection of a pharmacy program; the reader is referred to *Pharmacy School Admission Requirements* (American Association of Colleges of Pharmacy 1995) and the catalogs of individual colleges and schools of pharmacy for more information.

It is instructive, however, to view general and professional competencies in the context of curricular content and educational process since both are critical to the achievement of the educational outcomes described above. The content of the curriculum is "owned" by the faculty, and a strength of pharmaceutical education lies in the specific curriculums found in each college and school of pharmacy. The Commission to Implement Change in Pharmaceutical Education presented a core curriculum for academic pharmacy's consideration (See Table 14-1.); it cannot be overemphasized that the fact that an item is listed in the core does not necessarily mean that a specific course should be offered to cover the specified content.

What is critical, however, is the need to change the educational processes by which material contained in the curriculum is translated, delivered to, and learned by contemporary learners. Most of us were taught by a passive, dependent process; that is, the teacher transmitted information and the learner memorized it and recalled it to respond to examination items. Memorization, however, is not strongly linked to retention and, therefore, the material is not learned. Most individuals learn more effectively and efficiently if they are actively involved in the learning process. In practice, much more than recall of facts is required of the practitioner—patient's drug-related problems must be solved, facts need to be known as they relate to processes, and new material must be integrated with information already known. The responsibility for learning must be shifted away from the teacher and more directly toward the learner or student; teachers must view themselves as coaches and facilitators. Such teaching and learning processes can be described as follows:

Problem solving focuses on process, not the content or nature of the problems themselves. Skills necessary for problem solving include an adequate knowledge base; the ability to obtain and evaluate missing information; self-learning, motivation, and perseverance; interpersonal and group skills; coping ability; communication skills; and creativity.

Fundamental information places emphasis on biological, chemical, and social mechanisms and systems rather than isolated facts. Although practitioners and students must have knowledge of facts as they apply to specific patient needs, the learning environment must focus on the concepts on which science and practice are based and on the importance of scientific and social processes in solving patient-specific problems.

Communications must be integrated in all the practitioner and student do.

Practice skills build experience and, subsequently, efficiency and proficiency. Practice provides the opportunity to experience, first hand, the application of knowledge, attitudes, skills, and behaviors. When the practitioner or student sees something new in practice, it is desirable to translate the experience to learning by performing the same or similar function; the opportunity to teach the concept or demonstrate the skill to another individual further heightens the learning experience.

Methods which facilitate the implementation of these processes go beyond traditional didactic and experiential approaches; they include small group discussions,

Table 14-1. Core Curriculum

This curriculum outline should be viewed as a guide to pharmacy school faculty about the content of the curriculum. An item listed in the Core Curriculum does not necessarily mean that a course should be required to cover the indicated item.

1. General Education—The purpose of general education in the curriculum is to prepare educated, professional practitioners who are capable of understanding and appreciating society and their role in it as health care providers. General education, traditionally, has been provided to students in the initial phases of their education (pre-pharmacy). More recently, it has been recommended that elements of general education be interspersed throughout the professional pharmaceutical curriculum.
   a. Oral and Written Communication Skills
   b. Social Sciences
   c. Behavioral Sciences
   d. Humanities
   e. Computer Literacy and Information Technology
   f. General Science—Students must learn how knowledge is created and be introduced to the scientific method.
2. Basic Physical and Biological Sciences and Mathematics. Chemistry, physics, biology and microbiology course elements should contain associated laboratories or field experiments.
   a. Mathematics Including Calculus
   b. General Chemistry
   c. Organic Chemistry
   d. Physics
   e. Cell Biology and Microbiology
3. Biomedical Sciences
   a. Anatomy
   b. Physiology
   c. Biochemistry/Molecular Biology
   d. Immunology
   e. Biostatistics
4. Pharmaceutical Sciences
   a. Medicinal and Natural Products Chemistry
   b. Pharmaceutics and Pharmaceutical Chemistry (includes basic principles and applications of dosage forms, drug standards, quality control, biopharmaceutics, and pharmacokinetics)
   c. Pharmacology and Toxicology
   d. Pharmacy Administration (includes management, marketing, leadership, behavioral science, and knowledge of drug distribution and health care delivery systems)
5. Clinical Sciences
   a. Epidemiology
   b. Health Promotion and Disease Prevention
   c. Pathophysiology
   d. Clinical Laboratory Medicine
   e. Clinical Pharmacokinetics
   f. Clinical Pharmacology and Therapeutics
   g. Physical Assessment
6. Practice Experiences (All Students)
   a. Drug Information and Literature Evaluation
   b. Ethical Principles Pertaining to Professional Practice
   c. Laws
   d. Experiences in Ambulatory, Inpatient and Managed Care Environments
7. Practice Experiences (Optional Tracking Opportunities)
   a. Differentiated Practices (long term care, home health care, hospice)
   b. Specialized Practices (nuclear pharmacy, pharmacotherapy, nutrition support)
   c. Outpatient Health Care Settings (community health clinics, satellite settings)
   d. Medical Specialties (outpatient or inpatient)
   e. Nontraditional Experiences (industry, wholesale, management)

computer simulations, role playing, presentations, case studies, reading assignments, problem sets, laboratories, and research experiences.

Postgraduate Professional Education and Training

Postgraduate professional education and training provides new and expanded competencies for pharmacists and practice faculty. Two major approaches have been identified: residencies and mid-career education and training. Mid-career education and training includes certificate programs, non-traditional degree programs, and continuing education.

Pharmacy practice residencies are organized, postgraduate experiences in defined areas of practice. Residencies exist primarily to train pharmacists in professional practice and management activities. Residencies provide experience in integrating pharmacy services with the comprehensive needs of individual practice settings and provide in-depth experiences leading to advanced practice skills and knowledge. A residency is typically 12 months in duration. Pharmacy practice residencies offer major benefits to the profession and society—as a mechanism to prepare practitioners to meet patient's needs; as an efficient way to explore and develop new roles; as a way to test innovation; and for the development of practitioner/educators. Most residency programs are currently institution-based, although several exist in long-term care and community pharmacy practices. The American Society of Hospital Pharmacists, a pioneer in the accreditation of pharmacy practice residency programs, currently recognizes two types of programs: residencies in pharmacy practice (with emphasis on pharmaceutical care), and specialized pharmacy residency training.

Mid-career education and training programs are focused on the professional needs of individuals seeking formal programs that prepare them for new practice and educational roles. In the past, these programs have focused primarily on journal articles and one-day seminars. Today, these traditional approaches offer only one avenue for developing new knowledge and skills. For example, certificate programs are structured and systematic postgraduate educational and training experiences for pharmacists that are generally smaller in magnitude and shorter in duration than degree programs and that impart knowledge, skills, attitudes, and performance behaviors designed to meet specific practice objectives.

Degree programs, specifically programs leading to the doctor of pharmacy (Pharm.D.), are another mechanism in which practitioners acquire contemporary competencies. Non-traditional degree programs, which are accessible and innovative, hold promise for practitioners to pursue contemporary knowledge and skills which build on their experience. Currently, non-traditional programs provide the opportunity for pharmacists to pursue the didactic portion of their education via distance learning methods. Little progress has been made in assessing and awarding academic credit for prior learning and there are limited substitutes for returning to the academic institution for completing the experiential component of the curriculum. A priority of American Association of Colleges of Pharmacy (AACP) Center for the Advancement of Pharmaceutical Education (CAPE) is to identify contemporary competencies and appropriate assessment methods for those competencies in order to facilitate the awarding of the Pharm.D. degree to baccalaureate-degreed practitioners.

Traditional approaches will continue to play an important role in assisting practitioners in keeping up with developments in areas where they are already competent. This is in contrast to the development of new competencies such as those offered through curricular approaches to continuing education (certificate programs).

Among the general competencies desired of all practitioners is that of being a self-learner. Therefore, self-guided learning and documentation of practice experience is a fundamental method to maintain competence. Many practitioners experience this form of learning every day; most perhaps do not realize it or value the impact it has on their practices.

Maintaining disciplinary competence is important, especially for those educator/practitioners who have focused on one particular practice area and developed a specialized competence. Often, this specialized competence is maintained and further developed by participating in scholarly research. Experienced faculty may develop, maintain, or fine-tune disciplinary competence through participation in a sabbatical—a paid leave from normal employment responsibilities to participate in a concentrated study of or research in a particular area. New faculty or those intending to become faculty who wish to develop a particular disciplinary and research competence may complete a fellowship, often two years in length. Practice faculty, like other pharmacists, maintain and evolve their competence, both in their discipline and in practice, through interaction and scholarly discussion with colleagues, that is, other practice faculty, pharmacists, and students.

In addition to their responsibility to maintain competence as practitioners, practice faculty (educator/practitioners) also have a responsibility to maintain their competence as educators. Teaching competence may be developed and maintained through a variety of mechanisms. Many schools and colleges are located on university campuses with instructional development centers. These centers often offer faculty development programs and college teaching workshops on instructional design and development, particular instructional strategies, assessment methods, student advising, and curriculum development. As institutional and curricular changes occur to meet the challenge of educating future practitioners, so too must the educational processes used change. These changes necessitate faculty development and maintenance of teaching competence in the context of new educational paradigms.

Programs and resources to facilitate faculty development and teaching competence are also offered by associations in higher education, such as the American Association for Higher Education (AAHE) and the American Association of Colleges of Pharmacy (AACP). AACP programs, such as the annual Teachers

Seminar, focus on teaching skill development within the context of pharmaceutical education. AACP, through its Center for the Advancement of Pharmaceutical Education (CAPE), will also offer a Master Teacher program. This program will focus on the development of teaching competencies and recognition of teaching excellence in pharmaceutical education. Graduate students intending to become faculty members, college-based faculty, and practice faculty will be encouraged to participate in the Master Teacher program.

How Can Your Professional Competence be Recognized?

A mobile, complex society supported by a technological economy is, by nature, dependent on formal recognition of competence to identify qualified individuals, to protect against incompetence and fraudulent professional behavior, and to encourage learning and continuing competence. These are important professional reasons for practitioners to have their competence to practice recognized publicly.

In the United States, licensure by government agency, credentialing by educational institutions, and certification by voluntary and professional associations serve these social needs. Formal credentials fall into three categories.

- *Documents of certification, licensure, or registration* are issued by agencies of government to persons who meet specific requirements. In pharmacy, the most common example is the license to practice pharmacy granted by a state board of pharmacy. Such a license provides evidence that the state has granted a person permission to engage in a specified activity; practice by the uncredentialed is prohibited.

- *Documents of certification or registration awarded by a professional organization* attest that the holder meets certain requisites or professional standards. This credential represents an advisory opinion by the issuing agency that the holder is qualified to engage in specified practices. Professional certification may duplicate, complement, or supplement credentials offered by government agencies or institutions of higher learning. In pharmacy, the Board of Pharmaceutical Specialties recognizes competence in specialized areas of pharmacy practice.

- *Diplomas attesting to degree or certificate status conferred by educational institutions for successful completion of an organized program of study or for equivalent educational achievement* may, in some cases, be a requirement for governmental or professional credentialing. The doctor of pharmacy degree in pharmacy is such an example.

The credentialing process for all three categories are essentially the same. Each process involves three parties: the authority issuing the credential; the person to whom the credential is issued; and the persons, groups, or agencies benefitting from or using the judgments of the credentialing authority. Each process also involves the same three steps: definition of the competencies (knowledge, attitudes, skills, behaviors, and values) to be recognized; assessment of each individual to determine whether he or she meets the requisites; and the issuance of a document to attest the individual's possession of the requisites. A fourth step, periodic recredentialing, is often required. The credential is not a guarantee that the holder will perform satisfactorily or well in every situation; it indicates that those who are credentialed have the capability to deliver adequate services with substantially more consistency than those who do not hold the credential. In other words, credentialing cannot be expected to provide absolute protection to society, but it has social utility because it increases the likelihood that satisfactory services will be delivered.

An important distinction between the terms "certification" and "certificate" can be made. Certification is the process of credentialing individuals for possession of defined competencies. As such, certification attests to the achievement of a specified outcome. Examples of certification include certification in specialty pharmacy practices such as nuclear pharmacy or pharmacotherapy, as recognized by the Board of Pharmaceutical Specialties, and certification as a Master Teacher, as proposed by the American Association of Colleges of Pharmacy. Certificates, on the other hand, attest to the completion of a process. Certificates document completion of programs which provide the opportunity to acquire new knowledge and skills. For example, a residency certificate is awarded by hospital pharmacy departments with American Society of Hospital Pharmacists'-accredited residency programs and a certificate of Home Health Care is awarded by NARD for completion of its course in this subject area.

To the practitioner, public recognition of competence through credentialing confers pride in accomplishment and the knowledge that the mastery of requisite knowledge and skills is in the public interest. Further, credentialing is substantially interlinked with economic and social rewards in society. The overall social good of the credential, however, is to minimize risks to the public health, safety, and welfare by identifying those qualified to practice pharmacy.

The competencies associated with rendering pharmaceutical care do indeed respond to this social need. Practitioners can document their competency, and be publicly recognized as competent for practice, via any or all of the mechanisms described above.

In summary, all pharmacy practitioners must be capable of rendering pharmaceutical care—this statement represents both a societal and professional mandate. Competence for practice must be demonstrated and documented regularly by pharmacist, practice faculty, and student. Contemporary competence for practice is dynamic and requires individual efforts aimed at life-long learning and assessment of competence. Public and professional recognition of such contemporary competence to render pharmaceutical care serve as both safeguards and motivations for self-improvement.

References

American Association of Colleges of Pharmacy. 1995. Papers I, II, and III of the AACP Commission to Implement Change in Pharmaceutical Education. Alexandria, VA: AACP.

American Association of Colleges of Pharmacy. 1995. Pharmacy School Admission Requirements. Alexandria, VA: AACP.

Miller, J. W., and O. Mills. 1978. *Credentialing Educational Accomplishment*. Washington, DC: American Council on Education.

Pew Health Professions Commission. 1991. Healthy America: Practitioners for 2005, An Agenda for Action for US Health Professional Schools, eds. D. A. Shugars, E. H., O'Neil, and J. D., Bader. Durham, NC: Pew Health Professions Commission.

15

Organizing Practices for Pharmaceutical Care

Heidi M. Anderson-Harper, Ph.D.

> ". . . would you tell me, please which way I ought to [go] from here?"
> "That depends a good deal on where you want to get to," said the Cat.
> "I don't much care where——," said Alice.
> "Then it doesn't matter which way you [go]," said the Cat.
>
> Lewis Carroll
> Alice's Adventures in Wonderland[1]

Strand, Cipolle, and Morley (1992) state, "for the profession of pharmacy to accept the responsibility associated with the delivery of pharmaceutical care, an evolutionary process needs to occur." They suggest that the few individual practitioner models that already exist for delivering pharmaceutical care to patients can serve as useful prototypes for the implementation of pharmaceutical care. However, it must be emphasized that each pharmacist and each practice site begins at a different point in the evolutionary process of providing pharmaceutical care. Therefore, the pharmacy services that develop will be unique for each practice site. Because the types of patients served by each pharmacy can differ as well, patients' needs should be considered in establishing the priority for adding a new service that incorporates the pharmaceutical care philosophy into a particular site. For example, one setting might have patients who require a pharmacokinetics dosing service, and another site might require a diabetes teaching service.

This chapter describes how various pioneer pharmacists have organized their practices to provide pharmaceutical care. Practices in acute care institutions and in community, long term care, and managed care pharmacies are described and discussed. The chapter develops the theme that manager practitioners have a responsibility to develop practicing systems that facilitate the delivery of pharmaceutical care. Summaries of a mailed questionnaire and subsequent telephone interviews (Anderson-Harper 1993) with pharmacists in several prototype practice sites (see Table 15-1) are included to demonstrate how some pharmacists have organized their practices to provide pharmaceutical care. Finally, this chapter assumes the organization has adopted the pharmaceutical care philosophy and is beginning to reorganize or design a practice model for their organization. Each pharmacy organization will need to develop a plan based on their specific needs and may want to use the views, plans, and suggestions made by these pioneers to help with this process.

Table 15-1. Prototype Pharmacies Used in Interview

Type of Pharmacy Practice	Pharmacist Interviewed	Location
Independent	Ray Marcrom	Marcrom's Pharmacy Manchester, Tennessee
Independent	Arnold Gammaitori	Trooper's Pharmacy & Health Education Center Norristown, Pennsylvania
Office Practice	Beatrice Adreon	Pharmacy Counseling Services, Inc. Arlington, Virginia
Ambulatory Practice	Dennis J. McCallian	Family PharmaCare West Lafayette, Indiana
Services Community Ambulatory Pharmacies	Jeanne Ann Stasny	Pharmaceutical Care Services, Inc. Waco, Texas
Hospital	Christine Chatatas	St. John's Hospital Detroit, Michigan
Hospital	Max Ray	University of California-San Diego (UCSD) Medical Center San Diego, California
Hospital	Michael Melby	Blodgett Memorial Hospital Grand Rapids, Michigan
Nursing Home	Armon Neel	Institutional Pharmacy Consultant Griffin, Georgia
Managed Care	Bill Boyce	Chemawa Indian Health Center Salem, Oregon
Managed Care	Carey Cotterell	Kaiser Permanente Medical Care Program Anaheim, California
Managed Care	John Hopkins	Rocky Mountain HMO Grand Junction, Colorado
Managed Care	Kristin Young	HealthPartners Minneapolis, Minnesota

Source: Mailed questionnaire and telephone interviews conducted by H.M. Anderson-Harper, August–October, 1993.

The process of reorganizing or redesigning the pharmacy should follow a series of steps:

1. Explore the needs of the community the practice serves.
2. Develop a mission statement for the practice that reflects a commitment to pharmaceutical care.
3. Define the short-term and long-term goals of the pharmacy based on the new mission statement.
4. Determine the organizational structure (work analysis, technology, etc.) and resources that are needed to support the mission.
5. Develop minimum competencies and retrain the staff (technicians, pharmacists, etc.) to perform the new roles.
6. Develop procedures for implementing the new plan.
7. Use evaluation measures and techniques to determine if the plan is effective.

Mission Statement

The initial step in organizing the practice is to articulate the mission of the practice; this statement of the fundamental reason for the practice's existence should reflect the practice's commitment to pharmaceutical care. A mission statement is a broad declaration of the basic, unique purpose and scope of operations that distinguishes this practice from others of its type (Pearce and Robinson 1988). A statement of purpose broadly defines the ends or results an organization hopes to attain. Expressed in terms of an input-throughput-output model, purposes define a practice's outputs.

In highlighting the importance of the mission statement, Peter Drucker asserts that it defines the organization (Drucker 1973). Preparing a mission statement requires asking, "what is our business and what should it be?" Drucker points out that while nothing should be more obvious than knowing what business one is in, the actual determination of purpose of the business is difficult and what it should be is usually not obvious. In some organizations, the mission statement is explicit in the sense that it is a formal written document; in others, the mission may be more implicitly understood. Of course in the latter case, there is the danger that some of the organization's members may have different perceptions of the organization's mission, perhaps without realizing it (Want 1986).

Drucker believes that, "only a clear definition of the mission and purpose of the business makes possible clear and realistic business objectives. It is the foundation for priorities, strategies, plans and work assignments (Drucker 1973, 75)." The mission statement and organization purpose are the starting points for the designing of the organizational structure and jobs within that structure.

The mission statement serves several purposes. Useful statements provide a degree of specificity that allows differentiation of the organization from all others. Statements of purpose provide guidance to managers in judging the appropriateness of organizational arrangements and management practices. They provide a focus and direction for managerial attention and effort. Furthermore, for the manager, the statements can be a benchmark against which to evaluate success. For employees, a mission statement defines a common purpose, nurtures organizational loyalty, and fosters a sense of community (Nash 1988, 155–156).

The pharmaceutical care mission statement should highlight a patient-centered focus in which pharmacists accept responsibility for patient drug-related problems and outcomes. The pharmacy practice developing or redefining its mission statement may want to include some or all of the following components (David 1989):

1. Customers. Who are the organization's customers?

2. Products or services. What are the practice's major products or services?

3. Location. Where does the practice compete?

4. Technology. What is the practice's basic technology?

5. Concern for survival. What is the practice's commitment to economic objectives?

6. Philosophy. What are the basic beliefs, values, aspirations, and philosophical priorities of the professionals that make up the practice?

7. Self-concept. What are the practice's major strengths and competitive advantages?

8. Concern for public image. What are the practice's public responsibilities and what image is desired?

9. Concern for associates. What are the attitudes of the technical and professional staff toward each other?

Table 15-2 shows how the prototype pharmacies have addressed these components in their mission statements. Figures 15-1 and 15-2 show an example of a brochure

Table 15-2. Major Components of Mission Statements and Sample Excerpts

Major Components	Sample Excerpts
Customers	The Department of Pharmacy within the University of California San Diego (UCSD) Medical Center provides services to patients and to the San Diego community, educates health care professionals and the public, and pursue of new knowledge through research. *UCSD Medical Center*
Products or services	The UCSD Department of Pharmacy has established the following as its mission: to provide pharmaceutical care to all our patients. *UCSD Medical Center*
Location	Pharmacy Services in the Indian Health Service (IHS) are an integral part of a comprehensive, community-based health care delivery system. *Chemawa Indian Health Center*
Technology	Even though the nature of our practice is very diverse, we have striven to build it around the idea that patients deserve and need to know about their medical conditions and the medications or therapies they are receiving. We have attempted this integrated approach through the use of printed and computer-generated drug information to support counseling efforts. *Marcrom's Pharmacy*
Concern for survival	Attempting to consistently provide quality patient information has been a standard for our practice and a driving force in the growth of our business. *Marcrom's Pharmacy*
Philosophy	The mission of Family PharmaCare is to improve the health of our patrons by delivering patient-centered pharmaceutical care in a caring, convenient, cost-effective, and confidential manner. *Family PharmaCare*
Self-concept	To exercise leadership in the UCSD Medical Center in all matters related to the use of drugs. *UCSD Medical Center*
Concern for public image	Pharmacists in the IHS serve as role models for persons within the communities who may wish to pursue careers in the health field. *Chemawa Indian Health Center*
Concern for employees	Pharmacy services are fully integrated into the health system. Therefore pharmacists may be called upon to perform other extended functions such as primary patient care and program management. *Chemawa Indian Health Center*

Four words embrace our philosophy. We call them the 4-C's:

CARE our defining principle. It is so important that we made it part of our name. We are committed to a patient-centered approach which fosters a caring, personal relationship between the pharmacist and the patient.

CONVENIENCE is our second key principle. Patients deserve timely, accessible and efficient care. our policies and procedures are designed to minimize unnecessary waiting, while still ensuring the highest level of quality.

COST-EFFECTIVENESS is our third guiding principle. We recognize our obligation to achieve the highest possible quality of care at the lowest possible cost.

CONFIDENTIALITY is our fourth guiding principle. The medical information our patients and their physicians share with us represents a sacred trust. We pledge to safeguard that information and to use it exclusively in the fulfillment of our professional responsibilities.

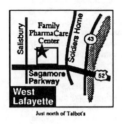

Just north of Talbot's

Family PharmaCare
Center, Inc.
University Square
Shopping Center
500 Sagamore
Parkway, West
Office Suite 5W
West Lafayette, IN 47906

Telephone Numbers

Monday - Friday 9 am - 6 pm
Saturday 9 am - 1 pm

Your health is our business.

Family PharmaCare

An independent community pharmacy unlike any other

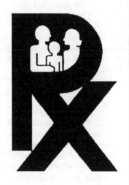

Your health is our business

Figure 15.1. Front of Family PharmaCare Brochure (used with permission).

used by one of the prototype pharmacies in marketing their philosophy to their patients.

Goals

Next the pharmacy needs to develop short-range and long-range organizational goals that are consistent with the mission of the practice and address targets to

What's different about Family PharmaCare?

In some ways Family PharmaCare is much like other pharmacies. We fill prescriptions and offer a complete line of non-prescription remedies.

But the similarity stops there. We go beyond the boundaries of traditional community pharmacy by offering a wide complement of services to better serve the health care needs of our patients:

- **EXTENDED CONSULTATION**
We believe the more you know about your medication therapy, the better you'll feel. That's why we offer personalized, private counseling sessions designed to provide you with the knowledge and the confidence to better manage your therapy.

- **MEDICATION PROFILE & REVIEW**
Every time you receive a prescription at Family PharmaCare we review all of your medications with you. We will ensure that your medications are working together with no adverse effects. We also provide you with a complete written summary.

- **BROWN BAG REVIEW**
As a new patient at Family PharmaCare, you may wish to start your medication profile with a "brown bag review." This service allows you the opportunity to bring in and discuss every prescription and over-the-counter remedy you are currently using.

- **SELF-CARE ADVICE**
Our pharmacists know which non-prescription drug products are right for you. Backed by our state-of-the-art computer technology and information you provide, we'll work with you to select the best treatment for your symptoms.

- **COMPOUNDING LABORATORY**
We maintain a complete prescription compounding service for the preparation of custom dosage formulations tailored to you and your needs.

- **HEALTH INFORMATION SERVICE**
We maintain a computerized health information service rivaling that of many hospitals. Our pharmacists are committed to achieving and maintaining the highest standards of professional knowledge and expertise.

- **24-HOUR EMERGENCY SERVICE**
We realize that your health care needs may arise outside of our regular business hours. That's why we have a 24-hour emergency number to provide you with the care you need, when you need it.

Patient Bill of Rights

As a Family PharmaCare patient, you have the right:

To be treated with courtesy and respect

To actively participate in your care

To accurate and complete information about your medication therapy

To speak to your pharmacist in private upon request

To complete confidentiality of your medical information

To review your medication records upon request

To authorize any substitution of prescribed medication

To receive a full explanation of all charges for pharmacy services

Dennis J. McCallian
Dennis J. McCallian,
President

Figure 15.2. Back of Family PharmaCare Brochure (used with permission).

be achieved by the group as a whole. Examples of goals include identifying drug-related problems and attaining specific increases in patient compliance or patient satisfaction. Research over several decades has highlighted the importance of goals in enhancing organizational efficiency and effectiveness (Lee, Locke, and Latham 1989). Specific goals should be established for each department, subunit, and individual.

A goal-oriented approach to reorganization has several major benefits (Roth et al. 1988). First, goals help clarify expectations, which can lead to increased performance. When goals are set, group members are more likely to have a clear idea of the major outcomes that they are expected to achieve. Goals also provide benchmarks against which progress can be assessed so that corrective action can be taken. An additional benefit of goal-setting is increased motivation, which develops from meeting goals, feeling a sense of accomplishment, and receiving recognition and other rewards for reaching targeted outcomes.

The goals experts, Edwin A. Locke and his associates (Locke and Latham 1990), state that goals should be challenging, attainable, specific and measurable, time-limited, and relevant. Extensive research indicates that, within reasonable limits, challenging goals lead to higher performance. Goals usually work best when they are attainable because they allow the individual a feeling of accomplishment. To be effective, goals need to be specific and measurable so that it is clear what is expected and when the goal has been achieved. Measurable goals are of two types: quantitative and qualitative. Quantitative goals encompass objective numerical standards that are relatively easy to verify. For example, a pharmacist may try to identify 60 drug-related problems daily. However, for some purposes qualitative goals are more appropriate. Qualitative goals involve subjective judgement about whether or not a goal is reached. An example of a qualitative goal could be increasing the quality of patient care or the patients' satisfaction with pharmacy services. Goals need be to time-limited. That is, there should be a defined period of time within which the goals must be accomplished. Otherwise, goals have little meaning, because individuals may continually put off achieving them. Finally, goals are more likely to generate support when they are clearly relevant to the major work of the practice (Locke and Latham 1984).

Linking Goals and Plans

Goals and plans are closely related. While goals are the desired ends, plans are the means that will be used to bring about the desired ends. Once goals are set, it is necessary to develop action plans that focus on the methods or activities necessary to reach particular goals. The plan describes what should be done, and how, when, where and by whom it should be done, in order to achieve a goal. Plans help make goal-attainment feasible by identifying problem areas, spelling out areas in which resources and assistance will be needed, and facilitating the search for more efficient and effective ways to achieve objectives. Such plans are usually developed by subordinates in conjunction with their supervisors (Bartol and Martin 1991, 181).

Clear goals provide a framework on which to design the pharmaceutical care practice model. Pharmaceutical care practices with different goals may have completely different components and structures. In some of the prototype pharmacies, the goals are presented in the form of Standards of Practice. The Standards of Practice demonstrate the knowledge required of a pharmacist and the level to which the pharmacist must participate with other health care professionals in order to provide the best care. The Standards of Practice also point to the conclusion that the standard of care owned by pharmacists is to be determined by the standards of the profession. Sample excerpts of Standards of Practice are listed in Tables 15-3 and 15-4.

The Analysis of Work

For any organization, even at a given point in time, there may be more than one appropriate structure which could serve equally well. Therefore, the organization needs to determine the work to be performed before addressing the issue of design. In Lewis Carroll's (1989) *Alice's Adventures in Wonderland,* the Cheshire cat reminds us of the importance of determining where it is you want to go before deciding how to get there. Any organizational design will do if it is not directed toward achieving any particular purpose. The purpose of work analysis is expressed succinctly in the motto, "work smarter, not harder." Work analysis uses logic and knowledge of how the human body functions in performing physical tasks to devise methods for task performance that are easier to learn, less fatiguing, quicker, safer, and more reliable than other methods.

The results of work analysis are often used to develop job descriptions, which are statements of the duties, working conditions, and other significant requirements associated with each job. Job descriptions are frequently combined with job specifications. A job specification is a statement of the skills, abilities, education, and previous work experience that are required to perform a particular job. Formats for job descriptions and job specifications tend to vary with the organization, but the information is often used extensively for activities that require a solid understanding of a job and the qualifications necessary for per-

Table 15-3. Abbreviated Example of Standards of Practice from a Prototype Pharmacy

United States Public Health Services, Indian Health Service,
Pharmacy Branch Standards of Practice

Standard 1. Assure appropriateness of drug therapy
Standard 2. Verify that patients understand their medications and appropriate outcomes of their drug therapy
Standard 3. Assure availability, preparation, and control of medications
Standard 4. Provide drug information, drug therapy consultation, and staff education relating to drug therapy
Standard 5. Provide health promotion and disease prevention activities relating to drug use and prevention therapy.
Standard 6. Manage therapy for selected patients in whom drugs are the primary method of treatment.

Used with permission from Bill Boyce, R.Ph., Chemawa Indian Health Center, Salem, Oregon

*Table 15-4. Abbreviated Example of Standards of Practice from a Prototype
Pharmacy*

Department of Pharmacy, University of California-San Diego (UCSD)
Medical Center Standards of Practice

Standard 1. Review of patient medication history, or establishment of a patient medication history if none exists.

Standard 2. Identification of drug-related problems (potential and actual problems) that the patient presents with.

Standard 3. Prevention or resolution of drug-related problems.

Standard 4. Decision about which problems (from the patient's health problem list) are treatable with drugs.

Standard 5. Establishment or clarification of goals and objectives of therapy (desired outcomes) in collaboration with physician or other primary provider, for each problem being treated.

Standard 6. Establishment of individualized treatment plan, with alternatives.

Standard 7. Facilitation of the implementation of the treatment plan.

Standard 8. Patient education and counseling, to assist the patient in making best use of his or her medication.

Standard 9. Monitoring of the patient's response to the treatment plan using appropriate clinical indicators.

Standard 10. Provision of a summary note for the benefit of the next pharmacist who cares for the patient.

Standard 11. Projecting an appropriate professional image to the public, to individual patients, and to health care associates.

Used with permission from Max Ray, Pharm. D., Department of Pharmacy, University of California-San Diego (UCSD) Medical Center, San Diego, California

forming it. Table 15-5 contrasts job descriptions for a pharmacist before and after the implementation of pharmaceutical care in a practice.

The process of analyzing work was described by Jeanne Stansy as one phase that *Pharmaceutical Care Services, Inc.* uses to help convert a traditional community pharmacy to one that provides pharmaceutical care. Specifically, this phase involves an analysis of the workflow of the pharmacy which results in revising the job descriptions of the professionals and technicians. Next, the pharmacy is remodeled based on the revised workflow to make the system more efficient. Finally, the technicians and pharmacists incrementally implement the new practices based on the revised job descriptions.

How to Conduct Work Analysis

The determination of the human resources needed to accomplish the organization's mission and goals is a process that often involves work analysis as a means of understanding the nature of jobs under consideration. *Work analysis* is the systematic collection and recording of information concerning the purpose of a job, its major duties, the conditions under which it is performed, the contacts

306 / Heidi M. Anderson-Harper, Ph.D.

Table 15-5. Sample Pharmacist Job Functions Before and After Implementing
Pharmaceutical Care

Before Pharmaceutical Care	After Pharmaceutical Care
Fill prescriptions in compliance with federal and state regulations in an accurate, timely, and courteous manner; and provide drug information and counseling to patients.	Interview patients to obtain information regarding medication use, medication allergies and sensitivities; document the information in the patient's medical record or pharmacy information system when appropriate; advise patients of directions for use, medication storage requirements, importance of compliance, precautions, and warnings for medication therapy; advise the patient on the use of related devices and the coordination of medication therapy with diet, according to established polices and procedures.
Adhere to departmental patient service standards.	Evaluate and resolve, using professional judgement and established policies and procedures, potential medication therapy problems identified through any and all available sources, including the patient and pharmacy information system.
Consult with health professionals.	Confer with medical personnel concerning pharmaceutical care and treatment of patients, related clinical diagnosis, drug combinations and dosage forms, and other factors that might influence the course of treatment and the activity of the medications; suggest changes in medication therapy and/or use as appropriate to assure optimum therapeutic results.
Maintain a professional image.	Exemplify pharmacy's mission and the organization's vision by contributing to the health and satisfaction of patients by providing appropriate medications, information, and professional services in a helpful, caring, courteous, and efficient manner.

with others that performance of the job requires, and the knowledge, skills, and abilities needed for performing the job effectively. Work analysis information can be collected by observing individuals doing the job, conducting interviews with individuals and their supervisors, having individuals keep diaries of job-related activities, and distributing questionnaires to be completed by job incumbents and their supervisors (Milkovich and Boudreau 1988).

Analyzing work consists of answering four separate but related questions which are briefly discussed in the next section (Drucker 1973).

1. What are the component parts of work and the characteristics and requirements of each part?

2. How do the component parts fit together?
3. What resources are needed to do the work?
4. What controls are needed to determine and evaluate the direction, quantity, and quality of work?

Determining the component parts of work will help in redefining the roles of all those involved in the pharmaceutical care practice to be as appropriate as possible.

The Parts of Work

To determine the component parts of work it is helpful first to ask simply, "what are the things that need to be done?" In most cases, the answer to this question will yield the basic components of work, and their inherent natural boundaries will be evident. For example, the different work performed by different professional groups (i.e., pharmacist vs. technician or nurse vs. pharmacist) is a natural place to look for inherent boundaries. A guideline to identifying boundaries of components of work is to look for differences along the following three general dimensions: time, technology, and territory (Charns and Schaefer 1983).

Along the dimension of time, the important question is whether work is done at distinctly different points in time. For example, the components of nursing care, medical care, or other health care may be performed for a patient during different visits to a clinic or office setting, or perhaps on different days while the person is hospitalized. Regarding territory, different elements of work can often be recognized by their performance in different places. For example, in a multiple clinic system, each clinic site forms a natural boundary around many types of work. Similarly, neighborhoods form boundaries for work done by home health care teams. Legal and broader community expectations form another type of boundary that must be accounted for early in the planning process. Technology should be considered broadly to include not only hardware but also skills and training, personality characteristics and interpersonal orientations, and different practices associated with performing different work.

Differences that identify natural internal boundaries among elements of work may also be associated with segments of an organization's environment. For example, it is important to ask what differences are inherent in working with different types of patients with different diseases, with those in pursuit of health maintenance and prevention of illness, or with people of different ethnic or socioeconomic backgrounds.

Interconnectedness

The second activity in work analysis is determining how the pieces fit together to form a coherent whole. To accomplish this, a manager should examine each work element to each other element to see if the pieces of work can be performed independently of each other or if their dependence upon each other requires that they be performed sequentially or simultaneously. For example, diagnosis of an illness is interconnected with treatment. Treatment plans follow directly from diagnosis; alterations in diagnosis result in changes in treatment; and errors in diagnosis directly affect the success of treatment. This example demonstrates the need to realize the interconnectedness of the physician and the pharmacist in establishing an appropriate therapeutic regimen.

Resource Requirements

Next, the manager needs to estimate what the total task requires in terms of staff, money, space, equipment, supplies, and information. Analysis of staff requirements consists of assessing the numbers and types of personnel, together with their skill requirements, and then determining what competencies and behaviors are required in order for tasks to be performed.

Control Requirements

To determine how well work is being performed—the quantity, quality and timeliness of output—and also to assess resource utilization, managers need information. In order to make decisions about what measures to use and when to use them, the costs and other effects of the measures on the practice need to be determined.

Training and Development

The implementation of the pharmaceutical care model requires a reorientation in the way pharmacists and technicians think and the duties they perform. All professional and technical staff who will be involved in the practice must be personally committed to providing pharmaceutical care and technically proficient at delivering it with consistently high quality. He asserts that the input from the staff allows the pharmacist manager to accomplish several objectives. First, staff can provide insight into how best to integrate the services into existing operations with minimal disruption in routine. Second, they can become comfortable with what they will be expected to do and how they will do it. Third, including staff in the planning of a new practice makes it *their* plan and increases their committment to making the service successful.

The training and development process can be used to redefine the role of these professionals. In essence, the tasks of the technician and pharmacist need to be redefined in terms of the new role. Training and development is a planned effort to facilitate employee's learning of job-related behaviors in order to improve their performance (Hall and Goodale 1986). Training must be directed toward the accomplishment of some organizational objective, such as more efficient identification of drug-related problems, improved quality of health care, or reduced health care costs. This means that a practice should commit its resources only to those training activities that can best help in achieving its objectives (Byars and Rue 1991, 206).

Phases of the Training Process

Training efforts generally encompass three main phases: assessment phase, training design and implementation phase, and evaluation phase (Cascio 1989). The *assessment phase* involves identifying training needs, setting training objectives, and developing criteria against which to evaluate the results of the training program. Within the assessment phase, training requirements are determined by conducting a needs analysis. A needs analysis is an assessment of an organization's training needs that considers overall organizational requirements, tasks (identified through job analysis) associated with jobs for which training is needed, and the degree to which individuals are able to perform those tasks effectively (Wexley and Latham 1981). The practice may want to have outside consultants help with various aspects in this phase. Additionally, establishing a relationship with local schools and colleges of pharmacy, disease specific patient organizations, and the national associations can help.

After training needs have been determined, objectives must be established for meeting these needs. Effective training objectives should state what the organization, department or individual is to be like when the training is completed. The objectives should demonstrate what the trainee must be taught in order to do the job efficiently, safely, economically, and intelligently. The desired outcomes, as minimum competencies to be performed, should be expressed in writing. Training objectives can be categorized as one of three types (Byars and Rue 1991, 208):

1. Instructional objectives. What principles, facts, and concepts are to be learned in the training? Who is to be taught?

2. Practice objectives. What impact will the training have on practice outcomes, such as improved patient quality of life?

3. Individual performance and growth objectives. What impact will the training have on the behavioral and attitudinal outcomes and personal growth of the pharmacist or technician?

The second phase of training, the *training design and implementation phase,* involves determining training methods, developing training materials, and actually conducting the training. Within this phase there are a number of training methods that can be used, which fall into three main categories: information presentation, simulation training, and on-the-job training (Scarpello and Ledvinka 1988). *Information presentation methods* entail teaching facts, skills, attitudes, or concepts without expecting trainees to put what they are learning into practice during the training. Examples are lectures, reading lists, videotapes, and most computerized instruction. *Simulation training methods* involve providing artificial situations that offer trainees a means of practicing their learning during the training. Examples include case analysis, role playing, and simulated computer cases. *On-the-job training methods* focus on having the trainee learn while actually performing a job, usually with the help of a mentor or preceptor. Examples include job rotation, vestibule training (in which the individual learns in a separate area that is set up to approximate as closely as possible the actual job situation), and on-the-job coaching (in which the individual performs the job under the direct guidance of a trainer).

One form of training that might be considered in the pharmacy setting is job rotation, also called cross training. In job rotation, the individual learns several different jobs within a work unit or department and performs each for a specified time period. One of the main advantages of job rotation is that it makes flexibility possible in the department. For example, when one member of a work unit is absent, another can perform that job. In training the employee on the job, several steps can be taken to ensure that the training is effective.

The third phase of the training process, the *evaluation phase,* entails assessing the results of the training against the criteria developed during the assessment phase. Major ways to evaluate training include measuring participants' reactions to the training to determine how useful they thought it was, assessing actual learning (perhaps through tests before and after the training), determining the extent of behavioral change (possibly by having the supervisor or subordinates of a trainee assess changes in the individual's behavior), and measuring actual results on the job (such as increased output) (Kirkpatrick 1967).

Examples of Training and Development

Stansy described the technician community pharmacy training seminar that is part of the *Pharmaceutical Care Services, Inc.* program (Table 15-6). The technicians complete a one-day, nine-hour training conference. Stansy states that the major role of the technician seminar is to assure that "the technicians understand the critical role that they play in the overall process of patient care." In this seminar, technicians learn to understand that if they take in false, assumed, or incorrect data, a pharmacist can not complete a proper drug regimen review and patient management will be hindered. The technicians learn various processes: the difference between objective and subjective thought; appropriate communication skills; important mathematical formulas; patient interview skills; and how to assist the pharmacist in completing pharmaceutical care. Stansy uses the following learning techniques in the technician seminar to accomplish the objectives: lectures, reading lists, videotapes, simulated case analysis, and on-the-job training. She states,

Table 15-6.   Technician Training Conference by Pharmaceutical Care Services, Inc.

Goal: To teach the pharmacy technician how to convert from the traditional role of pharmacy to the pharmaceutical care era of pharmacy.

Objectives:

1. To allow the technician to truly understand the new dual purpose of pharmacy and their role in that purpose.
2. To understand the importance of communication with patients.
3. To be able to interview patients without creating barriers or making assumptions.
4. To understand present pharmacy law.
5. To understand a workflow that accommodates the pharmacist performing cognitive services in a cost effective manner.

Used with permission from Jeanne Ann Stasny, R.Ph., CEO, Pharmaceutical Care Services, Inc., Waco, Texas

"the key to the whole process is proper training and proper preparation for the task at hand."

Another example of the training process is the Indian Health Service (IHS) clinical pharmacy training program. Pharmacists entering the IHS pharmacy practice find an active program with a strong emphasis on the clinical aspects of patient care; they are immediately challenged to make full use of their knowledge and skills. To further develop the skills of the pharmacists who practice in this environment, a clinical pharmacy training program series was developed, and it has become an important part of the staff development process. The first segment of the training program is a home study course. The course reviews the pathophysiology and pharmacotherapy of the most common acute and chronic diseases seen in the IHS ambulatory care settings and stresses the critical information necessary for providing quality care. The second component, which follows eight weeks later, is an intensive workshop consisting of didactic material and practical experience that covers patient interviewing techniques, patient and physician communication skills, patient consultation and education techniques, and medical chart screening techniques. This approach has been effective in developing and maintaining the skills of IHS pharmacists (Church 1987).

A final example involves the Pharmacy Department at Blodgett Memorial Medical Center in Grand Rapids, Michigan. Melby describes a two-phase pharmacist training program that includes a didactic self-taught component and on-the-job training. In the didactic phase, the pharmacists complete the Pharmacotherapy Self-Assessment Program (PSAP) (American College of Clinical Pharmacy 1991). PSAP is a unique, comprehensive series of self-study modules designed to develop, update, and assess pharmacists' knowledge in the science and application of pharmacotherapy. The second phase involves on-the-job training in pharmaceutical care. This is accomplished using weekly meetings in which pharmacists present actual cases and develop their skills at identifying drug problems and solutions.

Implementation

The goal of the implementation phase is to make the transition from the program design or plan to the successfully operating program. An effectively managed implementation plan is as important to the overall success of the program as an effective program design. In fact, the implementation phase requires more precise supervision than the design phase. If errors are made during the design phase, they can be corrected by redoing that portion of the design. When errors are committed during the implementation phase, the damage caused by those errors must be corrected before that portion of the implementation is revised (O'Donnell 1987, 42).

The implementation phase actually has two steps: planning the implementation of the program and executing the implementation plan. O'Donnell (1987) suggests using the following questions as a guide to planning the implementation:

1. What are the components that need to be implemented?
2. What are the steps required to implement each component?
3. What are the major milestones and the timetable for each of the steps, and how do they relate to other components being developed?
4. What resources, including funding, space, technological assistance, and people, are required for each step?
5. What are the progress monitors and measures of success?

The components that make a program successful include: strong support from top management, involvement of staff in developing the program, and competence of staff. The steps required to achieve each of the elements necessary for a successful program will be different in each case. For example, top management support will be achieved through a completely different set of steps than bringing the staff knowledge level to minimal competencies. Major milestones can be identified, and an implementation schedule can be outlined. This provides a specific guide to aim toward and against which to measure progress. It also helps coordinate the interaction among the different efforts.

During the executing of the implementation plan, the focus is on keeping the plan on track. This is done by monitoring the progress of the effort through predetermined mechanisms and measuring successes against previously established standards. Progress can be monitored by a weekly comparison of tasks completed to tasks planned. Specific assignment of this responsibility will facilitate these progress reports. Specific criteria for success can help redefine targets, for example, identifying 25 percent of the drug-related problems in one week or 50 percent by week four.

Periodic reviews are important to ensure that plans are implemented as expected and that goals will ultimately be met. Such reviews provide a good opportunity for checking performance to date, identifying and removing obstacles, solving problems, and altering action plans that are not achieving the expected results. Reviews also make it possible to assess the continuing appropriateness of the goals, to change the goals if necessary, or to add new goals if required by changing conditions.

Evaluation of the New Practice

The general aim of the evaluative efforts is to provide answers to questions and to determine the extent to which program objectives are being met. Evaluation of the pharmaceutical care practice involves a compilation of information which results in decisions that must be interpreted and acted upon by appropriate members of the pharmacy organization. The number and types of studies conducted at a given time depend upon the practices' needs and the resources available for evaluation. Evaluation may range from studies primarily descriptive of what is in existence, to those employing a strict research design methodology. Evaluation is a set of procedures used to appraise a program's merit and to provide information about its goals, activities, outcomes, impact, and costs.

Ideally, evaluation is an ongoing activity that begins at the first identification of the need for a new program, proceeds throughout the planning and implementing phases, and extends well beyond the length of the program itself. It is a vital part of developing a new program, results from systematic planning, involves a regular and comprehensive review of all phases of the program (including subsequent activities of those who participate), and serves as a mechanism for improving present and future programs and participants.

The evaluation process itself must undergo continuous scrutiny and be capable of refinement and improvement. Thus, procedures used for evaluation should include techniques for revising evaluation methodologies in response to questions raised in using them.

Types of Evaluation

There are two kinds of evaluation: formative evaluation and summative evaluation. *Formative evaluations* focus on finding out what goes on within a program, how well the program has been implemented, and how well the program is achieving its goals. The purpose of formative evaluation is to determine how a program can be upgraded and refined. Formative evaluation is conducted during the planning and operation of a program to provide those involved with evaluative information they can use in improving the program. In a community pharmacy attempting to develop a curriculum package to train new pharmacists about pharmaceutical care techniques that involve patient assessments, for example, formative evaluation might involve content inspection by experts, early tryouts with small numbers of patients, and so forth. Each step would provide immediate feedback to the developers, who could use such information to make necessary revisions.

Summative evaluations determine the effectiveness of and provide information about all potential program participants and all comparable programs. The purpose of summative evaluation is to appraise a program's overall impact and to determine the consistency with which it produces certain outcomes. Summative evaluation occurs after a program is considered for regular use and provides evidence for potential consumers about the program's worth. In the example, after the pharmaceutical care curriculum was developed, a summative evaluation might determine how effective the program was in identifying, resolving, and preventing patients' drug-related problems, using a broad sample of patients in the practice for which it was developed. The findings of that summative evaluation could indicate whether it is necessary to continue, revise, or terminate the particular program.

Steps in the Evaluation Process

The principles that govern the evaluation process of a program in pharmacy are the same as those that apply to the evaluation of any programmatic endeavor. Regardless of the setting, the steps of the process are the same. This is not to imply that evaluation is not specific to the setting in which it occurs. The uniqueness of a particular setting will affect the evaluation in terms of how the steps are actually implemented.

Essentially, five steps are involved in conducting a comprehensive evaluation. First, it is necessary to determine who is to be involved in the evaluation and to build in mechanisms for assuring that input will be obtained from all who will be affected by the decisions made on the basis of the evaluation findings. Evaluation is most relevant when it builds upon and involves the people directly and indirectly affected by its results.

If evaluation is to accomplish its purposes, those who collect and analyze evaluative information should be involved in decision making as well. When a distinction is implicitly or explicitly made between those conducting the evaluation and those making the decisions, evaluation is generally limited in scope, irrelevant to the needs of the audience, and, thus, unsuccessful (Staropoli and Waltz 1978, 85).

Second, the purposes for conducting the evaluation are made explicit. This involves stating the rationale for the evaluation as well as specifying the potential audiences for the evaluation results. This step will also determine the type of evaluation that needs to be completed (i.e., formative or summative).

Third, specific objectives need to be identified about the program inputs, operations, and outputs. Evaluation should focus on securing answers to specific questions regarding program efficiency and participant effectiveness that are of concern to the audiences for the evaluation results.

Fourth, evaluation methodology is determined. The tasks involved in this step are the identification of evaluation activities that will create a description of the program; answering the evaluation questions posed by planners, participants, clients and public; and providing evidence regarding the successful accomplishment of program objectives. Standards such as establishing a goal to resolve 80 percent of patients' drug-related problems must be established and agreed upon before data is collected.

Information collected for decision making will be useless unless specifications are made regarding what outcome leads to what action. Decision rules always exist when decisions are made, but they are often unstated, unsystematically formulated, and invented after the data are in. When this is the case, the construction of measuring instruments and analysis of data take place in a vacuum without guides to assure their usefulness (Staropoli and Waltz 1978, 85).

In determining the types of information to be collected to answer the specific questions regarding program inputs, operations, and outputs, it is necessary to plan for the collection of information that will be deemed acceptable by the various audiences for the results. Different audiences will seek different types of evidence for making decisions. Unless this fact is taken into account, the evaluator may find—after data collection is complete—that people are unwilling to base decisions on the information available.

Instruments employed for the collection of data should have the characteristics deemed essential to a "good" tool:

1. Reliability

2. Validity and specificity

3. Practical design

4. Utility in diagnosing strengths and weaknesses

5. Inclusion of factors crucial to making distinctions between individuals possessing differing amounts of the characteristic being measured. That is, not all movements carried out by a subject are crucial to the measurement of a given characteristic.

The fifth step in the evaluation process is determining when evaluation will occur and the points in the program where it is most advantageous to evaluate performance. To assess the accomplishment of program objectives, participants should be evaluated prior to, during, and immediately after the program, and at later intervals. In order to construct an accurate picture of participants' progress, evaluative efforts should reflect a progression in learning from simple to complex and from one stage of learning to the next. Inherent in each of these steps are procedures and techniques whereby an iterative process is established, meaning that evaluative information and results are fed back into the pharmacy program.

Internal and External Evaluation

The terms internal and external refer to whether the evaluation is conducted by someone employed within the pharmacy in which the program is based or by someone outside it. Regular staff members who take responsibility for evaluation activities are called internal evaluators, while outside consultants are called external evaluators. Internal evaluators have the advantage of being closer to the program and its staff and consequently less obtrusive. They are less likely to be objective than an outside evaluator, however, because they are personally involved in the program and because their job depends upon it. External evaluators, on the other hand, have the advantage of being objective and of having a fresh perspective. Disadvantages include their image as outsider-critics and sometimes their physical isolation from the program.

In formative evaluations, it is possible to use either an internal or external evaluator since the evaluation is likely to require close contact with the project and staff. In summative evaluations, however, use an external evaluator. The external evaluator is more likely to be objective and have an independent perspective, and, as a result, the evaluation's findings are more likely to be accepted.

Chapter Summary

Each pharmacist and each practice site begins at a different point in the evolutionary process of providing pharmaceutical care. The pharmacy services that develop will be different for each practice site and each site will have different types of patients. Therefore, patients' needs should be used to establish the priority for adding a new service that incorporates the pharmaceutical care philosophy into a particular site. The steps in organizing the pharmacy practice include:

- Developing a mission statement that reflects a commitment to pharmaceutical care
- Defining the short-term and long-term goals of the pharmacy based on the new mission statement
- Determining the organizational structure (work analysis, technology, etc.) and resources that are needed to support the mission
- Developing minimum competencies and re-training the staff (technicians, pharmacists, etc.) to perform the new roles
- Developing procedures for implementing the new plan
- Using evaluation measures and techniques to determine if the plan is effective

Finally, the pharmacy should evaluate the new program to obtain information about its goals, activities, outcomes, impact and costs to make decisions about the future of the program.

Acknowledgements

I would like to acknowledge and give public praising to *Beatrice Adreon, Bill Boyce, Christine Chatatas, Carey Cotterell, Arnold Gammaitori, John Hopkins, Ray Marcrom, Dennis J. McCallian, Michael Melby, Armon Neel, Max Ray, Jeanne Ann Stasny and Kristin Young* for completing the questionnaire, participating in the telephone interviews, and permitting me to use materials from their practices in the chapter. They provided valuable information about how they redesigned their pharmacy practices. Their openness will benefit us all. I would also like to express my sincere gratitude to *Taki May-Sasser* and *Larry James Harper* for their editorial advice and for helping me organize thoughts and clarify ideas in the chapter.

References

American College of Clinical Pharmacy. 1991. *Pharmacotherapy Self-Assessment Program*. Kansas City: American College of Clinical Pharmacy.

Anderson-Harper, H. M. Personal communication August-October, 1993.

Bartol, K. M., and D. C. Martin. 1991. *Management*. New York: McGraw-Hill.

Byars, L. L., and L. W. Rue. 1991. *Human Resource Management*. Illinois: Irwin.

Carroll, L. 1989. *Alice's Adventures in Wonderland: The Ultimate Illustrated Edition*. New York: Bantam Books.

Cascio, W. F. 1989. *Managing Human Resources*, 2nd ed. New York: McGraw-Hill.

Charns, M. P., and M. J. Schaefer. 1983. *Health Care Organizations: A Model for Management*. New Jersey: Prentice-Hall.

Church, R. M. 1987. Pharmacy Practice in the Indian Health Service. *American Journal of Hospital Pharmacy*. 44: 771–5.

David, F. R. 1989. How Companies Define Their Mission. *Long Range Planning*. 22: 90–7.

Drucker, P. F. 1973. *Management: Tasks, Responsibilities and Practices*. New York: Harper & Row.

Hall, D. T., and J. G. Goodale. 1986. *Human Resource Management*. Illinois: Scott Foresman.

Kirkpatrick, D. L. 1967. Evaluation of Training. In *Training and Development Handbook*, ed. R.L. Craig, and L.R. Bittel. New York: McGraw-Hill.

Lee, T. W., E. A. Locke, and G. P. Latham. 1989. Goal Setting Theory and Job

Performance. In *Goal Concepts in Personality and Social Psychology*, ed. L. A. Pervin, 291–326. New Jersey: Lawrence Erlbaum, Hillsdale.

Locke, E. A., and G. P. Latham. 1984. *Goal Setting: A Motivational Technique That Works!* New Jersey: Prentice-Hall.

Locke, E. A., and G. P. Latham. 1990. *A Theory of Goal Setting & Task Performance*. New Jersey: Prentice-Hall.

Milkovich, G. T., and J. W. Boudreau. 1988. *Personnel/Human Resource Management*. 5th ed. Texas: Business Publications.

Nash, L. 1988. Mission Statements—Mirrors and Windows. *Harvard Business Review*. March-April: 155–6.

O'Donnell, M. P. 1987. *Design of Workplace Health Promotion Programs*. American Journal of Health Promotion.

Pearce, J. A., II, and R. B. Robinson, Jr. 1988. *Strategic Management*. Illinois: Irwin.

Roth, P. L., et al. 1988. Designing a Goal-Setting System to Enhance Performance: A Practical Guide. *Organizational Dynamics*. (Summer): 69–78.

Scarpello, V. G., and J. Ledvinka. 1988. *Personnel/Human Resource Management*. Boston: PWS-Kent.

Staropoli, C. J., and C. F. Waltz. 1978. *Developing and Evaluating Educational Programs for Health Care Providers*. Philadelphia: F.A. Davis Company.

Strand, L. M., R. J. Cipolle, and P. C. Morley. 1992. *Pharmaceutical Care: An Introduction*. Michigan: Current Concepts. The Upjohn Company.

Want, J. H. 1986. Corporate Mission: The Intangible Contributor to Performance. *Management Review*. August: 46–50.

Wexley, K. N., and G. P. Latham. 1981. *Developing and Training Human Resources in Organizations*. Illinois: Scott Foresman.

16

The Ethics of Pharmaceutical Care

Bruce D. Weinstein, Ph.D.
Amy M. Haddad, Ph.D.

Introduction

Consider the following scenario:

> Accompanied by her middle-aged daughter, an elderly patient named Agnes Williams goes into a pharmacy to fill a prescription for an antianxiety drug. Ms. Williams appears a little confused. Pharmacist John Jones knows that Ms. Williams visits multiple pharmacies and that her physician has a habit of overprescribing painkillers and antianxiety medications for his elderly patients. The pharmacist wonders what he should do.
>
> Ethical hot spots. *Drug Topics* (April 25, 1994): 52

Whenever we ask the question, "What should I do?," and our choices concern the rights or welfare of other people, we are asking an ethical question. Pharmacists have always been faced with such questions, because the practice of pharmacy is a moral practice. That is, the mission of the pharmacist is to promote the well-being of others and to do for them what they wish to have done. John Jones' question is but one of many that pharmacists have been asking themselves throughout the long and rich history of the profession.

In reflecting upon the sorts of questions faced by John Jones, many pharmacists have relied upon a model for making ethical decisions that focuses on moral rules and principles. Although this model has served pharmacists well, it may not be sufficient to address the new challenges facing pharmacists in their delivery of pharmaceutical care. In this chapter we review the conventional model of ethical decision making and apply it to the case above. This model is useful in organizing one's thinking about a pharmacist's moral responsibilities, but, as we will show, one may be left wondering whether the pharmacist has adequately met his or her responsibilities in providing pharmaceutical care. We then briefly discuss the role that virtue plays in the moral life of the pharmacist and consider how pharmaceutical care will require taking into account moral rules and principles as well as virtues. The metaphor of the covenant, which takes a central place in definitions of pharmaceutical care, draws upon both the moral and virtue approaches to responding to ethical challenges. We use a second case to demonstrate why providers of pharmaceutical care should take both approaches seriously.[1]

Ethical Decision Making: A Conventional Approach to "Doing" Pharmacy Ethics

Let us investigate the case that introduced the chapter. We have already stated that the question facing John Jones, "What should I do?," or specifically, "Should I dispense this medication?," is an ethical one, because it concerns the pharmacist's conduct and has direct reference to the rights and welfare of the patient. Good ethical decision making begins with identifying the relevant facts, and it is not clear why the physician tends to prescribe anxiolytic drugs more often than is indicated. There are several reasons why this may be so, including the possibility that the physician may be unduly influenced by a drug company representative, a reason that is not grounded in a concern for the patient's well being. It is also not clear that the patient has provided informed consent to this medication, yet the adverse reactions to antianxiety medications such as lorazepam include sedation, dizziness, weakness, and unsteadiness, and most patients would want to have this information. The difficulty the pharmacist has in taking action is understandable, given his ignorance with respect to these important pieces of the clinical picture.

Values

Even though facts are necessary for addressing ethical questions, they are not sufficient; values also play an important role. The term "value" here refers to elements of the case that the pharmacist *ought* to consider important. As a member of the health care team, pharmacist Jones takes seriously his professional relationship with the prescribing physician. This value gives rise to the moral rule, "Maintain a good relationship with physician colleagues." If being faithful to colleagues were valuable only for its own sake, and if it were the only value that played a role in the case, Jones would not be faced with an ethical dilemma, because it would be clear that he ought to fill the prescription.

There are other relevant values, however. Chief among them are protecting the patient from harm and promoting the patient's welfare, as well as respecting her right to self-determination. The first two values correspond to the principle of beneficence, and the second corresponds to the principle of respect for autonomy. The term "beneficence" means literally, "doing the good," and this principle

---

[1]We will use the terms "ethical" and "moral" synonymously.

requires us to prevent harm, to remove harm, and to promote or restore the good. "Autonomy" means "self-ruling," and the corresponding principle requires us to respect the free choices of others. These two principles, and the values they support, appear to give rise to a moral dilemma for the pharmacist. Taking seriously the importance of honoring the relationship with the physician suggests that he ought to dispense the medication, while honoring his obligation to secure the patient's welfare and respect her autonomy suggests that he ought *not* to dispense it, at least for the time being. Is there a rational way to decide between these two alternatives?

One of the unfortunate aspects of most moral debates is that we tend to polarize the options open to us: *either* we should do X, *or* we should not do X. Moral problems are much richer than this, however, and do not admit to only two solutions. In fact, the ideal way to resolve a moral problem is to identify an option that would enable us to fulfill *all* of the relevant values.

In this case, that option would be to contact the prescribing physician *first* and learn more about the patient's history and why the physician believes that an antianxiety medication is indicated. The pharmacist has not only a right but also a duty to ask whether the patient has provided informed consent to receive this medication. In having an open and honest conversation with the prescribing physician, Dr. Jones will be taking seriously his obligations to other members of the health care team as well as to the patient. Only if this conversation suggests that the prescription was not written with this particular patient in mind and is unlikely to yield consequences that the patient would consider beneficial would the pharmacist be justified in refusing to dispense it.

Virtues

This approach to pharmacy ethics is not entirely satisfactory, because its focus on what the pharmacist ought to *do* neglects another element of the moral life that is important: virtues, or the excellences of character that make someone a good pharmacist. In other words, ethics is the attempt to answer not only the question, "What should I do?," but also the question, "Who should I be?" If John Jones used the perspective of virtue ethics, he would find himself reasoning in a different way. He would think not of actions that are required of him, but of kinds of dispositions and qualities of character that are consistent with moral excellence. Some of the virtues of pharmacy practice are truthfulness, charitableness, temperance, and friendship. Virtue ethics takes as its central concern the larger context of the pharmacist's life and, in so doing, goes beyond construing the moral life as a series of puzzles to be solved.

The virtuous pharmacist acts not merely from a sense of obligation, but from a deeply-ingrained disposition towards and a love of doing the right thing. In other words, a virtue-based approach to ethical decision making takes into account the motivations of the pharmacist and not merely what he or she decides to do.

The term "virtue," as it is used today, suggests an extraordinarily high standard for living morally, so that only a very few are capable of rightly being considered virtuous. This is not an accurate description of what an appeal to virtues has traditionally meant, and indeed, virtue ethics accounts for the way in which many people approach moral problems in their lives. Rather than teasing out the morally relevant values and their respective rules and principles, many of us ask ourselves instead, "How would a person I respect rise to this challenge?" That is, we imagine how a virtuous person we know would respond to the problem and try to follow her or his example. Returning to the case study, a virtue-based approach might lead Dr. Jones not only to refuse to dispense the prescription, but to spend the time necessary to both prevent harm to this patient and ensure that the health care needs of all of the prescribing physicians' patients are met. The pharmacist might think of his mentor from pharmacy school and recall that when faced with similar situation, the senior pharmacist rose to the challenge with kindness, charitableness, and a commitment to social justice, and that this disposition provided the basis for all of her conduct as a pharmacist.

In summary, the conventional way of approaching a moral question focuses on identifying one's obligations, and a virtue-based approach attends to the character of the person faced with the question. A virtue-based approach may even recast the kind of question that he or she asks. As Beauchamp and Childress note, these two approaches

> have different emphases, but they are compatible and mutually reinforcing. . . .
> To look at acts without also looking at the moral appropriateness and desirability
> of feelings, attitudes, forms of sympathy, and the like is to miss a large area
> of the moral picture. We do not merely expect persons to act in certain ways.
> We also expect them to have certain emotions, certain forms of responsiveness,
> and a trustworthy character. (Beauchamp and Childress 1994)

We now turn to an examination of the notion of covenant, the central role it plays in pharmaceutical care, and the ways in which this notion both draws from and enriches the approaches of conventional, ethical decision making and virtue ethics to thinking about the moral life of the pharmacist.

The Role of Covenant (See also Chapter 8)

Pharmaceutical care, the new standard of pharmacy practice, suggests a more proactive role for pharmacists, that includes participating in drug use decisions, determining dose and dosage schedule, providing drug information to the patient, and monitoring adverse drug reactions. This shift from the more distant, consulta-tive role of traditional pharmacy practice to one that places the pharmacist squarely in the center of a professional-patient relationship will present ethical challenges to pharmacists that heretofore were concerns only to health profession-als with more direct patient interaction and traditionally ascribed responsibilities.

Pharmacists, more than in the past, will have to deal with conflicts in loyalties between patients and colleagues, as case #2 illustrates.

Rhonda Spain, Pharm. D., works in the outpatient pharmacy of Pleasant Hills Community Hospital. Dr. Spain often comments to her colleagues that she has the best of both worlds, professionally speaking. She is involved in the traditional dispensing functions of a busy outpatient clinic, but she is also involved in the infusion program of the hospital's home care/hospice unit. Dr. Spain's work in the home infusion program requires more in-depth patient contact than her work in the traditional outpatient pharmacy. Dr. Spain considers herself an integral member of the home care team and, whenever possible, makes home visits to instruct patients and families about the use of an ambulatory pump or drug side effect.

During a home visit to Marian Busskohl, a 45-year-old woman with metastatic cancer of the breast, Dr. Spain asks Ms. Busskohl about the adequacy of her pain management. Dr. Spain can see the dark circles under Ms. Busskohl's eyes and the drawn expression on her face that indicates sleeplessness and pain. Ms. Busskohl responds, "I can sleep only for an hour or two, and then I have to take another pill. It's just not enough. I'm driving my family crazy. None of us is getting any sleep. Can't Dr. Olson order something better for the pain? Does he know what he's doing?"

Dr. Spain wishes that Ms. Busskohl hadn't asked these questions, since the pharmacist has already tried many times to convince Dr. Bernard Olson, Ms. Busskohl's primary physician, that morphine wasn't a drug of "last resort" and that addiction wasn't an issue in the case of terminally ill patients in pain. She has never been successful in these efforts. Dr. Spain has worked with many other physicians who successfully manage their patients' pain, and it seems wrong that Ms. Busskohl has to suffer unnecessarily because Dr. Olson appears incompetent in the area of pain management. Dr. Spain feels it would be inappropriate to express her misgivings about Dr. Olson to Ms. Busskohl. However, she also feels that she would be untruthful with Ms. Busskohl if she does not answer her questions.

Let us analyze Dr. Spain's moral problem in light of the standard of pharmaceutical care. Hepler and Strand describe the fundamental relationship in pharmaceutical care as a "covenant, a mutually beneficial exchange in which a patient promises to grant authority to the provider, and the provider promises competence and commitment (responsibility) to the patient (Hepler and Strand 1989)." According to convenantal ethics, the nature of the relationship between pharmacist and patient is a covenant, defined by Hepler and Strand as a "mutually beneficial exchange." The patient makes a promise to the provider "to grant authority," although the authority to do what is not made explicit. The provider promises to be competent and responsible in return. Others have interpreted the covenantal relationship differently. Manasse claims that, "the recipients of the services of a professional give up a certain degree of their autonomy in decision making and judgment in exchange for the knowledge, skills, and practice of the professional. The client or patient will also allow the engagement of the professional in certain behaviors that under other circumstances and with any other outsider would not be allowed (Manasse 1992)."

These definitions of covenant stray significantly from those found in the work of William F. May, whose application of Protestant moral theology to health care gave rise to the notion of covenant in the patient-provider relationship. It is beyond the scope of this chapter to determine *which* definition of covenant best describes the relationship between patient and pharmacist or, more basically, if covenant is being used in a descriptive manner (attending to the way the relationship *is*) or in a prescriptive one (attending to the way the relationship *ought to be*). However, it is important to distinguish among the various interpretations of covenant and to begin to ask questions about its fittingness for pharmacy practice and its application to ethical decision making.

A covenant, in the traditional biblical meaning, is an unconditional agreement that includes command, promise, and threat (McCoy 1991). As May writes,

> In its ancient and most influential form, a covenant usually included the following elements: (1) an original experience of gift between the soon-to-be covenanted partners; (2) a covenant promise based on this original or anticipated exchange of gifts, labors, or services; and (3) the shaping of subsequent life for each partner by the promissory event (May 1989).

A principal image of the covenant is found in the Torah, in which the Jews bind themselves to God at Mt. Sinai. The three elements described by May are clear in this episode. The gift from God is the deliverance of the Jews from Egypt; the promises are the vows at Mt. Sinai; and the consequences are the rituals and moral obligations that the Jews adopt as their way of life (May 1983). The traditional meaning of covenant thus emphasizes the gifts that each party brings to the relationship, the promises that each makes to the other, and the transformative effect of the covenant on each.

In applying this meaning of covenant to the relationship between patient and pharmacist, we begin by noting the gifts that each brings to the alliance. Patients give to pharmacists in at least three ways. First, they give themselves. Without the consent of many patients to the awkward ministrations of student learners, no one would be able to become a health professional. Without patients to whom to provide a service, no one could remain a health professional. Pharmacists, like other health care professionals, owe their education to the patients they serve. Second, patients, as taxpayers, invest in health care education, and as patients they provide professionals with an opportunity to repay debts to society. Third, patients provide health care providers with the opportunity for personal and professional growth. Pharmacists become transformed by the very act of providing care to patients. The therapeutic relationship changes not only the recipient of care, but the provider as well, in ways that are not immediately transparent, but are often profound and long lasting.

Pharmacists bring to the relationship their clinical knowledge and skill in promoting the health of patients and protecting patients from the potential harm of "drug misadventuring (Manasse 1989)." Indeed, pharmacists pledge to use their expertise for the benefit of others, and this promise is what distinguishes pharmacy, and other professions, from occupations like business. To be a professional in general, and a health care professional in particular, is to make a public promise to serve the interests of others. Because patients are often vulnerable when they present to pharmacists, a key challenge for pharmacists is to know what constitutes the good of the patient; without knowing the patient's narrative, it is difficult to help patients in the way in which they want to be helped. The promise that the pharmacist makes to the patient, then, is shaped not only by the pharmacist's clinical expertise but also by what the patient considers to be a good therapeutic outcome. The only way to fulfill one's obligations as a provider of pharmaceutical care is to know the patient as a person.

In its focus on the complexity of the relationship between patient and pharmacist, the metaphor of the covenant offers a richness lacking from the concept of moral life which presents morality simply as a matter of rules and principles to be balanced. The prominence to which covenant assigns loyalty shows its natural kinship with virtue ethics. Still, the religious roots of covenant may limit its appropriateness for the secular contexts in which most pharmacists practice. May clearly emphasizes the sacred meaning of covenant and contrasts it with various other types of professional relationships or professional obligations to patients, such as codes of ethics, philanthropy, and contract. Even if May is correct is holding that, unlike contracts, "covenants cut deeper into personal identity (May 1983)," the religious trappings of a covenant make it a less-than-ideal model in a world in which we come from different moral and religious traditions.

In a secular society like the United States, perhaps a more fitting metaphor for the patient-pharmacist relationship may be the contract rather than the covenant. A contract emphasizes the importance of obtaining informed consent and engaging in other practices that promote respect for patient autonomy. Contracts, unlike covenants, do not presume that the parties in the relationship are bound by the same moral and cultural traditions. However, the parties in a contractual relationship meet not only as strangers, but also as primarily self-interested individuals. Contracts are forged, after all, to guard against one party's abuse of another. This is not how one likes to think of the patient-pharmacist relationship. Also, contracts presume equality among the parties, and, although efforts like obtaining informed consent seek to promote more enlightened patients, there remains an imbalance of power and authority between health care provider and patient. Therefore, like the covenant metaphor, the metaphor of the contract has limitations when applied to the patient-pharmacist relationship.

Let us now revisit the case of Rhonda Spain and Marian Busskohl. If we think of the relationship between patient and pharmacist as covenantal (with the above limitations in mind), the pharmacist should not only tell the truth but also *be* true. Accordingly, it would not be morally sufficient to give her patient accurate information about her medications, side effects, and so forth; Dr. Spain also ought to be available to the patient through the difficulties that lie ahead. Doing a follow-up consultation might be considered "above and beyond the call of duty" if we approach this moral problem from the perspective of discrete ethical obligations, but, by using the metaphor of the covenant and recalling the insights of virtue ethics, we can see that this act flows naturally from the patient-pharmacist relationship.

In addition, Dr. Spain has personal experience with Dr. Olson's incompetence in the area of pain management, so it would be difficult for her to justify remaining silent in response to Ms. Busskohl's question. Ms. Busskohl is in need of Dr. Spain's expertise and support. Ms. Busskohl is suffering unnecessarily, and there are numerous adverse outcomes from unrelenting pain for patients and their families. Telling the truth about pain control would help to promote the value of minimizing the patient's suffering and avoiding adverse outcomes.

Promise-keeping also plays a role in this case. As a health professional, Dr. Spain has made an implied promise to patients to promote their welfare, and this promise may require supplying information that Ms. Busskohl needs to make a competent choice of physician. Dr. Spain may be able to communicate indirectly to Ms. Busskohl that there are other physicians in the area who are more expert at pain management than Dr. Olson. Dr. Spain might say, "It is possible to manage your pain more effectively. If I were in your position, I would consider Drs. Smith or Suzuki." Dr. Spain has also made a professional promise to the physicians with whom she works to be cooperative and loyal. This tacit understanding among professionals is violated when false accusations are made about a colleague's competence, but if a colleague is incompetent, then there is an ethical obligation to intervene appropriately (Parker and Manolakis 1995).

Dr. Spain has obligations that extend beyond her duties to Ms. Busskohl. Other patients in the hospice program require the same information that Ms. Busskohl does to make sound decisions. Dr. Spain should think about a course of action that not only attends to Ms. Busskohl's needs, but also to the needs of all patients who might be affected by Dr. Olson's apparent incompetence in the area of pain management. Dr. Olson's unwillingness to take Dr. Spain's suggestions seriously could be the result of a lack of education about the best modes of pain management currently available; it may also be an example of his lack of respect of the pharmacist's expertise generally. If Dr. Olson is not amenable to learning about current therapies, Dr. Spain could work with others in the hospice program to establish guidelines or policies about pain management that apply to all physicians in the program. These are only a few examples of how Dr. Spain might fulfill her obligation to make certain that all patients are protected from unnecessary harm.

Most of these facets of covenantal ethics have a counterpart in the conventional model of ethical decision making that introduced this chapter. However, the notion of covenant highlights the complexities of the relationship between health care provider and patient that are often absent from the conventional model when applied to ethical questions in health care. Pharmaceutical care, with the primacy it has given to the concept of covenant, places pharmacists in more intimate contact with patients, so it will be helpful to employ a variety of ethical perspectives in thinking about pharmacists' moral responsibilities. Taken together, the conventional model's concern with the ethics of action, coupled with virtue ethics' attention to role of moral character and motivation and also with the covenantal emphasis on the complex web of relationships, will help the pharmacist not only to do the right thing but to be the best pharmacist he or she can be.

Suggestions for Future Research

An emerging literature, much of it from a feminist perspective, draws attention to the role that care has played in the lives of women (Gilligan, 1993; Larrabee, 1993; Manning, 1992; Sherwin, 1992; Tong, 1993; Wood, 1994). Future research on the ethics of pharmaceutical care might consider this literature and the insights it has to offer to this new standard of pharmacy practice.

Acknowledgment

The authors gratefully acknowledge the assistance of Dr. Michael L. Manolakis, who provided useful comments on an earlier version of this chapter.

References

Anon. 1994. Ethical hot spots. *Drug Topics* 52.

Beauchamp, T. L., and Childress J. F. 1994. *Principles of Biomedical Ethics*. 4th ed. New York: Oxford University Press.

Gilligan, C. 1993. *In a Different Voice*. Cambridge, MA: Harvard University Press.

Hepler, C. D., and Strand, L. M. 1989. Opportunities and responsibilities in pharmaceutical care. *American Journal of Pharmaceutical Education* 53 (Winter Supplement): 7S–15S.

Larrabee M. J., ed. 1993. *An Ethic of Care: Feminist and Interdisciplinary Perspectives*. New York, NY: Routledge.

Manasse, H. R., Jr. 1989. Medication use in an imperfect world: Drug misadventuring as an issue of public policy, Part 1. *American Journal of Hospital Pharmacy*, 46:929–944.

Manasse, H. R., Jr. 1992. The CARE in pharmaceutical care. *Journal of Pharmacy Teaching*, 3(3): 39–52.

Manning, R. C. 1992. *Speaking From the Heart: A Feminist Perspective on Ethics.* Lanham, MD: Rowman & Littlefield Publishers.

May, W. F. 1983. *The Physician's Covenant.* Philadelphia, PA: Westminster Press, p. 108.

May, W. F. 1989. Code, covenant, contract, or philanthropy. In: Veatch R. M. (ed.) *Cross Cultural Perspectives in Medical Ethics: Readings.* Boston, MA: Jones and Bartlett Publishers.

McCoy, C. S. 1991. Creation and covenant: A comprehensive vision for environmental ethics. In C. S. Robb and C. J. Casebolt (eds.) *Covenant for a New Creation.* Maryknoll, NY: Orbis Books.

Parker, L. S., and Manolakis, M. 1995. Professional responsibilities toward incompetent or chemically dependent colleagues. In B. D. Weinstein (ed.) *Ethical Issues in Pharmacy.* Vancouver, WA: Applied Therapeutics.

Sherwin, S. 1992. *No Longer Patient: Feminist Ethics and Health Care.* Philadelphia, PA: Temple University Press.

Tong, R. 1993. *Feminine and Feminist Ethics.* Belmont, CA: Wadsworth Publishing.

Wood, J. T. 1994. *Who Cares? Women, Care, and Culture.* Carbondale, IL: Southern Illinois University Press.

Index